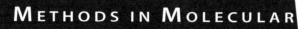

Series Editor
**John M. Walker**
**School of Life and Medical Sciences**
**University of Hertfordshire**
**Hatfield, Hertfordshire, UK**

For further volumes:
http://www.springer.com/series/7651

For over 35 years, biological scientists have come to rely on the research protocols and methodologies in the critically acclaimed *Methods in Molecular Biology* series. The series was the first to introduce the step-by-step protocols approach that has become the standard in all biomedical protocol publishing. Each protocol is provided in readily-reproducible step-by-step fashion, opening with an introductory overview, a list of the materials and reagents needed to complete the experiment, and followed by a detailed procedure that is supported with a helpful notes section offering tips and tricks of the trade as well as troubleshooting advice. These hallmark features were introduced by series editor Dr. John Walker and constitute the key ingredient in each and every volume of the *Methods in Molecular Biology* series. Tested and trusted, comprehensive and reliable, all protocols from the series are indexed in PubMed.

# Long Non-Coding RNAs in Cancer

Edited by

## Alfons Navarro

*Faculty of Medicine and Health Sciences, University of Barcelona, Barcelona, Spain*

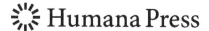 Humana Press

*Editor*
Alfons Navarro
Faculty of Medicine and Health
Sciences
University of Barcelona
Barcelona, Spain

ISSN 1064-3745          ISSN 1940-6029   (electronic)
Methods in Molecular Biology
ISBN 978-1-0716-1583-6      ISBN 978-1-0716-1581-2   (eBook)
https://doi.org/10.1007/978-1-0716-1581-2

© Springer Science+Business Media, LLC, part of Springer Nature 2021, corrected publication 2021
This work is subject to copyright. All rights are reserved by the Publisher, whether the whole or part of the material is concerned, specifically the rights of translation, reprinting, reuse of illustrations, recitation, broadcasting, reproduction on microfilms or in any other physical way, and transmission or information storage and retrieval, electronic adaptation, computer software, or by similar or dissimilar methodology now known or hereafter developed.
The use of general descriptive names, registered names, trademarks, service marks, etc. in this publication does not imply, even in the absence of a specific statement, that such names are exempt from the relevant protective laws and regulations and therefore free for general use.
The publisher, the authors, and the editors are safe to assume that the advice and information in this book are believed to be true and accurate at the date of publication. Neither the publisher nor the authors or the editors give a warranty, expressed or implied, with respect to the material contained herein or for any errors or omissions that may have been made. The publisher remains neutral with regard to jurisdictional claims in published maps and institutional affiliations.

This Humana imprint is published by the registered company Springer Science+Business Media, LLC part of Springer Nature.
The registered company address is: 1 New York Plaza, New York, NY 10004, U.S.A.

# Preface

In recent years, the relevance of the non-protein-coding portion of the genome, the so-called non-coding RNAs, has been more than demonstrated. They are key elements in all the normal regulatory processes of the cell, and their dysregulation is associated with pathogenesis. The boom in the study of non-coding RNAs began around 2005 with the discovery and association of microRNAs with cancer, which has led to thousands of publications demonstrating their relevance. Other groups of non-coding RNAs have been described and studied for the last few years, and they have been classified into two main groups according to their size: small and long non-coding RNAs (lncRNAs). This volume focuses on the study of lncRNAs, which is a heterogeneous group that includes all the non-coding RNAs longer than 200 nucleotides. They can be classified according to their genomic position in intergenic, exonic, intronic, or overlapping lncRNAs. Their sequence is poorly conserved, and some of them may be post-processed into smaller RNAs or to circular RNAs (circRNAs). Although they are usually expressed at very low levels, their expression is more tissue-specific than protein-coding genes. LncRNAs are involved in the regulation of various cell processes, including transcription, intracellular trafficking, and chromosome remodeling. Their dysregulation has been associated with the development and progression of various types of cancers. For all this, we can consider them promising cancer biomarkers.

The present book is focused on the main techniques needed for the study of lncRNAs in cancer from a translational research point of view. It covers from profiling of lncRNA expression in cancer tissue, tumor cells, or liquid biopsies to functional analysis to decipher the role of the deregulated lncRNAs identified. The book is organized into six parts. It begins with a description of the different types of lncRNAs, the main databases in charge of their registry, and the description of the main rules for using lncRNAs as cancer biomarkers. The second part covers lncRNA profiling by arrays and RNAseq. Since most of the techniques associated with arrays and RNAseq processes are nowadays mainly performed in specialized services, we included here only the necessary bioinformatic pipelines to analyze the raw data provided for most of the scientific facilities. Moreover, this part also provides a laboratory protocol for performing single cell RNAseq. The third part is dedicated to techniques used to validate the data obtained in the profiling phase of the study, including real-time PCR, digital PCR, and in situ hybridization. In the fourth part, the most relevant techniques used for performing functional studies with selected lncRNAs are described. *In vitro* and *in vivo* lncRNA silencing or overexpression using different methods such as siRNAs or CRISPR/CAS9 is discussed in this part. This part also includes chapters dedicated to lncRNA-protein interactions and to viral lncRNAs. In Part V, we focus on protocols for the study of lncRNAs in liquid biopsies, and the last part is committed to the special group of circRNAs.

This book attempts to summarize with laboratory protocols, bioinformatics pipelines, and review chapters, the main steps that translational researchers who decide to identify and study tumorigenic lncRNAs from a patient's tumor tissue or tumor cells need to perform. Starting with the identification (profiling phase) of candidate lncRNAs and ending with the decoding of the tumor function of each lncRNA. Hopefully all these contents will be of interest to researchers in the field of non-coding RNAs in cancer.

Lastly, I would like to thank all the authors for contributing to this book, for being generous enough to share the secrets and tricks of their most precious techniques, and for taking the time to write chapters to this book even during this difficult phase of the global COVID-19 pandemic. Moreover, I would like to thank the editorial staff from Springer for all their work and especially to John M. Walker, who has been pushing me to move on with the development of this book and that without his motivation probably this book would not have been published.

*Barcelona, Spain*                                                                                    *Alfons Navarro*

# Contents

# Contributors

LUCA AGNELLI • *Department of Oncology and Hemato-oncology, University of Milan, Milan, Italy; Hematology, Fondazione IRCCS Ca' Granda Ospedale Maggiore Policlinico, Milan, Italy; Department of Pathology, IRCCS Istituto Nazionale dei Tumori, Milan, Italy*

ENRICO ALESSIO • *Department of Biology, University of Padova, Padova, Italy*

NICOLA AMODIO • *Department of Experimental and Clinical Medicine, Magna Graecia University, Salvatore Venuta University Campus, Catanzaro, Italy*

LUIS ARNES • *Biotech Research & Innovation Centre (BRIC), Novo Nordisk Foundation Center for Stem Cell Biology (DanStem), University of Copenhagen, Copenhagen, Denmark*

JENNIFER BINTZ • *Biotech Research & Innovation Centre (BRIC), Novo Nordisk Foundation Center for Stem Cell Biology (DanStem), University of Copenhagen, Copenhagen, Denmark*

RAPHAEL SEVERINO BONADIO • *Department of Biology, University of Padova, Padova, Italy*

STEFANIA BORTOLUZZI • *Department of Molecular Medicine, University of Padova, Padova, Italy; Interdepartmental Research Center for Innovative Biotechnologies (CRIBI), University of Padova, Padova, Italy*

ALESSIA BURATIN • *Department of Molecular Medicine, University of Padova, Padova, Italy; Department of Biology, University of Padova, Padova, Italy*

STEFANO CAGNIN • *Department of Biology, University of Padova, Padova, Italy; CRIBI Biotechnology Center, University of Padova, Padova, Italy; CIR-Myo Myology Center, University of Padova, Padova, Italy*

GEORGE A. CALIN • *Department of Translational Molecular Pathology, The University of Texas MD Anderson Cancer Center, Houston, TX, USA; The Center for RNA Interference and Non-Coding RNAs, The University of Texas MD Anderson Cancer Center, Houston, TX, USA*

JORDI CANALS • *Molecular Oncology and Embryology Laboratory, Human Anatomy Unit, Faculty of Medicine and Health Sciences, University of Barcelona, IDIBAPS, Barcelona, Spain*

JOAN J. CASTELLANO • *Molecular Oncology and Embryology Laboratory, Human Anatomy Unit, Faculty of Medicine and Health Sciences, University of Barcelona, IDIBAPS, Barcelona, Spain*

ELEONORA D'AMBRA • *Department of Biology and Biotechnology 'Charles Darwin', Sapienza University of Rome, Rome, Italy*

ANNA DAL MOLIN • *Department of Molecular Medicine, University of Padova, Padova, Italy*

EMILY A. DANGELMAIER • *Regulatory RNAs and Cancer Section, Genetics Branch, Center for Cancer Research (CCR), National Cancer Institute (NCI), National Institutes of Health (NIH), Bethesda, MD, USA*

SONAM DHAMIJA • *CSIR Institute of Genomics and Integrative Biology, New Delhi, India*

TANIA DÍAZ • *Molecular Oncology and Embryology Laboratory, Human Anatomy Unit, Faculty of Medicine and Health Sciences, University of Barcelona, IDIBAPS, Barcelona, Spain*

MIHNEA P. DRAGOMIR • *Institute of Pathology, Charité-Universitätsmedizin Berlin, corporate member of Freie Universität Berlin, Humboldt-Universität zu Berlin and Berlin Institute of Health, Berlin, Germany*

VANESSA FAVASULI • *Department of Oncology and Hemato-oncology, University of Milan, Milan, Italy; Hematology, Fondazione Cà Granda IRCCS Policlinico, Milan, Italy*

MARIATERESA FULCINITI • *Department of Medical Oncology, Dana Farber Cancer Institute, Harvard Medical School, Boston, MA, USA*

ENRICO GAFFO • *Department of Molecular Medicine, University of Padova, Padova, Italy*

RAMIRO GARZON • *Division of Hematology, Department of Medicine, Comprehensive Cancer Center, The Ohio State University, Columbus, OH, USA*

MARIA D. GIRALDEZ • *Institute of Biomedicine of Seville (IBiS), Seville, Spain; Unit of Digestive Diseases, Virgen del Rocio University Hospital, Seville, Spain; University of Seville, Seville, Spain*

ANNAMARIA GULLA' • *Department of Medical Oncology, Dana Farber Cancer Institute, Harvard Medical School, Boston, MA, USA*

BING HAN • *Molecular Oncology and Embryology Laboratory, Human Anatomy Unit, Faculty of Medicine and Health Sciences, University of Barcelona, IDIBAPS, Barcelona, Spain*

JAKOB HØFFDING • *Bioneer A/S, Hørsholm, Denmark; Københavns Professionshøjskole, København, Denmark*

KIM HOLMSTRØM • *Bioneer A/S, Hørsholm, Denmark*

BJØRN HOLST • *Bioneer A/S, Hørsholm, Denmark*

YING HU • *Harbin Institute of Technology, School of Life Sciences and Technology, Harbin, China*

INGRAM IACCARINO • *Hematopathology Section and Lymph Node Registry, University of Kiel, Kiel, Germany*

MEHMET KARA • *Department of Molecular Biology and Genetics, College of Arts and Sciences, Uludağ University, Bursa, Turkey; Department of Molecular Genetics & Microbiology, College of Medicine, UF Health Cancer Center, University of Florida, Gainesville, FL, USA*

WOLFRAM KLAPPER • *Hematopathology Section and Lymph Node Registry, University of Kiel, Kiel, Germany*

ERIK KNUTSEN • *Department of Medical Biology, Faculty of Health Sciences, UiT—The Arctic University of Norway, Tromsø, Norway*

CHUN-TIEN KUO • *Division of Pharmaceutics and Pharmacology, College of Pharmacy, The Ohio State University, Columbus, USA*

ASHISH LAL • *Regulatory RNAs and Cancer Section, Genetics Branch, Center for Cancer Research (CCR), National Cancer Institute (NCI), National Institutes of Health (NIH), Bethesda, MD, USA*

JESPER LARSEN • *Bioneer A/S, Hørsholm, Denmark*

CHARLES H. LAWRIE • *Molecular Oncology Group, Biodonostia Research Institute, San Sebastián, Spain; IKERBASQUE, Basque Foundation for Science, Bilbao, Spain; Radcliffe Department of Medicine, University of Oxford, Oxford, UK*

ROBERT J. LEE • *Division of Pharmaceutics and Pharmacology, College of Pharmacy, The Ohio State University, Columbus, USA*

JENNIFER LINDEMANN • *Mayo Clinic, Jacksonville, FL, USA*

NATASHA HELLEBERG MADSEN • *Bioneer A/S, Hørsholm, Denmark*

MARTINA MANZONI • *Department of Oncology and Hemato-oncology, University of Milan, Milan, Italy; Hematology, Fondazione IRCCS Ca' Granda Ospedale Maggiore Policlinico, Milan, Italy*

MANOJ B. MENON • *Kusuma School of Biological Sciences, Indian Institute of Technology Delhi, New Delhi, India*

GARTZE MENTXAKA • *Molecular Oncology Group, Biodonostia Research Institute, San Sebastián, Spain*

TRINE MØLLER • *Bioneer A/S, Hørsholm, Denmark*

MARIANO MONZO • *Molecular Oncology and Embryology Laboratory, Human Anatomy Unit, Faculty of Medicine and Health Sciences, University of Barcelona, IDIBAPS, Barcelona, Spain; Thoracic Oncology Unit, Hospital Clinic, Barcelona, Spain*

EUGENIO MORELLI • *Department of Medical Oncology, Dana Farber Cancer Institute, Harvard Medical School, Boston, MA, USA*

MARIANGELA MORLANDO • *Department of Pharmaceutical Sciences, "Department of Excellence 2018-2022", University of Perugia, Perugia, Italy*

NIKHIL C. MUNSHI • *Department of Medical Oncology, Dana Farber Cancer Institute, Harvard Medical School, Boston, MA, USA; VA Boston Healthcare System, Boston, MA, USA*

SARA NAPOLI • *Faculty of Biomedical Sciences, Institute of Oncology Research, USI, Bellinzona, Switzerland*

ALFONS NAVARRO • *Molecular Oncology and Embryology Laboratory, Human Anatomy Unit, Faculty of Medicine and Health Sciences, University of Barcelona, IDIBAPS, Barcelona, Spain; Thoracic Oncology Unit, Hospital Clinic, Barcelona, Spain*

ANTONINO NERI • *Department of Oncology and Hemato-oncology, University of Milan, Milan, Italy; Hematology, Fondazione IRCCS Ca' Granda Ospedale Maggiore Policlinico, Milan, Italy*

SON LY NHAT • *Bioneer A/S, Hørsholm, Denmark*

BOYE SCHNACK NIELSEN • *Bioneer A/S, Hørsholm, Denmark*

YU OTA • *Mayo Clinic, Jacksonville, FL, USA*

PIER PAOLO PANDOLFI • *Department of Molecular Biotechnologies & Health Sciences, Molecular Biotechnology Center, University of Turin, Turin, Italy; Renown Institute for Cancer, Nevada System of Higher Education, Reno, NV, USA*

TUSHAR PATEL • *Mayo Clinic, Jacksonville, FL, USA*

LAURA POLISENO • *Oncogenomics Unit, CRL-ISPRO, Pisa, Italy; Institute of Clinical Physiology, CNR, Pisa, Italy*

GIANCARLO PRUNERI • *Department of Pathology, IRCCS Istituto Nazionale dei Tumori, Milan, Italy; Department of Oncology and Hemato-oncology, University of Milan, Milan, Italy*

DOMENICA RONCHETTI • *Department of Oncology and Hemato-oncology, University of Milan, Milan, Italy; Hematology, Fondazione IRCCS Ca' Granda Ospedale Maggiore Policlinico, Milan, Italy*

INGRID ARCTANDER ROSENLUND • *Department of Medical Biology, Faculty of Health Sciences, UiT—The Arctic University of Norway, Tromsø, Norway*

GABRIELE SALES • *Department of Biology, University of Padova, Padova, Italy*

CARLA SOLÉ • *Molecular Oncology Group, Biodonostia Research Institute, San Sebastián, Spain*

ELISA TAIANA • *Department of Oncology and Hemato-oncology, University of Milan, Milan, Italy; Hematology, Fondazione IRCCS Ca' Granda Ospedale Maggiore Policlinico, Milan, Italy*

PIERFRANCESCO TASSONE • *Department of Experimental and Clinical Medicine, Magna Graecia University of Catanzaro, Catanzaro, Italy*

MUNEESH TEWARI • *Hematology/Oncology Division, Department of Internal Medicine, University of Michigan, Ann Arbor, MI, USA; Center for Computational Medicine and Bioinformatics, University of Michigan, Ann Arbor, MI, USA; Department of Biomedical Engineering, University of Michigan, Ann Arbor, MI, USA*

MEIKE S. THIJSSEN • *Biotech Research & Innovation Centre (BRIC), Novo Nordisk Foundation Center for Stem Cell Biology (DanStem), University of Copenhagen, Copenhagen, Denmark*

SCOTT A. TIBBETTS • *Department of Molecular Genetics & Microbiology, College of Medicine, UF Health Cancer Center, University of Florida, Gainesville, FL, USA*

KATIA TODOERTI • *Department of Oncology and Hemato-oncology, University of Milan, Milan, Italy; Hematology, Fondazione IRCCS Ca' Granda Ospedale Maggiore Policlinico, Milan, Italy*

GIUSEPPE VIGLIETTO • *Department of Experimental and Clinical Medicine, Magna Graecia University of Catanzaro, Catanzaro, Italy*

MARIANNA VITIELLO • *Oncogenomics Unit, CRL-ISPRO, Pisa, Italy; Institute of Clinical Physiology, CNR, Pisa, Italy*

XINGWEN WANG • *Harbin Institute of Technology, School of Life Sciences and Technology, Harbin, China*

IRENE K. YAN • *Mayo Clinic, Jacksonville, FL, USA*

KUNMING ZHAO • *Harbin Institute of Technology, School of Life Sciences and Technology, Harbin, China*

# Part I

LncRNA Classification and Utility in Cancer

# Chapter 1

# LncRNAs and Available Databases

## Sara Napoli

### Abstract

Long noncoding RNAs (lncRNAs) are involved in many regulatory mechanisms in practically every step of the RNA cycle, from transcription to RNA stability and translation. They are a highly heterogeneous class of molecules in terms of site of production, interaction networks, and functions. More and more databases are available on the web with the aim to make public information about lncRNA accessible to the scientific community. Here we review the most interesting resources with the purpose to organize a compendium of useful tools to interrogate before studying a lncRNA of interest.

**Key words** lncRNA, Database, In silico prediction, Protein interaction, miRNA interaction, Disease association

## 1 Introduction

The human genome is pervasively transcribed, producing vast amounts of RNA transcripts, of which the majority does not encode proteins [1]. Many of them are long noncoding RNA (lncRNA), RNA molecules with low or no coding potential, usually longer than 200 nucleotides [2]. The primary sequence of lncRNA is poorly conserved [3], but the secondary and tertiary structure is highly conserved suggesting their regulatory function [4]. Recent studies have shown that lncRNA secondary structures serve as regulatory factors in biological processes and influence practically every step of the RNA life cycle, including RNA transcription, splicing, cellular localization, translation, and turnover [5]. LncRNAs are a highly heterogenic class of RNAs, such as intergenic lncRNAs, antisense transcripts, and enhancer RNAs [6]. Consistently with their heterogeneity, lncRNAs can play several different regulatory roles, such as sensory, guiding, scaffolding, and allosteric [7]. A function of lncRNA particularly studied is the epigenetic regulation, because lncRNAs can bind to chromatin-modifying proteins and modulate chromatin states [8].

Alfons Navarro (ed.), *Long Non-Coding RNAs in Cancer*, Methods in Molecular Biology, vol. 2348, https://doi.org/10.1007/978-1-0716-1581-2_1, © Springer Science+Business Media, LLC, part of Springer Nature 2021

LncRNAs plays a variety of functions in many important biological processes [9] and they are often expressed in tissue specific and development stage specific manner [10]. Concordantly, they are associated with several diseases [11].

## 2    Classification of lncRNAs

Several lncRNA classifications have been proposed until now, taking in consideration different lncRNA common features, as the site of production, the relationship with protein coding genes or the function. LncRNA classification has been extensively reviewed [12–14] and here we want just to summarize the main categories of lncRNAs that researchers are used to consider.

### 2.1 Classification Based on lncRNA Position Respect Protein Coding Genes

LncRNA can be subdivided based on their location respect protein coding genes (PCG). Long intergenic noncoding RNA (lincRNA) [15], that do not intersect any PCG, are usually 5′cap, 3′ polyadenylated, spliced, and mainly nuclear located. On the other hand, intragenic lncRNAs, overlapping PCG, can be distinct in natural antisense RNAs (NATs) [16], bidirectional lncRNAs [17], intronic or overlapping sense transcripts. NATs can in turn be defined cis-NATs if affect the expression of overlapping PCG or trans-NATs if they affect a nonpaired transcript. Bidirectional lncRNAs, transcribed from the opposite strand of a PCG, just partially overlap to the 5′ end of the paired gene, are usually unstable, but often expressed in genes involved in specific biological processes that must be finely tuned. Intronic lncRNAs are transcribed in introns of PCGs and can be independent transcriptional units or can derive from processing of the pre-mRNA. Circular intronic RNAs [18] (ciRNAs) and precursors of small nucleolar RNA (snoRNAs) belong to this last class and are proposed to regulate transcription or splicing of the host gene, while the independently transcribed intronic lncRNAs are numerical prevalent, even though their function is still poorly understood. Overlapping sense transcripts are transcribed along exons or the whole PCG in sense direction, but lack coding potential.

Intronic and overlapping lncRNA can often form circular RNAs (circRNAs) [19] due to the presence of repetitive sequences that help in the circularization of the RNA molecule. Usually they behave as miRNA sponge and they are highly stable (Fig. 1).

### 2.2 Classification Based on lncRNA Genomic Location

LncRNAs can also be classified based on their association to specific DNA regulatory regions. Pseudogene derived lncRNA [20] are transcribed from superfluous copies of functional genes that lost their coding potential during evolution. Their sequence is highly similar to parental genes so usually they can interact with mRNA by

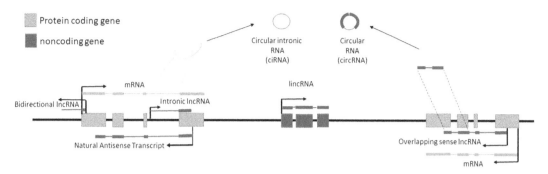

**Fig. 1** Schematic representation of the lncRNA classification based on the relationship with neighbor protein-coding genes

RNA:RNA pairing, acting as miRNA sponge or producing endogenous siRNAs.

T-UCR lncRNA are transcribed from ultraconserved (UCR) regions [21, 22], DNA sequences fully conserved among human, mouse, and rat. Those lncRNAs are aberrantly expressed in several cancer types and are proposed as molecular markers even though their function is still poorly understood.

Many enhancers and promoters are also transcribed in enhancer RNAs (eRNAs) [23] and promoter-associated lncRNAs (PALRs) [24], unstable transcripts that can interfere with the transcription of the neighbor gene. eRNAs in particular are highly tissue specific and can be activated by external stimuli, for instance inducing cell differentiation. Eventually they can affect transcription also of distal PCGs, contributing to the stabilization of complex 3D chromatin structure.

$3'$ UTR can be independently transcribed as well in lncRNAs called UTR-associated RNAs [25].

## 2.3 Classification Based on lncRNA Function

In the last years, the increased number of publications about molecular mechanism involving lncRNAs has allowed the classification of these transcripts on the basis of their biological function [26].

LncRNAs can behave as scaffold for RNP complexes. Their flexibility allows the formation of three-dimensional structures with affinity for proteins. The lncRNA structure is highly dynamic and can be modified by several events, in particular RNA modifications can alter conformation and RNA–protein interactions [27].

LncRNA scaffolds [28] often interacts with chromatin remodeling complexes or with transcription factors, regulating gene expression by epigenetic or transcriptional modulation.

Guide lncRNAs are particular scaffolds that are able to recruit RNP complexes to specific chromatin loci. Even though in some cases the presence of a triplex dsDNA–RNA was proven, the general mechanism of DNA target recognition is still to be fully elucidated [29, 30].

LncRNAs decoys are able to repress protein activity by allosteric modifications or blocking binding sites. The binding of a lncRNA to a protein can have also an activating function and such molecules are called rioboactivators. Among them, a specific subgroup of lncRNAs are called activating ncRNA (ncRNA-a) and are RNA molecules that bind Mediator protein at enhancer loci, facilitating chromatin looping and transcriptional activation [31].

Highly important is a class of lncRNAs called competing endogenous RNAs (ceRNAs) [32], which are lncRNAs and circRNAs with behavior of miRNA sponges because of high similarity of PCGs sequence. They are interesting regulators of post-transcriptional control.

LncRNAs can be precursor of smaller ncRNA as snoRNAs, miRNAs, piRNAs, or siRNAs. In particular, endo-siRNAs can be produced as effect of double strand RNAs forming as consequence of bidirectional transcription.

## 3   LncRNA Databases

Recently, in the attempt of unveiling the amount of still hidden components of this complex family of transcripts, many high-throughput experiments have been done in order to better define the different lncRNA classes, their function and the interaction networks they take part in.

The massive amount of sequencing data generates huge number of candidates of long noncoding RNAs but also creates big challenges for data analysis, such as identification of novel lncRNAs, their targets, their interactors, and statistical modeling [33, 34]. The relevant question of how many lncRNAs are present in the human genome is difficult to answer. While some studies report large transcriptomes containing over 90,000 lncRNAs [35], more conservative resources such as GENCODE annotate only 16,000 lncRNAs [36]. The challenges in the annotation of lncRNAs have led to the creation of several specialized lncRNAs databases. Since experimental methods to study this class of molecules are still limited in extensive screenings, a number of in silico tools and methods have been developed to analyze these data to interrogate the expression, variation, and function of ncRNA at the genomewide scale [37].

### 3.1 Identification of Known and Novel lncRNAs

Many databases are trying to collect all the lncRNAs in comprehensive catalogs (Table 1). Many of them rely on in silico annotation. The fragments of the transcribed RNA sequences, obtained by next-generation sequencing (NGS) technologies are mapped to the reference genome and reconstructed to obtain the transcribed units of the RNAs. To classify the transcribed units as coding or noncoding, the sequences of transcribed units are evaluated on the

**Table 1**
**LncRNA databases**

| LncRNA database | Web address | Brief description |
|---|---|---|
| *Identification of known and novel lncRNAs* | | |
| RNAcentral | https://rnacentral.org/ | Merge of all noncoding RNA annotation databases into a single compendium |
| LncBooK | http://bigd.big.ac.cn/lncbook | Expert-curated comprehensive collection of human lncRNAs, including a systematic curation of lncRNAs by multiomics data integration |
| LNCipedia | https://lncipedia.org | Merge of redundant transcripts across the different data sources, grouping the transcript into genes |
| FANTOMCAT | https://fantom.gsc.riken.jp/cat/v1/#/ | Comprehensive atlas of the human transcriptome, providing more accurate transcriptional start sites (TSSs) for coding and noncoding genes |
| NONCODE | http://www.noncode.org | Expression profiles from all human and mouse transcripts and genes, annotated with predicted functions. Includes relationships between lncRNAs and various diseases |
| LNCat | http://biocc.hrbmu.edu.cn/LNCat/ | Comprehensive database resource derived by manually curation of >205,000 annotated lncRNAs coming from available literature and GENCODE, LnCipedia, and NONCODE |
| *Prediction of function through subcellular distribution, structure analysis, interactions, coexpression* | | |
| LncATLAS | https://lncatlas.crg.eu/ | Subcellular localization for user-selected lncRNAs |
| lncRNome | http://genome.igib.res.in/lncRNome | Comprehensive biologically oriented knowledgebase for long noncoding RNAs in humans. Includes structure prediction and potential processing in small RNAs |
| LncTarD | http://biocc.hrbmu.edu.cn/LncTarD/ | Manually curated database of experimentally supported lncRNA–target regulations, lncRNA-influenced functions and lncRNA-mediated regulatory mechanisms in human diseases, from published literature |
| NPInter v4.0 | http://bigdata.ibp.ac.cn/npinter4 | ncRNA interactions with proteins and miRNAs, in 35 organisms, by manual literature mining and integration of high-throughput sequencing data |
| LncRInter | http://bioinfo.life.hust.edu.cn/lncRInter/ | High quality lncRNA interaction database containing experimentally validated data |
| DIANA-LncBase v3.0 | www.microrna.gr/LncBase | Database of experimentally verified miRNA targets on ncRNAs |
| LnCeDB | http://gyanxet-beta.com/lncedb | Database of human lncRNAs that can potentially act as ceRNAs |
| *Prediction of lncRNA–disease association* | | |

(continued)

**Table 1**
**(continued)**

| LncRNA database | Web address | Brief description |
|---|---|---|
| LncRNADisease | http://www.rnanut.net/lncrnadisease/ | Collection of curated experimentally supported lncRNA–disease association data |
| CCG | http://ccg.xingene.net | Manually curated database providing both known and candidate cancer protein-coding genes and lncRNAs |
| Lnc2Cancer | http://www.bio-bigdata.net/lnc2cancer | Experimentally supported associations between lncRNA or circRNA and human cancer |
| EVLncRNAs | http://biophy.dzu.edu.cn/EVLncRNAs | High-quality and integrated manually curated database of all kinds of experimentally validated lncRNAs |
| CLC | https://www.gold-lab.org/clc | Catalog of GENECODE-annotated lncRNA with demonstrated role in tumorigenesis or in cancer phenotype |
| LncRNASNP2 | http://bioinfo.life.hust.edu.cn/lncRNASNP2 | Impact of single nucleotide polymorphisms (SNPs) on lncRNA structure and function in human and mouse |
| LincSNP 3.0 | http://bioinfo.hrbmu.edu.cn/LincSNP | Annotation of disease or phenotype-associated variants including single nucleotide polymorphisms (SNPs), linkage disequilibrium SNP (LD SNP), somatic mutation and RNA editing in human long noncoding RNAs (lncRNAs) and circRNA |
| *Databases focused on specific features of lncRNAs* | | |
| Lnc2Meth | http://www.bio-bigdata.com/Lnc2Meth | Manually curated database of regulatory relationships between human lncRNAs and associated DNA methylation in diverse diseases |
| RMBase v2.0 | http://mirlab.sysu.edu.cn/rmbase | Comprehensive database of post-transcriptionally modifications of RNA as well as their relationship with microRNA bindings, disease related SNPs and RNA binding proteins |
| exoRBase | http://www.exoRBase.org | Repository of circular RNA (circRNA), long noncoding RNA (lncRNA), and messenger RNA (mRNA) derived from RNA-seq data analyses of human blood exosomes |

basis of codon statistics and similarity to known protein sequences. This annotation is cost and time effective, but unfortunately likely prone to errors. On the other hand, many other collections are based on literature, manual curation, and experimental validation.

*3.1.1 RNAcentral (https:/rnacentral.org/)*

RNAcentral aims to merge all noncoding RNA annotation databases into a single compendium. It is a free, public resource coordinated by European Bioinformatics Institute that offers integrated access to a comprehensive and up-to-date set of noncoding RNA sequences provided by a collaborating group of Expert Databases, representing a broad range of organisms and RNA types [38].

RNAcentral integrates data importing ncRNA sequences from multiple databases and enables integrated text search, sequence similarity search and bulk downloads. The sequences are mapped to reference genomes from more than 250 species, using blat when the genome mapping is not available. A genome browser allows to browse all mapped sequences, visualize individual sequences in their genomic context, or download genome coordinates. An important feature of RNA Central is the implementation of functional annotations. For instance, it imports modified nucleotides from Modomics [39], miRNA targets from TarBase [40], and Gene Ontology annotations from QuickGO [41]. It also provides secondary structure diagrams for a wide range of RNA types.

*3.1.2 LncBooK (http:/bigd.big.ac.cn/lncbook)*

LncBook is an expert curation–based resource, which is a complement to community curation–based LncRNAWiki [42–44]. LncBook constitutes a comprehensive collection of human lncRNAs and gives a systematic curation of lncRNAs by multiomics data integration, functional annotation and disease association. It includes a larger number of human lncRNAs derived from existing databases but also novel RNA assemblies based on RNA-seq data analysis. It includes community-contributed annotations from LncRNAWiki and expert-curated annotations from published literature. Particularly, it integrates a variety of multiomics data, including expression, methylation, genome variation, and lncRNA–miRNA interactions, conducts functional annotation and incorporates a collection of lncRNA–disease associations.

Currently, LncBook includes 270,044 lncRNAs and includes 1867 characterized lncRNAs with 3762 lncRNA–function associations. LncBook includes 3772 experimentally validated lncRNA–disease associations and identifies 97,998 lncRNAs putatively disease-associated. For any given lncRNA, LncBook profiles its expression levels across tissues and further identifies a total of 819 housekeeping lncRNAs, which are consistently expressed in almost all tissues and also 49,115 tissue-specific lncRNAs, which are expressed specifically in one or few tissues.

For each lncRNA, LncBook provides methylation levels of both promoter and body regions in normal and cancer samples across nine cancers. Only 583 lncRNAs are always hypermethylated in cancers, while 27,723 lncRNAs are always hypomethylated. LncBook also collects SNPs residing in lncRNA transcripts from dbSNP [45]. Among all these SNPs, there are 7571 pathogenic SNPs from ClinVar [46] overlapping 2280 lncRNA transcripts and 79,012 pathogenic SNPs from COSMIC [47] overlapping 26,008 lncRNA transcripts.

In addition, LncBook includes 145 lncRNA–miRNA interactions supported by experimental evidence from starBase [48], as well as many others predicted by TargetScan [49] and MiRanda [50].

LncBook integrates 3772 lncRNA–disease associations, derived from LncRNADisease [51] and LncRNAWiki [43] but also selected based on 2337 publications. LncRNAs in LncBook are associated with 462 diseases, but among all, the largest number is associated with cancer. Among the disease-associated lncRNAs, HOTAIR, MALAT1, H19, MEG3, CDKN2BAS1, PVT1, NEAT1, and GAS5 are extensively studied and each of them is associated with at least 30 different diseases. However, many other lncRNAs are predicted to be disease-associated, if any evidence for that can be obtained from methylation, genome variation and/or lncRNA–miRNA interaction [52].

### 3.1.3 LNCipedia (https:/lncipedia.org)

LNCipedia, released in 2012, is a database to collect human lncRNA sequences and annotation [53]. The main aim is the merging of redundant transcripts across the different data sources and grouping of the transcript into genes resulting in a highly consistent database, through regular updates. LNCipedia 5, the latest update of the database expanded the database with new lncRNAs, thanks to the release of valuable resources such as FANTOMCAT [54, 55] and improved the filtering pipeline. Importantly, an extensive manual literature curation resulted in the annotation of 2482 lncRNA publications, providing insights into functions of 1555 human lncRNAs.

LNCipedia 5 also introduced a new filtering pipeline to remove transcripts originating from protein coding genes. Transcripts with truncated or partial ORFs that overlap coding ORFs, often called processed transcripts, can be annotated as long noncoding RNA, even though they may originate from problems in the RNA sequencing analysis. LNCipedia 5 strictly disregards transcripts that have exons overlapping with coding ORFs in sense as lncRNAs. In this way, 9203 genes were removed. The high-confidence set, a subset of transcripts that lack coding potential by any metric [56], presently contains 49,372 genes.

Many lncRNAs have recently received an official gene symbol from the HUGO Gene Nomenclature Committee (HGNC). When the gene symbol is available, it is used as the primary identifier in LNCipedia; otherwise, they are identified with the nearest protein coding gene on the same strand. Currently, 23% of the transcripts and 6% of the genes in LNCipedia are annotated with an official gene symbol.

Recently the number of publications about functional characterization of lncRNAs is increasing enormously, even though the majority of them focus on few already well known lncRNAs. The lack of official names for the majority of lncRNAs had led authors to name the new molecules with their own identifiers. This is a big issue for annotators and manual curation is needed for functional annotation of lncRNAs. LNCipedia combines manual and programmatical curation of thousands of lncRNA papers in PubMed. In this way, 2482 PubMed articles were associated with lncRNAs in LNCipedia raising the number of lncRNA with at least one published article to 1555.

*3.1.4 FANTOMCAT*
*(https:/fantom.gsc.riken.jp/*
*cat/v1/#/)*

The FANTOM Consortium, through the use of Cap Analysis of Gene Expression sequencing (CAGE-seq), combined with public RNA-seq data, released a comprehensive atlas of the human transcriptome, providing more accurate transcriptional start sites (TSSs) for coding and noncoding genes, including numerous novel long noncoding genes: the FANTOM CAGE-Associated Transcriptome (FANTOM-CAT) [55]. Usually lncRNA catalogs are derived from RNA-seq and the 5′ ends of their transcript models are generally inaccurate. The 5′ complete transcript models allows to better categorizing lncRNA loci based on epigenetic marks at their transcription initiation regions (TIRs). Almost 30,000 high-confidence long noncoding RNA (lncRNA) genes are comprehensively annotated into categories based on their genomic and epigenomic features. Based on the expression profiles and genome-wide association studies, FANTOM CAT genes are associated with specific types of cell and traits respectively. Among all, 1970 lncRNA genes are associated with specific traits and expressed in the relevant cell-types and so potentially functional.

*3.1.5 NONCODE (http:/*
*www.noncode.org)*

NONCODE [57] contains 548,640 lncRNA transcripts from 17 species (human, mouse, cow, rat, chimpanzee, gorilla, orangutan, rhesus macaque, opossum, platypus, chicken, zebrafish, fruit fly, *Caenorhabditis elegans*, yeast, Arabidopsis, and pig). NONCODE v5 annotated the expression profiles from all human and mouse transcripts and genes, and some of these genes were annotated with predicted functions. Expression profiles in exosomes calculated for human species and the conservation of information between human and other species were also provided. The data sources of NONCODE include literature published and the latest versions of several public databases (Ensembl [58], RefSeq [59], lncRNAdb [60], and LNCipedia [56]). The number of transcripts in the last version, NONCODEv5, reached 548,640 after removal of false and redundant lncRNAs. The last version of NONCODE collected relationships between lncRNAs and various diseases using literature mining, differential lncRNA analysis by public RNA-seq data and microarray data and mutation analyses from public genomewide association study (GWAS) data. A total of 32,226 disease-related and 724,579 SNP-related genes were included in the

NONCODEv5 database and t majority of those associations is still unknown. One major advantage of NONCODE is the prediction of the RNA secondary structures of the human transcripts.

Currently, NONCODE covered the sequence, structure, expression, function, conservation, disease relevance, and many other aspects of lncRNAs. Compared to other lncRNA databases, NONCODE collected more lncRNA transcripts, and provided unique annotations of lncRNAs, such as RNA secondary structure, expression of exosome, and association between lncRNA and disease.

*3.1.6   LNCat (http:/biocc. hrbmu.edu.cn/LNCat/)*

LNCat [61] is a comprehensive database resource derived by manually curation of >205,000 annotated lncRNAs coming from available literatures, a collection of 19 articles corresponding to 21 resources that applied high-throughput sequencing data to identify lncRNAs. Three widely used lncRNA databases, including GENCODE (V19) [62], LNCipedia (version 2.1) [56] and NONCODE (version 4.0) [63], are also included, for a total of 24 lncRNA annotation resources. It provides genome browser of lncRNA structures for each resource and visualization of comparison analysis among these resources. LncRNAs from different annotation resources harbored specific characteristics in respect to genomic structure, conservation, tissue specificity, and chromatin state and function. Similar histone modification patterns across different lncRNA annotation resources and their tissue expression and functional specificity are evident, suggesting the need of integration of these resources. The resources focusing on specific tissues help to reveal many novel lncRNAs, generally critical to the biogenesis of specific tissues and tissue-related functions. LNCat is a tool that provides comparison and integration of different lncRNA annotation resources and allows researchers to achieve refined annotation of lncRNAs within the interested region.

Even though the main lncRNAs catalogs focus on human noncoding transcriptome, lncRNA annotation is not limited to human or laboratory animal species. For instance, the domestic-animal lncRNA database ALDB, stores pig, chicken, and cow lncRNAs [64]. Even though lncRNAs are considered evolutionary new, also plant lncRNAs have been discovered and are cataloged in few databases as CANTATA db [65] and GreenNC [66].

CANTATAdb 2.0 collects 239,631 lncRNAs predicted in 39 plant species. The database presents, among others, lncRNA sequences, expression values across RNA-Seq libraries, genomic locations, hypothetical peptides encoded by lncRNAs, BLAST search results against Swiss-Prot proteins, and noncoding RNAs from NONCODE.

The Green Non-Coding Database (GreeNC) is a repository of lncRNAs annotated in 37 plants and 6 algae. The GreeNC database provides information about sequence, genomic coordinates, coding potential and folding energy for all the identified lncRNAs.

## 3.2 Prediction of Function Through Subcellular Distribution, Structure Analysis, Interactions, Coexpression

Understanding the precise molecular mechanisms by which lncRNA regulates downstream key mediators to affect important biological functions is necessary to understand their roles in the pathogenesis of human diseases.

The location of lncRNAs in the cell provides a first clue about their function. For instance, lncRNAs that epigenetically regulate gene expression are mainly located in the nucleus and chromatin [28, 67–71]. However, a relevant population of lncRNAs is cytoplasmatic [15, 72, 73], and they can play a role in translation regulation [74], miRNA decoys [75], or protein trafficking [76, 77].

### 3.2.1 LncATLAS (https:/ lncatlas.crg.eu/)

It displays the subcellular localization for user-selected lncRNAs. It enables nonexpert users to quickly access a rich variety of easily interpreted data on their lncRNA of interest [78].

It takes advantage of large amounts of raw subcellular RNA sequencing (subcRNAseq) data, most notably from the ENCODE Consortium [1, 79]. SubcRNAseq is the only method currently capable of whole-genome localization mapping. In this process, cells are fractionated, RNA extracted and sequenced [1]. SubcRNAseq yields high-throughput and quantitative data, although does not provide the absolute counts of RNA molecules per cell [15]. RNA-seq experiments were obtained for 15 cell lines, from many different adult and embryonic organ sites and includes both transformed and normal cells. Only GENCODE-annotated lncRNA genes are present, and may be accessed using their identifier or official Gene Name. Several well-known lncRNAs with known localization are also available for reference.

### 3.2.2 lncRNome (http:/ genome.igib.res.in/ lncRNome)

LncRNome is a comprehensive searchable biologically oriented knowledgebase for long noncoding RNAs in humans [80]. It integrates annotations on a wide variety of biologically significant information. It is one of the largest catalogs for lncRNAs since it includes information on over 17,000 long noncoding RNAs in human. Each lncRNA gene has links to other relevant databases, annotation sets, and relevant categories of information as types, chromosomal locations, description on the biological functions, and disease associations of long noncoding RNAs. Sequence and structure prediction are also provided: the lncRNA sequences were downloaded from UCSC Genome Browser Database [81], and the structures were predicted using RNAfold version 1.8.5. Moreover, predictions of potential G-quadruplex forming motifs in lncRNA transcripts were obtained by Quadfinder [82] and potential hairpin structures by HairpinFetcher. An interesting analysis was also performed to derive information on potential lncRNAs that could be processed to smallRNAs, overlaying a comprehensive database of smallRNA annotations on the overall dataset of lncRNAs. In addition, it provides access to datasets on protein–lncRNA interactions, through experimental datasets of PAR-CLIP experiments but also by computational prediction method involving Support Vector Machine–based prediction of residues in RNA, which could have a chance to interact with proteins.

LncRNome also includes mapping of genomic variations in lncRNA loci, coming from dbSNP [45] and in particular it highlights which ones are disease associated variations from the NIH Catalog of published genomewide association studies. It also provides a comprehensive access to epigenetic marks in the promoters of lncRNAs.

Finally it predicts the possibility of lncRNA to be translated in peptides by the Sixpack (http://www.ebi.ac.uk/Tools/st/emboss_sixpack/) tool from EMBOSS.

*3.2.3 LncTarD (http:/biocc.hrbmu.edu.cn/LncTarD/)*

LncTarD is a manually curated database that provides a comprehensive resource of experimentally supported lncRNA–target regulations, lncRNA-influenced functions and lncRNA-mediated regulatory mechanisms in human diseases, coming from published literature [83].

Lnc-TarD provides key downstream targets and biological functions driven by disease-related lncRNAs in human diseases. It also indicates lncRNA-mediated regulatory mechanisms in human diseases, as transcriptional or epigenetic regulation, chromatin looping, ceRNA or sponge, interaction with mRNA and with proteins. It correlates the expression levels of disease-associated lncRNA and target genes. It identifies lncRNA–target regulations responsible for drug resistance or sensitivity involving 52 drugs in 41 human diseases, to suggest potential lncRNA–targeted strategies for overcoming drug resistance. Finally, LncTarD provides lncRNA microarray or sequencing data and TCGA [84] pan-cancer transcriptome data (33 cancer types), which were also integrated into LncTarD to characterize functional lncRNA–target regulations.

*3.2.4 NPInter v4.0 (http:/bigdata.ibp.ac.cn/npinter4)*

Several new methods have been developed to investigate interactions involving RNAs. CLIP-seq [85], PARIS [86], CLASH [87], ChIRP-seq [88], and GRID-seq [89] can find the interacting partners of ncRNAs specific target. NPInter database classified such ncRNA interactions in 35 organisms, mainly by manual literature mining and processing and integration of high-throughput sequencing data from different sources [90].

NPInter v4.0 reanalyzed 69 CLIP-seq datasets and 338 ENCODE eCLIP datasets [79]. RNA–protein binding sites are matched with ncRNA annotations from the NONCODEv5 database [57] and assigned a NONCODE ID to each binding site overlapping an ncRNA. The mean PhastCons sequence conservation score [91] was also calculated. NPInterv 4.0 also predicts miRNA–ncRNA interaction by TargetScan [49] and miRanda [50] inferring miRNA binding sites in Argonaute CLIPseq peaks. Finally 600,000 new experimentally identified ncRNA–DNA interactions derived from ChIRPseq data and circular RNA interactions have been included in the database. Information on diseases associated with each biomolecule and interaction were also included. It includes also functional modules such as binding prediction and network viewing.

### 3.2.5 LncRInter (http:/ bioinfo.life.hust.edu.cn/ lncRInter/)

LncRInter is reliable and high-quality lncRNA interaction database containing experimentally validated data [92]. Contrarily to NPInter [90], LncRInter does not infer lncRNA interactions from high-throughput sequencing experiments such as CLIP-seq and PAR-CLIP because they require careful computational analysis due to high rate of false positives. The lncRNA interaction datasets are all extracted from peer-reviewed publications by manual curation with strict criteria based on experimental evidences for direct lncRNA interactions (RNA pull-down, luciferase reporter assay, in vitro binding assay, etc.). They curated and categorized almost 1000 experimentally supported lncRNA interaction pairs in 15 organisms.

All the lncRNA interaction pairs are subdivided into seven interaction classes based on their molecule types (RNA–Protein, RNA–TF, RNA–RNA, RNA–DNA, DNA–Protein, DNA–TF, and DNA–DNA). Most of the lncRNA interactions are direct binding, even though some of the interaction pairs are reported as mediated by another intermediate molecule. LncRInter provides also user-friendly interfaces and graphic visualizations of lncRNA interaction networks. The lncRInter database is regularly updated with new experimentally supported lncRNA interaction data.

### 3.2.6 DIANA-LncBase v3.0 (www.microrna.gr/ LncBase)

LncBase is a database of experimentally verified miRNA targets on noncoding RNAs [93]. miRNAs can regulate the half-life of lncRNAs [94], but they can also be regulated by lncRNAs which act as miRNA sponge. In this case they reduce the suppressive activity of miRNAs on mRNAs and the lncRNA are called endogenous competing RNA (ceRNA) [95]. DIANA-LncBase v3.0 is a repository of ~240,000 experimentally supported tissue and cell type specific miRNA–lncRNA interactions in human and mouse species. The extensive collection of interactions has been derived from the manual curation of publications and the analysis of more than 300 high-throughput datasets. It employs an advanced CLIP-Seq analysis framework, microCLIP, to catalog highly confident miRNA binding [96]. It also catalogs direct miRNA–lncRNA chimeric fragments, derived from CLEAR-CLIP [97] and miRNA–lncRNA pairs, derived from the analysis of microarrays performed after miRNA perturbation experiments. Notably, also information about variants on 67,966 miRNA target sites, from the reference databases dbSNP [45], ClinVar [46], and COSMIC [47] are present.

### 3.2.7 LnCeDB (http:/gyanxet-beta.com/lncedb)

LnCeDB provides a database of human lncRNAs (from GEN-CODE 19 version) that can potentially act as ceRNAs [98]. Apart of the identification of lncRNA–miRNA pairs through AGO CLIP-seq data, LnCeDB provides lncRNA–mRNA pairs that can behave as ceRNA. This feature relies not only on the identification of common miRNA binding sites in lncRNA and mRNA but also on the number of these sites and on the relative abundance of miRNA, lncRNA. and mRNA, which is reported to be crucial for the ceRNA pairs [99]. LnCeDB offers the possibility to search the coexpression of ceRNA pairs and shared miRNAs in RNAseq datasets of 22 human tissues.

### 3.3 Prediction of lncRNA–Disease Association

A large number of studies have indicated that lncRNAs are highly associated with the progression of many kind of diseases and links between dysfunction of lncRNAs and diseases have been deeply investigated [100]. Many experimentally and/or computationally supported lncRNA–disease associations have been highlighted [101] and offer potential new clinical applications.

Here we review the most interesting resources linking lncRNA and diseases, in particular cancer.

### 3.3.1 LncRNADisease (http://www.rnanut.net/lncrnadisease/)

The LncRNADisease database collects curated experimentally supported lncRNA–disease association data but also integrates different tools for predicting novel lncRNA–disease associations [51]. In addition, LncRNADisease also reports lncRNA interactions at various levels, including protein, RNA, miRNA, and DNA. LncRNA-Disease 2.0 integrates experimentally and/or computationally supported data and provides the transcriptional regulatory relationships among lncRNA, mRNA, and miRNA. Particular attention is given to circular RNAs (circRNAs), a class of lncRNAs with miRNA sponging function and associated with a wide range of diseases. LncRNADisease 2.0 integrates experimentally supported circRNA–disease associations by manual literature curation [19, 102].

### 3.3.2 CCG (http:/ccg.xingene.net)

Catalogue of Cancer Genes/lncRNAs, is a manually curated database providing both known and candidate cancer protein-coding genes and lncRNAs [103]. It gives access to a comprehensive list of cancer genes as well as uniform genomic aberration information, as somatic mutation and copy number variation and drug–gene inter-actions. CCG integrates well supported and candidate cancer protein-coding and long noncoding RNA genes and takes advan-tages of high-throughput sequencing results on large populations to facilitate understanding of cancer mechanisms. In addition, drug–gene information is useful to the development of new anti-cancer drugs and selection of rational combination therapies.

### 3.3.3 Lnc2Cancer (http:/www.bio-bigdata.net/lnc2cancer)

Lnc2Cancer is a manually curated database that provides compre-hensive experimentally supported associations between lncRNA or circRNA and human cancer [104]. The current version of Lnc2Cancer documents 10,346 entries of associations between 2775 human lncRNAs, 743 circRNAs, and 226 human cancer subtypes through review of more than 1500 published papers.

### 3.3.4 EVLncRNAs (http:/biophy.dzu.edu.cn/EVLncRNAs)

EVLncRNAs is a high-quality and integrated database that manu-ally curated all kinds of experimentally validated lncRNAs [105]. Contrarily to other databases, EVLncRNAs collects all pub-lished experimentally validated lncRNAs of 77 species, including animals, plants, and microbes [106]. EVLncRNAs also provides the disease-associated and functional lncRNAs, as well as the interac-tions of lncRNAs with other molecules.

### 3.3.5 CLC (https:/www.gold-lab.org/clc)

The Cancer LncRNA Census is a catalog of GENECODE-annotated lncRNA with demonstrated role in tumorigenesis or in cancer phenotype [107]. Cancer lncRNAs are defined as those having direct experimental or genetic evidence supporting a causa-tive role in cancer. Information of more than 268,000 LncRNAs, including more than 3700 function and disease associations, expression and methylation data (normal vs. Cancer), SNPs and interactions of lncRNAs with miRNAs are present and includes target genes of lncRNAs confirmed by different types of experi-ments. The updated CLC2 includes lncRNAs from literature resources but also candidate cancer lncRNAs from mutagenesis and CRISPRi screens. The original CLC and the CLC2 can be used to analyze the genomic and functional properties of cancer-lncRNAs and to define lncRNA cancer-driver prediction, by ExI-nAtor. This is a tool for discovering cancer driver lncRNAs with excess of exonic mutations, compared to the expected local neutral rate estimated from surrounding regions. It requires as input a gene annotation and sets of somatic mutations [108].

### 3.3.6 LncRNASNP2 (http:/bioinfo.life.hust.edu.cn/lncRNASNP2)

LncRNASNP2 [109] is a database that focuses mainly on exploring the impact of single nucleotide polymorphisms (SNPs) on lncRNA structure and function in human and mouse. Along with SNP effects on lncRNA structure, it provides mutation in lncRNAs and lncRNA–miRNA binding, with lncRNA expression in cancer, as well.

In addition to what already provided by LncRNASNP2, LincSNP 3.0 annotates disease or phenotype-associated variants including single nucleotide polymorphisms (SNPs), linkage disequilibrium SNP (LD SNP), somatic mutation, and RNA editing in human long noncoding RNAs (lncRNAs) and circRNA [110]. Noteworthy, LincSNP 3.0 also includes disease-associated SNPs in lncRNA regulatory elements such as transcription factor binding sites (TFBSs), enhancer, DNase I hypersensitive site (DHS), topologically associated domain (TAD), footprints, and open chromatin region. In addition, the effects of SNP on methylation in lncRNAs and circRNAs are also included. Furthermore, it includes almost 60 experimentally supported SNP–lncRNA–disease associations.

## 3.4  Databases Focused on Specific Features of lncRNAs

The extensive study of the several functions of lncRNA pushed the researchers to explore also specific features that could help to clarify their role. So specialized databases have grown in number, collecting particular details about a considerable number of molecules. Here we review three of them focused on the epigenomics, epitranscriptomics, and the extracellular trafficking of lncRNAs.

LncRNAs play an important role in modulating gene expression or participating in some essential epigenetic regulation processes as chromatin modification or DNA methylation. DNA methylation is a fundamental feature of epigenomes that can affect the expression of protein-coding or noncoding transcripts. Lnc2Meth [111] is a manually curated database for clarifying the regulatory relationships between human lncRNAs and associated DNA methylation in diverse diseases. It can identify the lncRNAs dysmethylated in a specific disease or the diseases with a specific dysmethylated lncRNA. Furthermore, Lnc2Meth integrates tools to reannotate probes from the Illumina Infinium Human Methylation 450 k BeadChip (HM450k) array to lncRNA loci, in the different functional regions of the lncRNA of interest. Lnc2Meth is also able to identify differential methylation patterns of the lncRNAs with user-supplied external HM450k array datasets. Except for the lncRNAs with known gene symbol or Ensembl Gene ID, users could also reannotate and calculate methylation patterns for a newly assembled lncRNA by providing its genomic loci.

RMBase 2.0 is a comprehensive database to integrate epitranscriptomic sequencing data for exploring post-transcriptionally modifications of RNA as well as their relationship with microRNA bindings, disease related SNPs and RNA binding proteins [112].

By integrating and analyzing numerous high-throughput epitranscriptome sequencing data and collecting data from public resources, RMBase v2.0 provides a gallery of RNA modification marks that cover more than 100 types of them on transcript products in 13 species including humans, mice, zebrafish and yeast.

RMBase v 2.0 can help to investigate the potential functions and mechanisms of RNA modifications in lncRNAs in complex post-transcriptional regulatory networks.

*3.4.3 exoRBase (http://www.exoRBase.org)*

exoRBase is a repository of circular RNA (circRNA), long noncoding RNA (lncRNA) and messenger RNA (mRNA) derived from RNA-seq data analyses of human blood exosomes [113]. Several long RNA species, present in human blood exosomes, are potential regulators or biomarkers [114]. A compendium of these RNA species will help to identify molecular signatures in blood exosomes, new circulating biomarkers and functional implication for human diseases.

ExoRBase integrates RNA expression profiles based on normalized RNA-seq data of normal individuals and patients with different diseases. It contains 58,330 circRNAs, 15,501 lncRNAs and 18,333 mRNAs from 87 blood exosomal RNA-seq datasets. It also includes some experimental validations from published articles. The RNA-seq expression profiles of 30 tissues from the GTEx project [115] have been used to annotate possible original tissues of exosomal RNAs.

In addition, exoRBase allows researchers to submit new exosomal RNAs and their expression profiles in human blood exosomes.

# 4 Conclusions

In this review, we tried to collect and organize the most useful databases actually available, containing information about lncRNA annotation, structure, function, and clinical impact. The resources we described here are comprehensive collections of information manually curated or derived from public repositories of NGS datasets that can help researchers to orientate in the plenty of information already available about known or novel lncRNAs. Starting from features already reported or likely associated to specific molecules by experimental or in silico evidences, researchers may shortcut and reduce the efforts needed to elucidate new mechanisms and biological functions of lncRNAs.

# References

1. Djebali S, Davis CA, Merkel A, Dobin A, Lassmann T, Mortazavi A, Tanzer A, Lagarde J, Lin W, Schlesinger F, Xue C, Marinov GK, Khatun J, Williams BA, Zaleski C, Rozowsky J, Roder M, Kokocinski F, Abdelhamid RF, Alioto T, Antoshechkin I, Baer MT, Bar NS, Batut P, Bell K, Bell I, Chakrabortty S, Chen X, Chrast J, Curado J, Derrien T, Drenkow J, Dumais E, Dumais J, Duttagupta R, Falconnet E, Fastuca M, Fejes-Toth K, Ferreira P, Foissac S, Fullwood MJ, Gao H, Gonzalez D, Gordon A, Gunawardena H, Howald C, Jha S, Johnson R, Kapranov P, King B, Kingswood C, Luo OJ, Park E, Persaud K, Preall JB, Ribeca P, Risk B, Robyr D, Sammeth M, Schaffer L, See LH, Shahab A, Skancke J, Suzuki AM, Takahashi H,

Tilgner H, Trout D, Walters N, Wang H, Wrobel J, Yu Y, Ruan X, Hayashizaki Y, Harrow J, Gerstein M, Hubbard T, Reymond A, Antonarakis SE, Hannon G, Giddings MC, Ruan Y, Wold B, Carninci P, Guigo R, Gingeras TR (2012) Landscape of transcription in human cells. Nature 489 (7414):101–108. https://doi.org/10.1038/nature11233

2. Guttman M, Amit I, Garber M, French C, Lin MF, Feldser D, Huarte M, Zuk O, Carey BW, Cassady JP, Cabili MN, Jaenisch R, Mikkelsen TS, Jacks T, Hacohen N, Bernstein BE, Kellis M, Regev A, Rinn JL, Lander ES (2009) Chromatin signature reveals over a thousand highly conserved large non-coding RNAs in mammals. Nature 458 (7235):223–227. https://doi.org/10.1038/nature07672

3. Washietl S, Kellis M, Garber M (2014) Evolutionary dynamics and tissue specificity of human long noncoding RNAs in six mammals. Genome Res 24(4):616–628. https://doi.org/10.1101/gr.165035.113

4. Johnsson P, Lipovich L, Grander D, Morris KV (2014) Evolutionary conservation of long non-coding RNAs; sequence, structure, function. Biochim Biophys Acta 1840 (3):1063–1071. https://doi.org/10.1016/j.bbagen.2013.10.035

5. Wan Y, Kertesz M, Spitale RC, Segal E, Chang HY (2011) Understanding the transcriptome through RNA structure. Nat Rev Genet 12(9):641–655. https://doi.org/10.1038/nrg3049

6. Boon RA, Jae N, Holdt L, Dimmeler S (2016) Long noncoding RNAs: from clinical genetics to therapeutic targets? J Am Coll Cardiol 67(10):1214–1226. https://doi.org/10.1016/j.jacc.2015.12.051

7. Mattick JS (2018) The state of long non-coding RNA biology. Noncoding RNA 4(3):17. https://doi.org/10.3390/ncrna4030017

8. Gupta RA, Shah N, Wang KC, Kim J, Horlings HM, Wong DJ, Tsai MC, Hung T, Argani P, Rinn JL, Wang Y, Brzoska P, Kong B, Li R, West RB, van de Vijver MJ, Sukumar S, Chang HY (2010) Long non-coding RNA HOTAIR reprograms chromatin state to promote cancer metastasis. Nature 464(7291):1071–1076. https://doi.org/10.1038/nature08975

9. Dykes IM, Emanueli C (2017) Transcriptional and post-transcriptional gene regulation by long non-coding RNA. Genomics Proteomics Bioinformatics 15(3):177–186.

https://doi.org/10.1016/j.gpb.2016.12.005

10. Cabili MN, Trapnell C, Goff L, Koziol M, Tazon-Vega B, Regev A, Rinn JL (2011) Integrative annotation of human large intergenic noncoding RNAs reveals global properties and specific subclasses. Genes Dev 25 (18):1915–1927. https://doi.org/10.1101/gad.17446611

11. Chen YG, Satpathy AT, Chang HY (2017) Gene regulation in the immune system by long noncoding RNAs. Nat Immunol 18 (9):962–972. https://doi.org/10.1038/ni.3771

12. St Laurent G, Wahlestedt C, Kapranov P (2015) The landscape of long noncoding RNA classification. Trends Genet 31 (5):239–251. https://doi.org/10.1016/j.tig.2015.03.007

13. Kopp F, Mendell JT (2018) Functional classification and experimental dissection of long noncoding RNAs. Cell 172(3):393–407. https://doi.org/10.1016/j.cell.2018.01.011

14. Jarroux J, Morillon A, Pinskaya M (2017) History, discovery, and classification of lncRNAs. Adv Exp Med Biol 1008:1–46. https://doi.org/10.1007/978-981-10-5203-3_1

15. Ulitsky I, Bartel DP (2013) lincRNAs: genomics, evolution, and mechanisms. Cell 154 (1):26–46. https://doi.org/10.1016/j.cell.2013.06.020

16. Khorkova O, Myers AJ, Hsiao J, Wahlestedt C (2014) Natural antisense transcripts. Hum Mol Genet 23(R1):R54–R63. https://doi.org/10.1093/hmg/ddu207

17. Albrecht AS, Orom UA (2016) Bidirectional expression of long ncRNA/protein-coding gene pairs in cancer. Brief Funct Genomics 15(3):167–173. https://doi.org/10.1093/bfgp/elv048

18. Zhang Y, Zhang XO, Chen T, Xiang JF, Yin QF, Xing YH, Zhu S, Yang L, Chen LL (2013) Circular intronic long noncoding RNAs. Mol Cell 51(6):792–806. https://doi.org/10.1016/j.molcel.2013.08.017

19. Memczak S, Jens M, Elefsinioti A, Torti F, Krueger J, Rybak A, Maier L, Mackowiak SD, Gregersen LH, Munschauer M, Loewer A, Ziebold U, Landthaler M, Kocks C, le Noble F, Rajewsky N (2013) Circular RNAs are a large class of animal RNAs with regulatory potency. Nature 495 (7441):333–338. https://doi.org/10.1038/nature11928

20. Milligan MJ, Lipovich L (2014) Pseudogene-derived lncRNAs: emerging regulators of gene expression. Front Genet 5:476. https://doi.org/10.3389/fgene.2014.00476

21. Fabris L, Calin GA (2017) Understanding the genomic ultraconservations: T-UCRs and cancer. Int Rev Cell Mol Biol 333:159–172. https://doi.org/10.1016/bs.ircmb.2017.04.004

22. Pereira Zambalde E, Mathias C, Rodrigues AC, de Souza Fonseca Ribeiro EM, Fiori Gradia D, Calin GA, Carvalho de Oliveira J (2020) Highlighting transcribed ultraconserved regions in human diseases. Wiley Interdiscip Rev RNA 11(2):e1567. https://doi.org/10.1002/wrna.1567

23. Mikhaylichenko O, Bondarenko V, Harnett D, Schor IE, Males M, Viales RR, Furlong EEM (2018) The degree of enhancer or promoter activity is reflected by the levels and directionality of eRNA transcription. Genes Dev 32(1):42–57. https://doi.org/10.1101/gad.308619.117

24. Mapelli SN, Napoli S, Pisignano G, Garcia-Escudero R, Carbone GM, Catapano CV (2019) Deciphering the complexity of human non-coding promoter-proximal transcriptome. Bioinformatics 35(15):2529–2534. https://doi.org/10.1093/bioinformatics/bty981

25. Mayr C (2017) Regulation by 3′-untranslated regions. Annu Rev Genet 51:171–194. https://doi.org/10.1146/annurev-genet-120116-024704

26. Wang KC, Chang HY (2011) Molecular mechanisms of long noncoding RNAs. Mol Cell 43(6):904–914. https://doi.org/10.1016/j.molcel.2011.08.018

27. Liu N, Dai Q, Zheng G, He C, Parisien M, Pan T (2015) N(6)-methyladenosine-dependent RNA structural switches regulate RNA-protein interactions. Nature 518 (7540):560–564. https://doi.org/10.1038/nature14234

28. Tsai MC, Manor O, Wan Y, Mosammaparast N, Wang JK, Lan F, Shi Y, Segal E, Chang HY (2010) Long noncoding RNA as modular scaffold of histone modification complexes. Science 329(5992):689–693. https://doi.org/10.1126/science.1192002

29. Li Y, Syed J, Sugiyama H (2016) RNA-DNA triplex formation by long noncoding RNAs. Cell Chem Biol 23(11):1325–1333. https://doi.org/10.1016/j.chembiol.2016.09.011

30. Kuo CC, Hanzelmann S, Senturk Cetin N, Frank S, Zajzon B, Derks JP, Akhade VS, Ahuja G, Kanduri C, Grummt I, Kurian L, Costa IG (2019) Detection of RNA-DNA binding sites in long noncoding RNAs. Nucleic Acids Res 47(6):e32. https://doi.org/10.1093/nar/gkz037

31. Laham-Karam N, Laitinen P, Turunen TA, Yla-Herttuala S (2018) Activating the chromatin by noncoding RNAs. Antioxid Redox Signal 29(9):813–831. https://doi.org/10.1089/ars.2017.7248

32. Tay Y, Rinn J, Pandolfi PP (2014) The multi-layered complexity of ceRNA crosstalk and competition. Nature 505(7483):344–352. https://doi.org/10.1038/nature12986

33. Da Sacco L, Baldassarre A, Masotti A (2012) Bioinformatics tools and novel challenges in long non-coding RNAs (lncRNAs) functional analysis. Int J Mol Sci 13(1):97–114. https://doi.org/10.3390/ijms13010097

34. Robinson EK, Covarrubias S, Carpenter S (1863) The how and why of lncRNA function: an innate immune perspective. Biochim Biophys Acta Gene Regul Mech 2020 (4):194419. https://doi.org/10.1016/j.bbagrm.2019.194419

35. Iyer MK, Niknafs YS, Malik R, Singhal U, Sahu A, Hosono Y, Barrette TR, Prensner JR, Evans JR, Zhao S, Poliakov A, Cao X, Dhanasekaran SM, Wu YM, Robinson DR, Beer DG, Feng FY, Iyer HK, Chinnaiyan AM (2015) The landscape of long noncoding RNAs in the human transcriptome. Nat Genet 47(3):199–208. https://doi.org/10.1038/ng.3192

36. Frankish A, Diekhans M, Ferreira AM, Johnson R, Jungreis I, Loveland J, Mudge JM, Sisu C, Wright J, Armstrong J, Barnes I, Berry A, Bignell A, Carbonell Sala S, Chrast J, Cunningham F, Di Domenico T, Donaldson S, Fiddes IT, Garcia Giron C, Gonzalez JM, Grego T, Hardy M, Hourlier T, Hunt T, Izuogu OG, Lagarde J, Martin FJ, Martinez L, Mohanan S, Muir P, Navarro FCP, Parker A, Pei B, Pozo F, Ruffier M, Schmitt BM, Stapleton E, Suner MM, Sycheva I, Uszczynska-Ratajczak B, Xu J, Yates A, Zerbino D, Zhang Y, Aken B, Choudhary JS, Gerstein M, Guigo R, Hubbard TJP, Kellis M, Paten B, Reymond A, Tress ML, Flicek P (2019) GENCODE reference annotation for the human and mouse genomes. Nucleic Acids Res 47(D1):D766–D773. https://doi.org/10.1093/nar/gky955

37. Iwakiri J, Hamada M, Asai K (2016) Bioinformatics tools for lncRNA research. Biochim Biophys Acta 1859(1):23–30. https://doi.org/10.1016/j.bbagrm.2015.07.014

38. The RC (2019) RNAcentral: a hub of information for non-coding RNA sequences. Nucleic Acids Res 47(D1):D221–D229. https://doi.org/10.1093/nar/gky1034

39. Boccaletto P, Machnicka MA, Purta E, Piatkowski P, Baginski B, Wirecki TK, de Crecy-Lagard V, Ross R, Limbach PA, Kotter A, Helm M, Bujnicki JM (2018) MODOMICS: a database of RNA modification pathways. 2017 update. Nucleic Acids Res 46(D1):D303–D307. https://doi.org/10.1093/nar/gkx1030

40. Karagkouni D, Paraskevopoulou MD, Chatzopoulos S, Vlachos IS, Tastsoglou S, Kanellos I, Papadimitriou D, Kavakiotis I, Maniou S, Skoufos G, Vergoulis T, Dalamagas T, Hatzigeorgiou AG (2018) DIANA-TarBase v8: a decade-long collection of experimentally supported miRNA-gene interactions. Nucleic Acids Res 46(D1): D239–D245. https://doi.org/10.1093/nar/gkx1141

41. Binns D, Dimmer E, Huntley R, Barrell D, O'Donovan C, Apweiler R (2009) QuickGO: a web-based tool for gene ontology searching. Bioinformatics 25(22):3045–3046. https://doi.org/10.1093/bioinformatics/btp536

42. Ma L, Cao J, Liu L, Li Z, Shireen H, Pervaiz N, Batool F, Raza RZ, Zou D, Bao Y, Abbasi AA, Zhang Z (2019) Community curation and expert curation of human long noncoding RNAs with LncRNAWiki and LncBook. Curr Protoc Bioinformatics 67(1):e82. https://doi.org/10.1002/cpbi.82

43. Ma L, Li A, Zou D, Xu X, Xia L, Yu J, Bajic VB, Zhang Z (2015) LncRNAWiki: harnessing community knowledge in collaborative curation of human long non-coding RNAs. Nucleic Acids Res 43(Database issue): D187–D192. https://doi.org/10.1093/nar/gku1167

44. Ma L, Cao J, Liu L, Du Q, Li Z, Zou D, Bajic VB, Zhang Z (2019) LncBook: a curated knowledgebase of human long non-coding RNAs. Nucleic Acids Res 47(D1): D128–D134. https://doi.org/10.1093/nar/gky960

45. Sherry ST, Ward MH, Kholodov M, Baker J, Phan L, Smigielski EM, Sirotkin K (2001) dbSNP: the NCBI database of genetic variation. Nucleic Acids Res 29(1):308–311. https://doi.org/10.1093/nar/29.1.308

46. Landrum MJ, Lee JM, Benson M, Brown GR, Chao C, Chitipiralla S, Gu B, Hart J, Hoffman D, Jang W, Karapetyan K, Katz K, Liu C, Maddipatla Z, Malheiro A, McDaniel K, Ovetsky M, Riley G, Zhou G, Holmes JB, Kattman BL, Maglott DR (2018) ClinVar: improving access to variant interpretations and supporting evidence. Nucleic Acids Res 46(D1):D1062–D1067. https://doi.org/10.1093/nar/gkx1153

47. Tate JG, Bamford S, Jubb HC, Sondka Z, Beare DM, Bindal N, Boutselakis H, Cole CG, Creatore C, Dawson E, Fish P, Harsha B, Hathaway C, Jupe SC, Kok CY, Noble K, Ponting L, Ramshaw CC, Rye CE, Speedy HE, Stefancsik R, Thompson SL, Wang S, Ward S, Campbell PJ, Forbes SA (2019) COSMIC: the catalogue of somatic mutations in Cancer. Nucleic Acids Res 47 (D1):D941–D947. https://doi.org/10.1093/nar/gky1015

48. Li JH, Liu S, Zhou H, Qu LH, Yang JH (2014) starBase v2.0: decoding miRNA-ceRNA, miRNA-ncRNA and protein-RNA interaction networks from large-scale CLIP-Seq data. Nucleic Acids Res 42(Database issue):D92–D97. https://doi.org/10.1093/nar/gkt1248

49. Agarwal V, Bell GW, Nam JW, Bartel DP (2015) Predicting effective microRNA target sites in mammalian mRNAs. elife 4:e05005. https://doi.org/10.7554/eLife.05005

50. Betel D, Koppal A, Agius P, Sander C, Leslie C (2010) Comprehensive modeling of micro-RNA targets predicts functional non-conserved and non-canonical sites. Genome Biol 11(8):R90. https://doi.org/10.1186/gb-2010-11-8-r90

51. Bao Z, Yang Z, Huang Z, Zhou Y, Cui Q, Dong D (2019) LncRNADisease 2.0: an updated database of long non-coding RNA-associated diseases. Nucleic Acids Res 47(D1):D1034–D1037. https://doi.org/10.1093/nar/gky905

52. Ma L, Cao J, Liu L, Du Q, Li Z, Zou D, Bajic VB, Zhang Z (2019) LncBook: a curated knowledgebase of human long non-coding RNAs. Nucleic Acids Res 47(5):2699. https://doi.org/10.1093/nar/gkz073

53. Volders PJ, Anckaert J, Verheggen K, Nuytens J, Martens L, Mestdagh P, Vandesompele J (2019) LNCipedia 5: towards a reference set of human long non-coding RNAs. Nucleic Acids Res 47(D1): D135–D139. https://doi.org/10.1093/nar/gky1031

54. Imada EL, Sanchez DF, Collado-Torres L, Wilks C, Matam T, Dinalankara W, Stupnikov A, Lobo-Pereira F, Yip CW, Yasuzawa K, Kondo N, Itoh M, Suzuki H, Kasukawa T, Hon CC, de Hoon MJL, Shin JW, Carninci P, Jaffe AE, Leek JT, Favorov A, Franco GR, Langmead B, Marchionni L

(2020) Recounting the FANTOM CAGE-associated transcriptome. Genome Res 30 (7):1073–1081. https://doi.org/10.1101/gr.254656.119

55. Hon CC, Ramilowski JA, Harshbarger J, Bertin N, Rackham OJ, Gough J, Denisenko E, Schmeier S, Poulsen TM, Severin J, Lizio M, Kawaji H, Kasukawa T, Itoh M, Burroughs AM, Noma S, Djebali S, Alam T, Medvedeva YA, Testa AC, Lipovich L, Yip CW, Abugessaisa I, Mendez M, Hasegawa A, Tang D, Lassmann T, Heutink P, Babina M, Wells CA, Kojima S, Nakamura Y, Suzuki H, Daub CO, de Hoon MJ, Arner E, Hayashizaki Y, Carninci P, Forrest AR (2017) An atlas of human long non-coding RNAs with accurate 5′ ends. Nature 543(7644):199–204. https://doi.org/10.1038/nature21374

56. Volders PJ, Verheggen K, Menschaert G, Vandepoele K, Martens L, Vandesompele J, Mestdagh P (2015) An update on LNCipedia: a database for annotated human lncRNA sequences. Nucleic Acids Res 43(Database issue):D174–D180. https://doi.org/10.1093/nar/gku1060

57. Fang S, Zhang L, Guo J, Niu Y, Wu Y, Li H, Zhao L, Li X, Teng X, Sun X, Sun L, Zhang MQ, Chen R, Zhao Y (2018) NONCO-DEV5: a comprehensive annotation database for long non-coding RNAs. Nucleic Acids Res 46(D1):D308–D314. https://doi.org/10.1093/nar/gkx1107

58. Yates A, Akanni W, Amode MR, Barrell D, Billis K, Carvalho-Silva D, Cummins C, Clapham P, Fitzgerald S, Gil L, Giron CG, Gordon L, Hourlier T, Hunt SE, Janacek SH, Johnson N, Juettemann T, Keenan S, Lavidas I, Martin FJ, Maurel T, McLaren W, Murphy DN, Nag R, Nuhn M, Parker A, Patricio M, Pignatelli M, Rahtz M, Riat HS, Sheppard D, Taylor K, Thormann A, Vullo A, Wilder SP, Zadissa A, Birney E, Harrow J, Muffato M, Perry E, Ruffier M, Spudich G, Trevanion SJ, Cunningham F, Aken BL, Zerbino DR, Flicek P (2016) Ensembl 2016. Nucleic Acids Res 44(D1):D710–D716. https://doi.org/10.1093/nar/gkv1157

59. O'Leary NA, Wright MW, Brister JR, Ciufo S, Haddad D, McVeigh R, Rajput B, Robbertse B, Smith-White B, Ako-Adjei D, Astashyn A, Badretdin A, Bao Y, Blinkova O, Brover V, Chetvernin V, Choi J, Cox E, Ermolaeva O, Farrell CM, Goldfarb T, Gupta T, Haft D, Hatcher E, Hlavina W, Joardar VS, Kodali VK, Li W, Maglott D, Masterson P, McGarvey KM, Murphy MR, O'Neill K, Pujar S, Rangwala SH, Rausch D,

Riddick LD, Schoch C, Shkeda A, Storz SS, Sun H, Thibaud-Nissen F, Tolstoy I, Tully RE, Vatsan AR, Wallin C, Webb D, Wu W, Landrum MJ, Kimchi A, Tatusova T, DiCuccio M, Kitts P, Murphy TD, Pruitt KD (2016) Reference sequence (RefSeq) database at NCBI: current status, taxonomic expansion, and functional annotation. Nucleic Acids Res 44(D1):D733–D745. https://doi.org/10.1093/nar/gkv1189

60. Quek XC, Thomson DW, Maag JL, Bartonicek N, Signal B, Clark MB, Gloss BS, Dinger ME (2015) lncRNAdb v2.0: expanding the reference database for functional long noncoding RNAs. Nucleic Acids Res 43 (Database issue):D168–D173. https://doi.org/10.1093/nar/gku988

61. Xu J, Bai J, Zhang X, Lv Y, Gong Y, Liu L, Zhao H, Yu F, Ping Y, Zhang G, Lan Y, Xiao Y, Li X (2017) A comprehensive overview of lncRNA annotation resources. Brief Bioinform 18(2):236–249. https://doi.org/10.1093/bib/bbw015

62. Derrien T, Johnson R, Bussotti G, Tanzer A, Djebali S, Tilgner H, Guernec G, Martin D, Merkel A, Knowles DG, Lagarde J, Veeravalli L, Ruan X, Ruan Y, Lassmann T, Carninci P, Brown JB, Lipovich L, Gonzalez JM, Thomas M, Davis CA, Shiekhattar R, Gingeras TR, Hubbard TJ, Notredame C, Harrow J, Guigo R (2012) The GENCODE v7 catalog of human long noncoding RNAs: analysis of their gene structure, evolution, and expression. Genome Res 22(9):1775–1789. https://doi.org/10.1101/gr.132159.111

63. Xie C, Yuan J, Li H, Li M, Zhao G, Bu D, Zhu W, Wu W, Chen R, Zhao Y (2014) NONCODEv4: exploring the world of long non-coding RNA genes. Nucleic Acids Res 42 (Database issue):D98–D103. https://doi.org/10.1093/nar/gkt1222

64. Li A, Zhang J, Zhou Z, Wang L, Liu Y, Liu Y (2015) ALDB: a domestic-animal long non-coding RNA database. PLoS One 10(4): e0124003. https://doi.org/10.1371/journal.pone.0124003

65. Szczesniak MW, Rosikiewicz W, Makalowska I (2016) CANTATAdb: a collection of plant long non-coding RNAs. Plant Cell Physiol 57(1):e8. https://doi.org/10.1093/pcp/pcv201

66. Paytuvi Gallart A, Hermoso Pulido A, Anzar Martinez de Lagran I, Sanseverino W, Aiese Cigliano R (2016) GREENC: a wiki-based database of plant lncRNAs. Nucleic Acids Res 44(D1):D1161–D1166. https://doi.org/10.1093/nar/gkv1215

67. Hutchinson JN, Ensminger AW, Clemson CM, Lynch CR, Lawrence JB, Chess A (2007) A screen for nuclear transcripts identifies two linked noncoding RNAs associated with SC35 splicing domains. BMC Genomics 8:39. https://doi.org/10.1186/1471-2164-8-39

68. Rinn JL, Kertesz M, Wang JK, Squazzo SL, Xu X, Brugmann SA, Goodnough LH, Helms JA, Farnham PJ, Segal E, Chang HY (2007) Functional demarcation of active and silent chromatin domains in human HOX loci by noncoding RNAs. Cell 129(7):1311–1323. https://doi.org/10.1016/j.cell.2007.05.022

69. Zhao J, Sun BK, Erwin JA, Song JJ, Lee JT (2008) Polycomb proteins targeted by a short repeat RNA to the mouse X chromosome. Science 322(5902):750–756. https://doi.org/10.1126/science.1163045

70. Whitehead J, Pandey GK, Kanduri C (2009) Regulation of the mammalian epigenome by long noncoding RNAs. Biochim Biophys Acta 1790(9):936–947. https://doi.org/10.1016/j.bbagen.2008.10.007

71. Mondal T, Rasmussen M, Pandey GK, Isaksson A, Kanduri C (2010) Characterization of the RNA content of chromatin. Genome Res 20(7):899–907. https://doi.org/10.1101/gr.103473.109

72. van Heesch S, van Iterson M, Jacobi J, Boymans S, Essers PB, de Bruijn E, Hao W, MacInnes AW, Cuppen E, Simonis M (2014) Extensive localization of long noncoding RNAs to the cytosol and mono- and polyribosomal complexes. Genome Biol 15(1):R6. https://doi.org/10.1186/gb-2014-15-1-r6

73. Carlevaro-Fita J, Rahim A, Guigo R, Vardy LA, Johnson R (2016) Cytoplasmic long noncoding RNAs are frequently bound to and degraded at ribosomes in human cells. RNA 22(6):867–882. https://doi.org/10.1261/rna.053561.115

74. Schein A, Zucchelli S, Kauppinen S, Gustincich S, Carninci P (2016) Identification of antisense long noncoding RNAs that function as SINEUPs in human cells. Sci Rep 6:33605. https://doi.org/10.1038/srep33605

75. Cesana M, Cacchiarelli D, Legnini I, Santini T, Sthandier O, Chinappi M, Tramontano A, Bozzoni I (2011) A long noncoding RNA controls muscle differentiation by functioning as a competing endogenous RNA. Cell 147(2):358–369. https://doi.org/10.1016/j.cell.2011.09.028

76. Kino T, Hurt DE, Ichijo T, Nader N, Chrousos GP (2010) Noncoding RNA gas5 is a growth arrest- and starvation-associated repressor of the glucocorticoid receptor. Sci Signal 3(107):ra8. https://doi.org/10.1126/scisignal.2000568

77. Aoki K, Harashima A, Sano M, Yokoi T, Nakamura S, Kibata M, Hirose T (2010) A thymus-specific noncoding RNA, Thy-ncR1, is a cytoplasmic riboregulator of MFAP4 mRNA in immature T-cell lines. BMC Mol Biol 11:99. https://doi.org/10.1186/1471-2199-11-99

78. Mas-Ponte D, Carlevaro-Fita J, Palumbo E, Hermoso Pulido T, Guigo R, Johnson R (2017) LncATLAS database for subcellular localization of long noncoding RNAs. RNA 23(7):1080–1087. https://doi.org/10.1261/rna.060814.117

79. ENCODE Project Consortium (2012) An integrated encyclopedia of DNA elements in the human genome. Nature 489(7414):57–74. https://doi.org/10.1038/nature11247

80. Bhartiya D, Pal K, Ghosh S, Kapoor S, Jalali S, Panwar B, Jain S, Sati S, Sengupta S, Sachidanandan C, Raghava GP, Sivasubbu S, Scaria V (2013) lncRNome: a comprehensive knowledgebase of human long noncoding RNAs. Database (Oxford) 2013:bat034. https://doi.org/10.1093/database/bat034

81. Kent WJ, Sugnet CW, Furey TS, Roskin KM, Pringle TH, Zahler AM, Haussler D (2002) The human genome browser at UCSC. Genome Res 12(6):996–1006. https://doi.org/10.1101/gr.229102

82. Scaria V, Hariharan M, Arora A, Maiti S (2006) Quadfinder: server for identification and analysis of quadruplex-forming motifs in nucleotide sequences. Nucleic Acids Res 34(Web Server issue):W683–W685. https://doi.org/10.1093/nar/gkl299

83. Zhao H, Shi J, Zhang Y, Xie A, Yu L, Zhang C, Lei J, Xu H, Leng Z, Li T, Huang W, Lin S, Wang L, Xiao Y, Li X (2020) LncTarD: a manually-curated database of experimentally-supported functional lncRNA-target regulations in human diseases. Nucleic Acids Res 48(D1):D118–D126. https://doi.org/10.1093/nar/gkz985

84. Wang Z, Jensen MA, Zenklusen JC (2016) A practical guide to The Cancer Genome Atlas (TCGA). Methods Mol Biol 1418:111–141. https://doi.org/10.1007/978-1-4939-3578-9_6

85. Yeo GW, Coufal NG, Liang TY, Peng GE, Fu XD, Gage FH (2009) An RNA code for the FOX2 splicing regulator revealed by mapping RNA-protein interactions in stem cells. Nat

Struct Mol Biol 16(2):130–137. https://doi.org/10.1038/nsmb.1545

86. Lu Z, Zhang QC, Lee B, Flynn RA, Smith MA, Robinson JT, Davidovich C, Gooding AR, Goodrich KJ, Mattick JS, Mesirov JP, Cech TR, Chang HY (2016) RNA duplex map in living cells reveals higher-order transcriptome structure. Cell 165(5):1267–1279. https://doi.org/10.1016/j.cell.2016.04.028

87. Helwak A, Kudla G, Dudnakova T, Tollervey D (2013) Mapping the human miRNA interactome by CLASH reveals frequent noncanonical binding. Cell 153(3):654–665. https://doi.org/10.1016/j.cell.2013.03.043

88. Chu C, Qu K, Zhong FL, Artandi SE, Chang HY (2011) Genomic maps of long noncoding RNA occupancy reveal principles of RNA-chromatin interactions. Mol Cell 44(4):667–678. https://doi.org/10.1016/j.molcel.2011.08.027

89. Li X, Zhou B, Chen L, Gou LT, Li H, Fu XD (2017) GRID-seq reveals the global RNA-chromatin interactome. Nat Biotechnol 35(10):940–950. https://doi.org/10.1038/nbt.3968

90. Teng X, Chen X, Xue H, Tang Y, Zhang P, Kang Q, Hao Y, Chen R, Zhao Y, He S (2020) NPInter v4.0: an integrated database of ncRNA interactions. Nucleic Acids Res 48(D1):D160–D165. https://doi.org/10.1093/nar/gkz969

91. Siepel A, Bejerano G, Pedersen JS, Hinrichs AS, Hou M, Rosenbloom K, Clawson H, Spieth J, Hillier LW, Richards S, Weinstock GM, Wilson RK, Gibbs RA, Kent WJ, Miller W, Haussler D (2005) Evolutionarily conserved elements in vertebrate, insect, worm, and yeast genomes. Genome Res 15(8):1034–1050. https://doi.org/10.1101/gr.3715005

92. Liu CJ, Gao C, Ma Z, Cong R, Zhang Q, Guo AY (2017) lncRInter: a database of experimentally validated long non-coding RNA interaction. J Genet Genomics 44(5):265–268. https://doi.org/10.1016/j.jgg.2017.01.004

93. Karagkouni D, Paraskevopoulou MD, Tastsoglou S, Skoufos G, Karavangeli A, Pierros V, Zacharopoulou E, Hatzigeorgiou AG (2020) DIANA-LncBase v3: indexing experimentally supported miRNA targets on non-coding transcripts. Nucleic Acids Res 48(D1):D101–D110. https://doi.org/10.1093/nar/gkz1036

94. Wang X, Li M, Wang Z, Han S, Tang X, Ge Y, Zhou L, Zhou C, Yuan Q, Yang M (2015) Silencing of long noncoding RNA MALAT1 by miR-101 and miR-217 inhibits proliferation, migration, and invasion of esophageal squamous cell carcinoma cells. J Biol Chem 290(7):3925–3935. https://doi.org/10.1074/jbc.M114.596866

95. Smillie CL, Sirey T, Ponting CP (2018) Complexities of post-transcriptional regulation and the modeling of ceRNA crosstalk. Crit Rev Biochem Mol Biol 53(3):231–245. https://doi.org/10.1080/10409238.2018.1447542

96. Paraskevopoulou MD, Karagkouni D, Vlachos IS, Tastsoglou S, Hatzigeorgiou AG (2018) microCLIP super learning framework uncovers functional transcriptome-wide miRNA interactions. Nat Commun 9(1):3601. https://doi.org/10.1038/s41467-018-06046-y

97. Grosswendt S, Filipchyk A, Manzano M, Klironomos F, Schilling M, Herzog M, Gottwein E, Rajewsky N (2014) Unambiguous identification of miRNA:target site interactions by different types of ligation reactions. Mol Cell 54(6):1042–1054. https://doi.org/10.1016/j.molcel.2014.03.049

98. Das S, Ghosal S, Sen R, Chakrabarti J (2014) lnCeDB: database of human long noncoding RNA acting as competing endogenous RNA. PLoS One 9(6):e98965. https://doi.org/10.1371/journal.pone.0098965

99. Ala U, Karreth FA, Bosia C, Pagnani A, Taulli R, Leopold V, Tay Y, Provero P, Zecchina R, Pandolfi PP (2013) Integrated transcriptional and competitive endogenous RNA networks are cross-regulated in permissive molecular environments. Proc Natl Acad Sci U S A 110(18):7154–7159. https://doi.org/10.1073/pnas.1222509110

100. Kopp F (2019) Molecular functions and biological roles of long non-coding RNAs in human physiology and disease. J Gene Med 21(8):e3104. https://doi.org/10.1002/jgm.3104

101. Schmitz SU, Grote P, Herrmann BG (2016) Mechanisms of long noncoding RNA function in development and disease. Cell Mol Life Sci 73(13):2491–2509. https://doi.org/10.1007/s00018-016-2174-5

102. Haddad G, Lorenzen JM (2019) Biogenesis and function of circular RNAs in health and in disease. Front Pharmacol 10:428. https://doi.org/10.3389/fphar.2019.00428

103. Liu M, Yang YT, Xu G, Tan C, Lu ZJ (2016) CCG: an integrative resource of cancer protein-coding genes and long noncoding RNAs. Discov Med 22(123):351–359

104. Gao Y, Wang P, Wang Y, Ma X, Zhi H, Zhou D, Li X, Fang Y, Shen W, Xu Y, Shang S, Wang L, Wang L, Ning S, Li X (2019) Lnc2Cancer v2.0: updated database of experimentally supported long non-coding RNAs in human cancers. Nucleic Acids Res 47(D1):D1028–D1033. https://doi.org/10.1093/nar/gky1096

105. Zhou B, Zhao H, Yu J, Guo C, Dou X, Song F, Hu G, Cao Z, Qu Y, Yang Y, Zhou Y, Wang J (2018) EVLncRNAs: a manually curated database for long non-coding RNAs validated by low-throughput experiments. Nucleic Acids Res 46(D1):D100–D105. https://doi.org/10.1093/nar/gkx677

106. Zhou B, Zhao H, Yu J, Guo C, Dou X, Song F, Hu G, Cao Z, Qu Y, Yang Y, Zhou Y, Wang J (2019) Experimentally validated plant lncRNAs in EVLncRNAs database. Methods Mol Biol 1933:431–437. https://doi.org/10.1007/978-1-4939-9045-0_27

107. Carlevaro-Fita J, Lanzos A, Feuerbach L, Hong C, Mas-Ponte D, Pedersen JS, Drivers P, Functional Interpretation G, Johnson R, Consortium P (2020) Cancer LncRNA census reveals evidence for deep functional conservation of long noncoding RNAs in tumorigenesis. Commun Biol 3 (1):56. https://doi.org/10.1038/s42003-019-0741-7

108. Lanzos A, Carlevaro-Fita J, Mularoni L, Reverter F, Palumbo E, Guigo R, Johnson R (2017) Discovery of Cancer driver long non-coding RNAs across 1112 tumour genomes: new candidates and distinguishing features. Sci Rep 7:41544. https://doi.org/10.1038/srep41544

109. Miao YR, Liu W, Zhang Q, Guo AY (2018) lncRNASNP2: an updated database of functional SNPs and mutations in human and mouse lncRNAs. Nucleic Acids Res 46(D1):D276–D280. https://doi.org/10.1093/nar/gkx1004

110. Ning S, Yue M, Wang P, Liu Y, Zhi H, Zhang Y, Zhang J, Gao Y, Guo M, Zhou D, Li X, Li X (2017) LincSNP 2.0: an updated database for linking disease-associated SNPs to human long non-coding RNAs and their TFBSs. Nucleic Acids Res 45(D1):D74–D78. https://doi.org/10.1093/nar/gkw945

111. Zhi H, Li X, Wang P, Gao Y, Gao B, Zhou D, Zhang Y, Guo M, Yue M, Shen W, Ning S, Jin L, Li X (2018) Lnc2Meth: a manually curated database of regulatory relationships between long non-coding RNAs and DNA methylation associated with human disease. Nucleic Acids Res 46(D1):D133–D138. https://doi.org/10.1093/nar/gkx985

112. Xuan JJ, Sun WJ, Lin PH, Zhou KR, Liu S, Zheng LL, Qu LH, Yang JH (2018) RMBase v2.0: deciphering the map of RNA modifications from epitranscriptome sequencing data. Nucleic Acids Res 46(D1):D327–D334. https://doi.org/10.1093/nar/gkx934

113. Li S, Li Y, Chen B, Zhao J, Yu S, Tang Y, Zheng Q, Li Y, Wang P, He X, Huang S (2018) exoRBase: a database of circRNA, lncRNA and mRNA in human blood exosomes. Nucleic Acids Res 46(D1):D106–D112. https://doi.org/10.1093/nar/gkx891

114. Colombo M, Raposo G, Thery C (2014) Biogenesis, secretion, and intercellular interactions of exosomes and other extracellular vesicles. Annu Rev Cell Dev Biol 30:255–289. https://doi.org/10.1146/annurev-cellbio-101512-122326

115. GTEx Consortium (2013) The genotype-tissue expression (GTEx) project. Nat Genet 45(6):580–585. https://doi.org/10.1038/ng.2653

# Chapter 2

# LncRNA as Cancer Biomarkers

## Ingram Iaccarino and Wolfram Klapper

## Abstract

Although the great majority of cancers share a defined group of hallmarks that is responsible for the uncontrolled growth of particular cell types, it is today clear that under the name of cancer we refer to hundreds of different diseases. Furthermore, each of these diseases has an intrinsic variability due to the genetic background in which it develops. The ability to correctly identify these diseases is urgently needed, because each of them may require a specific therapeutic treatment for successful cure. Cancer biomarkers can be extremely valuable tools for efficient diagnosis and prognosis of cancers. In order to succeed in distinguishing between cancer types and progression-associated genetic backgrounds, cancer biomarkers need to have a strong specificity for a particular disease condition. With the development of novel sequencing technologies, it became clear that the set of genes transcribed from human cells is not limited to genes that code for proteins. On the contrary, our cells contain thousands of RNA without any protein-coding potential. The observation that these transcripts have a much higher cell/tissue specificity of expression in comparison to protein-coding genes makes them a potentially very valuable source of novel cancer biomarkers.

**Key words** lncRNAs, Cancer biomarker, Biomarker discovery, Diagnostic, Prognostic, Predictive

## 1 Introduction

A cancer biomarker is a molecule or a group of molecules that is specifically present or absent in patients affected by a particular type of cancer. It can be a protein, an mRNA, a mutated gene, or a metabolite. It can be produced directly from the tumor cells, it can be a reaction of the body to the presence of tumor cells or it can be produced by cellular components of the tumor microenvironment. It can be specifically expressed only in a cancer subtype, in a defined cancer developmental stage or by a cancer developing in a particular genetic context. The use of cancer biomarkers in cancer research can be diagnostic, if its use can help the diagnosis of the disease. A cancer biomarker expressed very early in cancer development, for instance, can be extremely useful for early cancer detection. A cancer biomarker expressed only in a subtype of the same tumor can be helpful in the diagnosis of that type of cancer. The use of

Alfons Navarro (ed.), *Long Non-Coding RNAs in Cancer*, Methods in Molecular Biology, vol. 2348,
https://doi.org/10.1007/978-1-0716-1581-2_2, © Springer Science+Business Media, LLC, part of Springer Nature 2021

cancer biomarkers can also be prognostic or predictive if informative on how aggressive the disease is or how well a patient will respond to treatment, respectively [1].

With the advent of modern molecular biology, scientists have been interested in defining patterns of gene expression peculiar for specific diseases and particularly cancer. The development of gene chips and RNA sequencing made the analysis of global gene expression of normal and diseased tissues much easier. Furthermore, scientists profit from the existence of published gene expression profiles stored in publicly available databases. Global gene expression profiling of cancer tissue gives a snapshot of the tumor status in that particular developmental stage. The pool of expressed genes in a particular tissue have embedded several expression signatures: they carry information on the origin of the tissue, the amount and quality of the tissue stromal cells as well as of particular metabolic conditions associated to hypoxic or nutrients stress. Single genes or group of genes that can signal each of these conditions could become useful cancer biomarkers. In order to be considered a useful cancer biomarker a gene expression signature or the expression of a single gene needs to have a good signal-to-noise ratio. An ideal biomarker would be, for instance, a gene not expressed usually in the normal tissue of origin whose expression is reactivated (either genetically or epigenetically) in the process of oncogenic transformation. The gene coding for *SOX11*, for instance is normally expressed in the developing neuronal tissue only, but it is reexpressed in mantle cell lymphoma (MCL), a rare type of B cell non-Hodgkin lymphoma [2]. Because of its complete absence of expression by hematopoietic cells, SOX11 became therefore a strong diagnostic cancer biomarker for a correct identification of MCL [3]. Genes with highly restricted tissue specificity have therefore better chance to become good cancer biomarkers if reexpressed in cancer tissues.

The development of novel sequencing technologies has been accompanied by a tremendous increase in our knowledge of the human genome and transcriptome. It is now clear that the human genome is able to produce at least as much RNA without protein-coding potential than RNAs coding for proteins. Among all noncoding transcripts present in human cells, those classified as long noncoding RNAs (lncRNAs) are emerging as crucial players in the control of gene expression [4–6]. By definition, lncRNAs are RNAs longer than 200 nucleotides and with no predicted coding potential. They can be divided in several subclasses according to their location relative to coding genes (intergenic, intronic, overlapping with exons of coding genes in antisense or sense orientations) [7–9] (*see* Chapter 1). Functional characterization of a fraction of existing lncRNAs suggests that they can work either as guides or scaffolds, exploiting their concomitant ability to fold in specific protein-binding domains and their ability to engage sequence specific base pairing with either DNA or other RNA molecules [6].

In an attempt to characterize the expression of these novel RNAs, one of the general feature that emerged was that lncRNAs exhibit more specific expression patterns than coding RNAs, meaning that there are more lncRNAs than protein-coding genes expressed in a single cell type or tissue type [7–9]. LncRNAs have also the tendency to have expression patterns specific for cancer subtypes and disease stages [10, 11]. These features make lncRNAs ideal targets for cancer biomarker discovery.

## 2  Guidelines for the Discovery of lncRNAs Behaving as Cancer Biomarkers

### 2.1  Cohort Selection

In order to identify lncRNAs that could end up being useful biomarkers for a certain type of cancer it is essential to set up a suitable experimental pipeline. Tumor samples must be selected from a cohort reflecting the final goal of the experiment: the cohort could include specimens from different subtypes of a cancer; different stages of the same type of cancer; samples form patients before and after treatment with a certain therapy or before and after relapsing after therapy. The cohort might reflect also an interest on the effect of a particular genotype on tumor development: in this case the cohort will include cancer samples from individuals carrying or not a specific mutation or chromosomal translocation or epigenetic signature. Each group should be represented by a reasonable number of samples to ensure statistical significance of the findings. LncRNA expression profiling could end up subdividing each group in two or more subgroups: if the initial group is not represented by enough samples the identification of the subgroup may not reach statistical significance. One possible approach is to use a relatively small cohort of samples (with each group consisting of up to 20 samples) as a discovery cohort and bigger cohort to validate the candidate lncRNAs identified in the discovery cohort.

### 2.2  Sample Source

Cancer biopsies are usually either provided as fresh frozen (FF) material or as formalin-fixed, paraffin-embedded (FFPE) blocks. The choice between FF and FFPE material might depend not only on sample availability but also on the type of technological platform the researcher intends to use for the analysis of lncRNA expression. Expression analyses based on RNA-sequencing (the most powerful approach, able to identify also unannotated transcripts) should preferably make use of FF material. Indeed the process of deparaffinization and reverse of fixation necessary to extract RNA from FFPE material induces relatively high levels of RNA fragmentation. This could create problems in transcripts quantification particularly when using a poly(A)-selection protocol. Nevertheless, in case only FFPE material is available, several studies have shown that there can be a good correlation between expression data obtained by RNA-seq from FFPE material with data obtained from FF material from the same samples [12]. On the contrary, expression analyses based on different technologies, like direct digital detection with nCounter® technology (NanoString), might produce quantitative data also from FFPE material. With the disadvantage that the nCounter® technology can detect the expression of predesigned or custom panels of no more than 700 genes and is therefore limited to a small selection of already known transcripts. Given that the most recent estimates of lncRNAs are in the range of the several thousands (see later), this could be a clear limitation. Nevertheless, the nCounter® technology could be a good choice for the analysis in a validation cohort of a limited set of transcripts identified by RNA-seq in a discovery cohort.

### 2.3 Sample Composition: Tumor Cell Content and Microenvironment

When processing tumor tissue samples for gene expression analysis it is important to keep in mind that the identified RNAs could derive either from the cancer cells or from cellular components of the tumor microenvironment, also referred as tumor stroma [13, 14]. The amount of stroma present in a tumor biopsy can strongly vary depending on the tumor type. Among B cell lymphomas, for instance, the difference in stroma content can be huge. Burkitt's lymphomas are known to have very high tumor cell content, up to 90%. At the same time Hodgkin lymphomas are characterized by a tumor mass where not more than 5% of the cells are malignant B cells, the rest being cellular component of the microenvironment, like T and B cells, macrophages, eosinophils and mast cells [15, 16]. It is important to keep in mind that these cells, although not neoplastically transformed, can also be an important source of cancer biomarker. Cancer cells have been shown to be capable to induce cellular differentiation in stroma cells, either through a direct cell-to-cell contact or through soluble secreted factors. The pool of lncRNAs expressed by stroma cells might therefore differ from that of normal tissue-infiltrating cellular components. Alternatively, the presence of cancer cells in a tissue might affect the local metabolite composition of the microenvironment inducing a differential transcription program also in stroma cells. It could be therefore an added value for lncRNA expression analysis of some kind of tumors to consider also the microenvironment in the choice of sample material. Independently if the scientific project is aimed at including the tumor stroma in the analysis, an important issue in selecting samples for the patient's cohort is to focus on specimens with similar tumor cell content. This will ensure that the differences in lncRNA expression identified will not be associated to the different ratios between tumor and stroma content.

**2.4 Integrating Patients Material with Cell Lines Samples**

One of the problem scientists face when analyzing lncRNAs expression changes in cohorts of cancer samples is connected with the complexity of the result. Complexity might be associated to the difficulty to define targets for further analyses or to differentiate lncRNAs expressed by the tumor cells or by the stroma cells. In order to address these issues it may be helpful to include in the experimental pipeline the analysis of samples derived from homogeneously purified cell lines. A simple way to define cancer cell specific genes is to run in parallel expression analysis of cancer cell lines established from the same cancer type. Because cancer cell lines are single clones derived from different individuals, their expression profiles might be quite heterogeneous. For this reason, it is advised to use more cell lines if available. It could be also particularly useful to include in the experimental setting immortalized nontransformed cell line of the same tissue of origin, to better establish the genes that are important for the oncogenic transformation of that particular tissue. If the interest of the cancer biomarker discovery project is focused on lncRNAs expressed in a defined genetic background, RNA-seq data from cancer cell lines carrying or not that particular genetic background may also be used. For tumor types where a transcription factor is known to play a strong role in tumor development a cell line expressing the transcription factor in an inducible manner could be informative [11]. Alternatively, if the cancer in question is known to be accompanied by specific changes in the metabolite composition of the microenvironment, the experimental pipeline could include cell lines cultivated in conditions that mimic the change in metabolite composition. Purified cellular component of the stroma might also be included in order to help deconvoluting the identified gene expression signature. It is important to keep in mind that the expression pattern of cancer cell lines or generally of cells grown in vitro can differ dramatically from that of cells growing in a tissue context. Data generated on cancer cell lines must therefore be carefully evaluated.

**2.5 Choice of the Technological Platform**

A major step forward the use of gene expression profiling for the identification of cancer biomarkers came with the introduction of microarrays and gene chips [17] (*see* Chapter 3). Initially microarrays included probes limited to protein-coding genes, but with the increase of information coming from the systematic sequencing of expressed sequence tags (ESTs), they lately included also sequences corresponding to lncRNAs. At the same time the number and nature of the lncRNAs represented on commercial microarrays is based on arbitrary selection that needs to be as general as possible for commercial purposes. Microarrays have therefore the potential to detect the expression of a limited set of known lncRNAs. Given the high specificity of lncRNA expression in tissues and disease conditions, there will be always the possibility of missing lncRNAs specifically expressed in the experimental setting of choice. With the advent of NGS and with the strong fall in sequencing prices, RNA-seq is today the technique of choice for the identification of lncRNAs as cancer biomarkers (*see* Chapter 4). Given that RNA-seq is not based on hybridization of RNAs to a defined set of probes but on the direct sequencing of all reverse transcribed RNAs present in a sample, it is capable to assess the quantitative expression of all transcripts produced by all cells present in the sample of interest. In a typical RNA-seq protocol, total RNA extracted from samples of interest is subjected to a selection protocol for the exclusion of ribosomal RNA (rRNA) from the analysis. rRNA constitutes 90% of total cellular RNA and if not removed from the input material before RNA-seq analysis it would strongly impair the ability to quantitatively assess changes in expression of all other genes. Contrary to rRNAs, protein-coding genes (mRNAs) are post-transcriptionally modified by polyadenylation at their 3′ end. RNA-seq protocols for the expression analysis of coding genes usually include a selection with oligo-dT primers, to ensure that only RNAs with a poly-A tail will be further processed and sequenced. An alternative to oligo-dT selection is the depletion of rRNAs from total RNA through hybridization capture and magnetic bead separation (Ribo-minus). This selection approach is a valid option if the interest of the sequencing experiment is not limited to polyadenylated RNAs. Although most lncRNAs do have a poly-A tail, there are some classes of lncRNAs, like enhancer associated lncRNAs, that are known to lack polyadenylation [18]. Other lncRNAs, like MALAT1, are subject to posttranscriptional processing that removes the poly-A tail [19]. All these transcripts will therefore be either missing or underrepresented in an RNA-seq analysis performed using oligo-dT selection [20]. At the same time it is important to keep in mind that, due to the increase in intronic sequences found in RNA-seq experiments performed with the rRNA depletion selection, the latter will end up requiring more sequencing depth respect to oligo-dT selection, increasing by up to 30% the total costs of the experiment [20]. If the budget is limiting, it is probably a better option to use an oligo-dT selection protocol than decreasing the number of samples to be sequenced reducing the overall statistical significance of the experiment. Finally, given that lncRNAs tend to be expressed at lower levels relative to protein-coding genes, for a comprehensive analysis of lncRNAs expression by RNA-seq it is highly recommended to increase samples sequencing depth, with an output of 50 M reads per sample being optimal.

**2.6   Data Analysis**

It is not in the aim of this chapter to discuss the bioinformatic tools available for the analysis of RNA-seq data (*see* Chapter 4). Generally speaking, the output of a sequencing experiment is a list of short sequences (also known as "reads") with or without strand information, depending on the sequencing protocol used. These sequences represent fragments of all transcripts expressed in the analyzed samples. Some of the tools used in the transcriptomics analyses will align these sequences to a reference genome. This task will add more information to the list of sequences obtained: the genomic coordinates. But in order to assign a sequence read to a particular protein-coding or lncRNA gene, the sequences obtained from each sample need to be aligned also to an annotated transcriptome, where the exon–intron structure is defined. The GENCODE project systematically classifies all gene features in the human genome, releasing these annotations for the benefit of the research community. The last GENECODE release, GENCODE 34, annotated 48,479 long noncoding RNA loci transcripts, belonging to 17,960 long noncoding RNA genes (https://www.gencodegenes.org/human/stats.html). Other annotations have been created with a particular focus on lncRNAs. The NONCODE annotation, for instance, in its last release includes up to 96,308 lncRNA genes (http://www.noncode.org/analysis.php). The use of an annotation file enables to assign each sequence read to a transcript providing a quantitative estimate of gene expression, based on counting the number of reads aligned with each transcript. A quantitative estimate of gene expression will be crucial to identify lncRNAs that are either upregulated or downregulated in the particular cancer of interest. At the same time, use of an annotation file will automatically exclude from the quantitative analysis all the transcripts that are not annotated in the reference transcriptome used. One way to overcome this problem is to use a de novo sequence assembly approach. De novo assembly is based on the fact that the short sequence reads generated by sequencing have usually overlapping ends. Programs for de novo assembly use the sequence information present in the overlapping ends of the shot fragments of a transcript to recreate the entire transcript [21]. The choice between de novo transcriptome assembly and the use of an annotation file to quantify the transcripts present in a sample may depend on the bioinformatics capabilities the biomarkers discovery project is able to count on.

Once lists of normalized read counts for all transcripts in all samples have been generated, the search for lncRNAs potentially behaving as cancer biomarkers can start. Even if our interest is exclusively focused on lncRNAs, it may be important not to exclude protein-coding genes at this stage. While for most of the protein-coding genes a lot of information on function or cellular specificity is present, the majority of lncRNAs will look like a list of letters and numbers with unknown significance. An unsupervised clustering analysis having lncRNAs clustering with genes of known function could be helpful in drawing hypotheses on the possible function, or cell of origin of the identified lncRNA. Unsupervised clustering and principal component analysis (PCA) are probably the first analyses that need to be performed on the quantitative expression data. Both analyses will divide the samples according to their similarity of expression pattern. These analyses are not only useful for the identification of novel subgroups of the same disease but can also help to perform a quality check on the cohort samples. Samples that could have been swapped by mistake between two groups will cluster with the group they belong to in PCA. These samples could be either excluded from further analyses or relabeled if the swapping event could be invariably identified. Unsupervised clustering analysis will define sets of lncRNAs with expression patterns specific for subgroups of the same disease. At this stage, a quantitative differential expression analysis among the newly defined groups will be important to select among the identified lncRNAs those with the highest expression difference.

*2.7 Databases Mining*

Once a group of lncRNAs differentially expressed in a disease condition has been identified, it will be important to assess the degree of cell/tissue specificity of their expression. Every tissue, either normal or neoplastic, is infiltrated with cellular components of the blood and lymphatic systems. In many cancers an active immune response, either productive or unproductive, takes place, increasing the number of infiltrating immune cells. Other cellular types, like cancer associated fibroblasts (CAFs), may also be present. We can therefore expect that the original patient sample will be a mixture of cancer cells and various components of the tumor stroma. Comparison of cancer-specific lncRNA expression signatures with cell type-specific signatures present in publicly available databases could be very helpful in defining the cell/tissue specificity of lncRNA expression. This analysis will be important also because stroma-expressed lncRNAs could end up being useful prognostic biomarkers. The use of checkpoint inhibitors to stimulate an active immune reaction against cancer cells, for instance, is one of the most promising therapeutic approaches in many types of tumors [22, 23]. The identification of lncRNAs that could signal either a quantitative or qualitative change in the intratumoral immune response could therefore have a strong prognostic value. Similarly, CAFs have been shown to play a major role in facilitating tumor dissemination [24]. Therefore, lncRNAs' expression signatures that potentially enable their quantitative and qualitative assessment could be highly valuable for the prediction of the metastatic power of a tumor.

Understanding the cell of origin of the identified lncRNA can be strongly facilitated by the mining of publicly available gene expression databases. Many of the available data have been made easy to enquire in online platforms like the Expression Atlas from the European Bioinformatics Institute (https://www.ebi.ac.uk/gxa/home), the Xena Functional Genomics Explorer from the Genomics Institute of the University of California Santa Cruz (https://xena.ucsc.edu) or the atlas of ncRNAs in cancer, TAN-RIC, from the MD Anderson Cancer Center of the University of Texas (https://www.tanric.org/). Most of the data found on these platforms derive from projects of scientific consortia involved in the analysis of gene expression in multiple cancers as well as normal tissues. The Genotype-Tissue Expression (GTEx) project has built a comprehensive public resource to study tissue-specific gene expression and regulation performing RNA-Seq on samples from 54 nondiseased tissue sites across nearly 1000 individuals. The GTEx database is therefore extremely useful to investigate normal tissue expression of the identified lncRNA. Expression in normal tissue can be useful for several reasons. If an lncRNA is highly expressed in multiple tissues, like MALAT1, contaminations from other tissues could impair its correct quantification from the cancer biopsy, reducing its sensitivity as a cancer biomarker. High expression of an lncRNA in blood could hinder its use in liquid biopsies. At the same time an lncRNA predominantly expressed in whole blood and spleen will strongly suggest that its expression is mainly associated with immune cells infiltrating the tumor sample. In the latter case, one may be interested in knowing which of the several cellular components of the whole blood expresses the identified lncRNA. The Blueprint project was founded to provide to the scientific community with a reference information on the epigenetic status of most of the cellular components of the hematopoietic system. In this context, RNA-seq profiles were also produced and are publicly available. Other research groups have also been focusing on investigating the gene expression profile of single cell components of the blood [25]. All these data are available and can be extremely useful to indicate the cell of origin of an identified lncRNA. The lncRNA LUCAT1, for instance, has been proposed as a novel prognostic biomarker for papillary thyroid cancer [26]. Interestingly, its GTEx expression profile shows that, although expressed also in thyroid, whole blood is the tissue with the highest expression of LUCAT1 (Fig. 1a). The analysis of the Blueprint data led us finally understand that LUCAT1 is indeed expressed specifically by the two phagocytic components of the innate immune system, namely, monocytes and neutrophils (Fig. 1b). Infiltrating monocytes and neutrophils can be a measure of tissue inflammation. This analysis may therefore suggest that either LUCAT1 expression is strongly increased in tumor thyroid cells or that the increase in LUCAT1 expression in thyroid cancer could be due to an increase in tissue inflammation. Another example is shown in Fig. 1. Let us imagine we have identified LINC01871 as one of the most differentially expressed lncRNAs comparing two patient groups with different disease progressions. The GTEx expression profile of the lncRNA LINC01871 shows high expression particularly in whole blood, spleen, small intestine, and lung. Together with blood, spleen is an organ rich in T

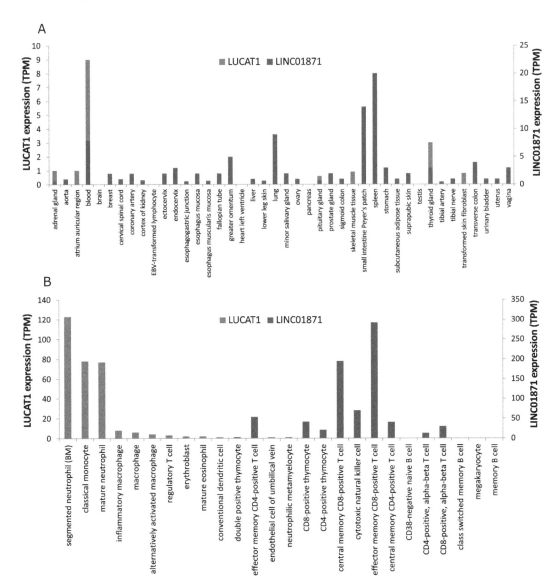

**Fig. 1** Examples of tissue- and cell-specific expression of two lncRNAs evaluated using publicly available data. (**a**) Expression of the lncRNAs LUCAT1 and LINC01871 in different human tissues using data from the Genotype-Tissue Expression (GTEx) project. (**b**) Expression of the lncRNAs LUCAT1 and LINC01871 in different cellular components of the blood using data from the Blueprint project. The data presented have been generated by the GTEx and Blueprint Consortia and downloaded from the Expression Atlas web site (https:/ www.ebi.ac.uk/gxa/home). The Blueprint project was funded by the European Union's Seventh Framework Programme (FP7/2007–2013) under grant agreement no 282510—BLUEPRINT. A full list of the investigators who contributed to the generation of the data is available from www.blueprint-epigenome.eu

lymphocytes involved in an active immune response through humoral and cell-mediated pathways. Small intestine and lung, being at the interface with the external environment are also rich in lymph nodes to readily respond to infections. This could suggest that LINC01871 may be expressed by T-lymphocytes. Indeed, looking at the Blueprint data LINC01871 seems to be predominantly expressed by memory CD8-positive T cells. LINC01871 could therefore represent a useful marker for the presence of intratumoral infiltrating memory CD8+ T cells. Given that the presence of intratumoral infiltrating memory T cells have been associated with a good outcome [27], LINC01871 could end up serving as prognostic cancer biomarker. Indeed high LINC01871 expression was associated with lower risk for cutaneous melanoma: together with two more lncRNAs, LINC01871 expression was shown to be able to significantly predict overall survival [28].

Publicly available expression data are not limited to normal tissues and cell types but have also been generated for many types of cancers. The above mentioned online platforms enable the researchers to search for the expression of genes of interest, including most of the annotated lncRNAs in data generated from the Cancer Genome Atlas (TCGA) and the International Cancer Genome Consortium (ICGC). For most of these samples also clinical data are available, enabling direct assessment of possible associations between lncRNA expression and patient's survival. Furthermore data from a high number of RNA-seq experiments is constantly deposited at the NCBI Sequence Read Archive (SRA), the largest publicly available repository of high throughput sequencing data. Scientists have the possibility to search the repository for data that could be integrated in their own experimental pipeline. Suitable data sets can be downloaded and reanalyzed using the same bioinformatic approach used for the analysis of the rest of the samples. Given that reproducibility is an extremely important concept in cancer biomarker discovery, the possibility to compare experimental data with data published by others on similar cancers or to extend findings to other cancer types can be very useful for the definition of an lncRNA as a novel cancer biomarker.

## 2.8 Validation of lncRNAs as Cancer Biomarkers

If a particular lncRNA will be used as a cancer biomarker, further validation experiments are mandatory. As all biomarkers, the lncRNA will need to be shown to have analytic validity [1], being able to be detected using different assays in different experimental conditions. This could be particularly important for an lncRNA. RNA is indeed particularly unstable as molecule and its detection might strongly fluctuate depending on the quality of the sample and the extraction method used. The development of a robust analytical assay will be essential to assess the clinical validity of the lncRNA. The best way to define the clinical significance of the identified lncRNA is to test its ability to discern the disease group in several independent cohorts of patients and possibly by independent groups of researchers. Finally, for an lncRNA to have clinical utility, the benefits brought from its identification in the sample must be clearly higher than the costs associated to its detection. If the only way to measure the expression of the lncRNA is through

RNA-seq of a biopsy that requires invasive surgery, the utility of such a cancer biomarker can be justified only by a strong diagnostic or prognostic power. If the expression of the identified lncRNA can be measured in liquid biopsies using a relatively inexpensive assay, its clinical use may be justified also in case of a relatively lower diagnostic potential.

## 3   Conclusions

In conclusion, given the high tissue specificity of expression, lncRNAs can be seen as a very valuable source of novel cancer biomarkers. With the advent of NGS and with the strong fall in sequencing costs, RNA-sequencing is a powerful tool for the identification of known or novel lncRNA transcripts that could end up being cancer biomarkers. The presence of an increasing amount of sequencing data from normal and diseased tissues that has been deposited in publicly available databases makes the identification and characterization of lncRNAs as potential cancer biomarkers much easier. The above described guidelines (also depicted in Fig. 2) will be useful for the identification of a set of lncRNAs differentially expressed in subsets of a certain cancer type or in patients that have the tendency to relapse or in patients with a specific genetic background. This analysis will also define if the lncRNAs of interest are expressed by the tumor cells or by some of the cellular components of the tumor stroma. However, only the setup of a robust detection assay and the establishment of its clinical utility will define if the identified lncRNA will really become a valuable cancer biomarker.

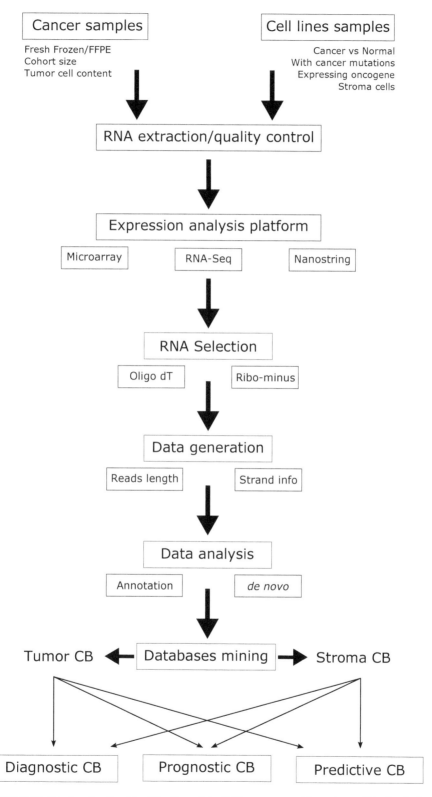

**Fig. 2** Experimental pipeline for the identification of lncRNA as cancer biomarkers. CB stands for cancer biomarker

## References

1. Henry NL, Hayes DF (2012) Cancer biomarkers. Mol Oncol 6(2):140–146. https://doi.org/10.1016/j.molonc.2012.01.010

2. Ek S, Dictor M, Jerkeman M, Jirstrom K, Borrebaeck CA (2008) Nuclear expression of the non B-cell lineage Sox11 transcription factor identifies mantle cell lymphoma. Blood 111 (2):800–805. https://doi.org/10.1182/blood-2007-06-093401

3. Mozos A, Royo C, Hartmann E, De Jong D, Baro C, Valera A, Fu K, Weisenburger DD, Delabie J, Chuang SS, Jaffe ES, Ruiz-Marcellan C, Dave S, Rimsza L, Braziel R, Gascoyne RD, Sole F, Lopez-Guillermo A, Colomer D, Staudt LM, Rosenwald A, Ott G, Jares P, Campo E (2009) SOX11 expression is highly specific for mantle cell lymphoma and identifies the cyclin D1-negative subtype. Haematologica 94(11):1555–1562. https://doi.org/10.3324/haematol.2009.010264

4. Rinn JL, Chang HY (2012) Genome regulation by long noncoding RNAs. Annu Rev Biochem 81:145–166. https://doi.org/10.1146/annurev-biochem-051410-092902

5. Iaccarino I (2017) lncRNAs and MYC: an intricate relationship. Int J Mol Sci 18 (7):1497. https://doi.org/10.3390/ijms18071497

6. Kopp F, Mendell JT (2018) Functional classification and experimental dissection of long noncoding RNAs. Cell 172(3):393–407. https://doi.org/10.1016/j.cell.2018.01.011

7. Cabili MN, Trapnell C, Goff L, Koziol M, Tazon-Vega B, Regev A, Rinn JL (2011) Integrative annotation of human large intergenic noncoding RNAs reveals global properties and specific subclasses. Genes Dev 25 (18):1915–1927. https://doi.org/10.1101/gad.17446611

8. Derrien T, Johnson R, Bussotti G, Tanzer A, Djebali S, Tilgner H, Guernec G, Martin D, Merkel A, Knowles DG, Lagarde J, Veeravalli L, Ruan X, Ruan Y, Lassmann T, Carninci P, Brown JB, Lipovich L, Gonzalez JM, Thomas M, Davis CA, Shiekhattar R, Gingeras TR, Hubbard TJ, Notredame C, Harrow J, Guigo R (2012) The GENCODE v7 catalog of human long noncoding RNAs: analysis of their gene structure, evolution, and expression. Genome Res 22(9):1775–1789. https://doi.org/10.1101/gr.132159.111

9. Djebali S, Davis CA, Merkel A, Dobin A, Lassmann T, Mortazavi A, Tanzer A, Lagarde J, Lin W, Schlesinger F, Xue C, Marinov GK, Khatun J, Williams BA, Zaleski C, Rozowsky J, Roder M, Kokocinski F, Abdelhamid RF, Alioto T, Antoshechkin I, Baer MT, Bar NS, Batut P, Bell K, Bell I, Chakrabortty S, Chen X, Chrast J, Curado J, Derrien T, Drenkow J, Dumais E, Dumais J, Duttagupta R, Falconnet E, Fastuca M, Fejes-Toth K, Ferreira P, Foissac S, Fullwood MJ, Gao H, Gonzalez D, Gordon A, Gunawardena H, Howald C, Jha S, Johnson R, Kapranov P, King B, Kingswood C, Luo OJ, Park E, Persaud K, Preall JB, Ribeca P, Risk B, Robyr D, Sammeth M, Schaffer L, See LH, Shahab A, Skancke J, Suzuki AM, Takahashi H, Tilgner H, Trout D, Walters N, Wang H, Wrobel J, Yu Y, Ruan X, Hayashizaki Y, Harrow J, Gerstein M, Hubbard T, Reymond A, Antonarakis SE, Hannon G, Giddings MC, Ruan Y, Wold B, Carninci P, Guigo R, Gingeras TR (2012) Landscape of transcription in human cells. Nature 489 (7414):101–108. https://doi.org/10.1038/nature11233

10. Prensner JR, Iyer MK, Balbin OA, Dhanasekaran SM, Cao Q, Brenner JC, Laxman B, Asangani IA, Grasso CS, Kominsky HD, Cao X, Jing X, Wang X, Siddiqui J, Wei JT, Robinson D, Iyer HK, Palanisamy N, Maher CA, Chinnaiyan AM (2011) Transcriptome sequencing across a prostate cancer cohort identifies PCAT-1, an unannotated lincRNA implicated in disease progression. Nat Biotechnol 29(8):742–749. https://doi.org/10.1038/nbt.1914

11. Doose G, Haake A, Bernhart SH, Lopez C, Duggimpudi S, Wojciech F, Bergmann AK, Borkhardt A, Burkhardt B, Claviez A, Dimitrova L, Haas S, Hoell JI, Hummel M, Karsch D, Klapper W, Kleo K, Kretzmer H, Kreuz M, Kuppers R, Lawerenz C, Lenze D, Loeffler M, Mantovani-Loffler L, Moller P, Ott G, Richter J, Rohde M, Rosenstiel P, Rosenwald A, Schilhabel M, Schneider M, Scholz I, Stilgenbauer S, Stunnenberg HG, Szczepanowski M, Trumper L, Weniger MA, Consortium IM-S, Hoffmann S, Siebert R, Iaccarino I (2015) MINCR is a MYC-induced lncRNA able to modulate MYC's transcriptional network in Burkitt lymphoma cells. Proc Natl Acad Sci U S A 112(38): E5261–E5270. https://doi.org/10.1073/pnas.1505753112

12. Bossel Ben-Moshe N, Gilad S, Perry G, Benjamin S, Balint-Lahat N, Pavlovsky A, Halperin S, Markus B, Yosepovich A, Barshack I, Gal-Yam EN, Domany E, Kaufman B, Dadiani M (2018) mRNA-seq whole transcriptome profiling of fresh frozen

versus archived fixed tissues. BMC Genomics 19(1):419. https://doi.org/10.1186/s12864-018-4761-3

13. Bissell MJ, Radisky D (2001) Putting tumours in context. Nat Rev Cancer 1(1):46–54. https://doi.org/10.1038/35094059

14. Sebens S, Schafer H (2012) The tumor stroma as mediator of drug resistance--a potential target to improve cancer therapy? Curr Pharm Biotechnol 13(11):2259–2272. https://doi.org/10.2174/138920112802501999

15. Scott DW, Gascoyne RD (2014) The tumour microenvironment in B cell lymphomas. Nat Rev Cancer 14(8):517–534. https://doi.org/10.1038/nrc3774

16. El-Daly SM, Bayraktar R, Anfossi S, Calin GA (2020) The interplay between MicroRNAs and the components of the tumor microenvironment in B-cell malignancies. Int J Mol Sci 21(9):3387. https://doi.org/10.3390/ijms21093387

17. Schulze A, Downward J (2001) Navigating gene expression using microarrays--a technology review. Nat Cell Biol 3(8):E190–E195. https://doi.org/10.1038/35087138

18. Kim TK, Hemberg M, Gray JM, Costa AM, Bear DM, Wu J, Harmin DA, Laptewicz M, Barbara-Haley K, Kuersten S, Markenscoff-Papadimitriou E, Kuhl D, Bito H, Worley PF, Kreiman G, Greenberg ME (2010) Widespread transcription at neuronal activity-regulated enhancers. Nature 465(7295):182–187. https://doi.org/10.1038/nature09033

19. Wilusz JE, Freier SM, Spector DL (2008) 3′ end processing of a long nuclear-retained non-coding RNA yields a tRNA-like cytoplasmic RNA. Cell 135(5):919–932. https://doi.org/10.1016/j.cell.2008.10.012

20. Zhao S, Zhang Y, Gamini R, Zhang B, von Schack D (2018) Evaluation of two main RNA-seq approaches for gene quantification in clinical RNA sequencing: polyA+ selection versus rRNA depletion. Sci Rep 8(1):4781. https://doi.org/10.1038/s41598-018-23226-4

21. Zerbino DR, Birney E (2008) Velvet: algorithms for de novo short read assembly using de Bruijn graphs. Genome Res 18(5):821–829. https://doi.org/10.1101/gr.074492.107

22. Pardoll DM (2012) The blockade of immune checkpoints in cancer immunotherapy. Nat Rev Cancer 12(4):252–264. https://doi.org/10.1038/nrc3239

23. Darvin P, Toor SM, Sasidharan Nair V, Elkord E (2018) Immune checkpoint inhibitors: recent progress and potential biomarkers. Exp Mol Med 50(12):1–11. https://doi.org/10.1038/s12276-018-0191-1

24. De Vincenzo A, Belli S, Franco P, Telesca M, Iaccarino I, Botti G, Carriero MV, Ranson M, Stoppelli MP (2019) Paracrine recruitment and activation of fibroblasts by c-Myc expressing breast epithelial cells through the IGFs/IGF-1R axis. Int J Cancer 145(10):2827–2839. https://doi.org/10.1002/ijc.32613

25. Monaco G, Lee B, Xu W, Mustafah S, Hwang YY, Carre C, Burdin N, Visan L, Ceccarelli M, Poidinger M, Zippelius A, Pedro de Magalhaes J, Larbi A (2019) RNA-Seq signatures normalized by mRNA abundance allow absolute deconvolution of human immune cell types. Cell Rep 26(6):1627–1640.e7. https://doi.org/10.1016/j.celrep.2019.01.041

26. Luzon-Toro B, Fernandez RM, Martos-Martinez JM, Rubio-Manzanares-Dorado M, Antinolo G, Borrego S (2019) LncRNA LUCAT1 as a novel prognostic biomarker for patients with papillary thyroid cancer. Sci Rep 9(1):14374. https://doi.org/10.1038/s41598-019-50913-7

27. Fridman WH, Pages F, Sautes-Fridman C, Galon J (2012) The immune contexture in human tumours: impact on clinical outcome. Nat Rev Cancer 12(4):298–306. https://doi.org/10.1038/nrc3245

28. Tian J, Yang Y, Li MY, Zhang Y (2020) A novel RNA sequencing-based prognostic nomogram to predict survival for patients with cutaneous melanoma: clinical trial/experimental study. Medicine (Baltimore) 99(3):e18868. https://doi.org/10.1097/MD.0000000000018868

# Part II

## LncRNA Profiling and Discovery

# Chapter 3

# Bioinformatics Pipeline to Analyze lncRNA Arrays

## Katia Todoerti, Domenica Ronchetti, Martina Manzoni, Elisa Taiana, Antonino Neri, and Luca Agnelli

## Abstract

Despite the fact that next-generation sequencing approaches, in particular RNA sequencing, provide deep genome-wide expression data that allow both careful annotations/mapping of long noncoding RNA (lncRNA) molecules and de-novo sequencing, lncRNA expression studies by microarray is a still cost-effective procedure that could allow to have a landscape of the most characterized lncRNA species. However, microarray design does not always correctly address the overlap between coding and noncoding samples to discriminate between the original transcript source. In order to overcome this issue, in this chapter we present a bioinformatics pipeline that enables accurate annotation of GeneChip® microarrays, to date the most commonly adopted among the commercial solutions. Overall, this approach holds two main advantages, a gain in specificity of transcript detection and the adaptability to the whole panel of GeneChip® arrays.

**Key words** lncRNA, Microarrays

## 1 Introduction

Long noncoding RNAs (lncRNAs) represent a wide class of non-coding transcripts with a length of more than 200 nucleotides. Compared with coding messenger RNAs, unless few exceptions lncRNAs are generally poorly expressed and have stronger tissue specificity. LncRNAs have fundamental role in a variety of physiological processes including the expression regulation of coding genes at various levels (i.e., epigenetic inheritance, transcription, and posttranscription), the organization of nuclear domains as well as the physical and functional interaction with proteins or RNAs [1, 2]. LncRNA deregulation is involved in many pathologies including cancer [3], this strongly prompting their study.

Katia Todoerti and Domenica Ronchetti contributed equally to this work. Antonino Neri and Luca Agnelli are co-last authors.

Alfons Navarro (ed.), *Long Non-Coding RNAs in Cancer*, Methods in Molecular Biology, vol. 2348, https://doi.org/10.1007/978-1-0716-1581-2_3, © Springer Science+Business Media, LLC, part of Springer Nature 2021

Next-generation sequencing approaches, in particular RNA sequencing, provide deep genome-wide expression data that allow both careful annotations and mapping of noncanonical transcripts, such as lncRNAs, and de novo sequencing [4]. However, lncRNA expression studies by microarray is still a cost-effective, reliable and with few lab-requirements procedure that could allow for depicting a portrait of the most characterized lncRNA species.

One important caveat of lncRNA expression studies is their annotations that lag considerably behind those of protein-coding genes [5]. Indeed, there are different factors that make lncRNA annotation challenging, first of all their relatively low expression, meaning that their transcripts will be weakly sampled in any unbiased transcriptomic data (e.g., in polyA-enriched samples); in addition, since our understanding of the lncRNA sequence–function relationship is still poor, sequence features or functional elements can hardly be used, at present, to identify novel lncRNAs. Moreover, lncRNAs tend to be weakly conserved during evolution, making it difficult to identify their orthologs or paralogs by sequence similarity [5]. Based on these considerations, it is not surprising that annotations are rapidly overdue, not always coherent between repositories (e.g., LNCipedia, lncRNAdb, NONCODE) that rely on different release of sources, and timely updates are needed.

Concerning the microarray approach, GeneChip® microarrays (currently hold by Thermo Fisher Scientific, Waltham, MA) represent to date the gold standard for custom microarray analysis; indeed, other array solutions are available but their low diffusion does not guarantee up-to-date tools and annotations, if not even in some cases analysis pipeline are private. For these reasons, the present chapter will discuss GeneChip® array annotation and analysis pipeline.

Microarray design and sample preparation for GeneChip® technology are currently consolidated procedures, which normally grant effective and reliable results. This is absolutely true if we considered, for example, expression arrays that are specifically designed to detect coding transcripts. However, in the last years several GeneChip® solutions for expression analysis have been designed to capture the whole RNA-ome scenario, spanning from short to long, coding to non-coding RNA fractions of the transcriptome: this demands high accuracy to avoid annotation biases.

Noteworthy, during our recent research studies, we have observed that microarray design does not always address correctly the overlap between coding and noncoding samples (Fig. 1), in virtue of (a) the natural overlapping between coding and antisense noncoding transcripts and contextually (b) the sample preparation that converts any strand to cDNA to labeled fragmented RNA. In other words, this means that if two transcripts shared the same sense/antisense sequence (which is a common feature for several

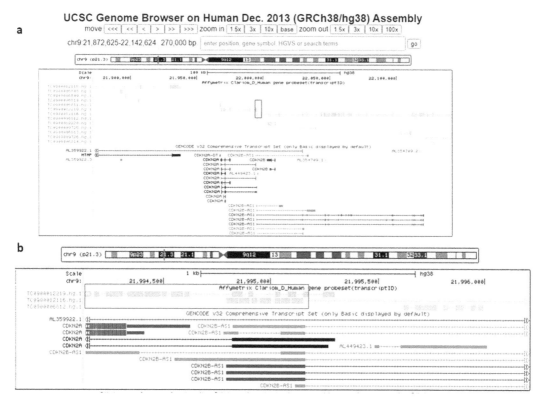

**Fig. 1** Example of how microarray design fails to discriminate between the original transcript source: (**a**) *CDKN2B-AS1* e *CDKN2A* overlap head to head on chromosome 9p21. The red box outlines the array probes that map within the shared sequence and will be discarded based on our pipeline. (**b**) Zoom view of the overlapping lncRNA–mRNA region

antisense lncRNA transcripts [6–8]) and the array probe mapped within the shared sequence, there will not be any possibility to discriminate between the original transcript source. As regards lncRNA expression analysis, we would consider that this represents the true tricky issue, since many valid solutions, likely gold-standard options for expression analysis such as RMA [9], could be chosen to import and normalize data. Therefore, we have chosen a conventional R procedure to annotate and normalize data, but here we propose a customized reannotation pipeline for Chip Definition Files (CDF) to escape errors. An example at the end of the chapter will better clarify the advantage of the procedure.

Several different annotations exist for the human genome, each with advantages and drawbacks that might not be immediately evident [5, 10]. They are based on two main strategies of automated and manual annotation. Automated annotation typically employs transcriptome assembly approaches, which are rapid and inexpensive but produce incomplete and inaccurate annotations. Manual annotation yields high-quality catalogs but at slow rates, and furthermore requires substantial long-term economic support. We have adopted the GENCODE curated gene set annotation (https://www.gencodegenes.org/pages/data_access.html), as it has been created by merging the results of manual and computational gene annotation methods. In addition, the GENCODE consortium continues to improve the quality of the reference gene annotation by refining the representation of existing loci and extending annotation coverage via the addition of entirely novel loci, as well as alternatively spliced transcripts [10].

Here, we report the pipeline that we are using to investigated lncRNA expression by GeneChip® microarrays.

## 2   Materials

The full procedure can be run on a common Unix-based up-to-date desktop solution for microarray analysis purposes. A 64-bit computer, running either Linux or MacOSX, with at least 8 GB RAM is suggested (*see* **Note 1**).

## 3   Methods

### 3.1  lncRNA Annotation GeneChip Microarrays

In line with previous considerations, we developed a procedure that allowed reannotating CDF files according to the principle "OPOG" (one probe, one gene).

The annotations can be downloaded at the "BrainArray" repository from the University of Michigan (*see* **Note 2**):

1. Go to http://brainarray.mbni.med.umich.edu/Brainarray/Database/CustomCDF/CDF_download.asp.

2. Download GENECODET package, for example, http://mbni.org/customcdf/24.0.0/gencodet.download/ClariomDHuman_Hs_GENCODET_24.0.0.zip.

3. Unzip to ClariomDHuman_Hs_GENCODET_24.0.0 folder.

### 3.2  Probe Filter Strategy

We applied two filters on the probe/probeset downloaded.

(a)  Probe mapping multiple ENSG elements will be filtered out.

(b)  Probesets with less than four probes will be filtered out.

To apply those filters and to produce a Flat file for the next procedure, for convenience we developed a script named brainArray2Flat.sh that can be downloaded here: https://github.com/emacgene/lncAnnot.

The script can be run from the shell of any unix-based system with the following command.

```
/brainArray2Flat.sh -p ClariomDHuman_Hs_GENCODET_probe_tab -d
ClariomDHuman_Hs_GENCODET_desc.txt -n 4 -o
ClariomDHuman_Hs_GENCODET_24
```

The syntax represents the exemplar application of the following function.

```
brainArray2Flat.sh -p <FILE.probe_tab> -d <FILE.desc.txt> -o
<OUT_FILENAME> [ -n <MIN_PROBES_NUMBER> ] [-h]
  Flag:
   -p/--probe_tab FILE Probe tab file from Brain Array CDF
package
   -d/--desc FILE Description file from Brain Array
CDF package
   -o/--out PREFIX Output prefix name
   Optional Flag:
   -n/--probe_th INT Min number of probes used as
threshold to select a probeset [DEFAULT = 4]
```

For example, −n 4 --> Probeset with less than 4 probe will be filtered out (*see* **Note 3**).

**3.3  Flat File Creation**    The **flat2Cdf** function from **affxparser** package for Bioconductor can now be run to create the newly annotated CDF file.

For convenience, a modified version of the **flat2Cdf** function that add tags with "." instead of "," is included as source file and can be downloaded at https://github.com/emacgene/lncAnnot.

Then, from an R environment, the following functions should be run.

```
if (!requireNamespace("BiocManager", quietly = TRUE))
install.packages("BiocManager")
BiocManager::install("affxparser")
library(affxparser)
source("./flat2Cdf.R") # Please note: set the correct path to the
downloaded file
flat2Cdf("./ClariomDHuman_Hs_GENCODET_24.0.0/ClariomD_GENECODET.flat",
chipType="ClariomD.ENSG",  tag="v24",  col.class=c("character","inte-
ger","integer","character","character","character"),  rows=2572,  cols=
2680,  xynames=c("X","Y"),  ucol=5,  gcol=6) # Please note: set the
correct path
```

1. Concerning this last function, please note that it works correctly only if the correct number of **rows** and **columns** is indicated in the parameters. To know the effective value, users can easily assess the header of *any* CEL files generated for the array of interest with the **affxparser::readCelHeader()** function.

2. `ucol` and `gcol` parameters represent, respectively, units and groups to be considered to associate the probe to a probeset (and consequently to the output). Ideally, starting from GEN ECODET data users could choose either to generate ENST, that is, transcript-based, or ENSG, that is, gene-based annotations.

This is a major aspect of lncRNA annotation, since it is a prerogative of the user to choose at which level the lncRNA transcripts would be investigated (*see* **Note 4**).

### 3.4 CDF File Creation

Later, a conventional procedure can be applied to transform the . CDF file into usable R package.

```
if (!requireNamespace("BiocManager", quietly = TRUE))
 install.packages("BiocManager")
BiocManager::install("makecdfenv")
library(makecdfenv)
pkgpath =("Set_the_Path_to_CDF_file")
make.cdf.package("ClariomDHuman_Hs_GENCODET.cdf", compress =
FALSE, species="Homo_sapiens", unlink=TRUE, cdf.path = pkgpath,
package.path = pkgpath)
```

Finally, the library can be installed and loaded into R (optionally, from the Unix shell with R CMD command).

```
# R CMD build --force clariomdhumanhsgencodetcdf
# R CMD INSTALL clariomdhumanhsgencodetcdf_1.64.0.tar.gz
library(clariomdhumanhsgencodetcdf)
```

At this point, users could virtually choose custom procedure to generate the expression data. However, here we prefer to indicate the usage of a conventional pipeline with `affy()` package and RMA normalization method, considering this last one as the gold standard for microarray data.

```
library(affy)
cel.data <-ReadAffy(celfile.path= "", cdfname=
"clariomdhumanhsgencodetcdf")# read raw data, CEL files, into an
Affybatch object
eset<-rma(cel.data) # convert the AffyBatch object into an
ExpressionSet object using the robust multi-array average (RMA)
expression measure
expr.data=as.data.frame(exprs(eset)) ) # save the expression data
object
```

For convenience, RMA normalized transcript expression data can be annotated using Biomart data mining tool (https://m. ensembl.org/info/data/biomart/index.html), applying the Ensembl transcript/gene stable ID with version as filter, and choosing the corresponding desired attributes, for example, "transcript name," "transcript type," "transcript start," "transcript end," "chromosome/scaffold name" or "gene name," "gene type," "gene start," "gene end" for gene-level analysis.

## 4  Notes

1. The procedure has been tested on an iMacPro equipped with MacOSX 10.15.6 through the UNIX shell (no graphical user interface is needed) and RStudio v1.3.959. However, the pipeline of generating the modified annotation file does not need to meet any specific hardware requirement: the bottleneck is conversely represented by the number of samples that should be managed during data import and normalization in R. In general, the brainArray2Flat.sh commands run on a single node. Using a 64-bit computer running either Linux or MacOSX with 8 GB RAM (16 GB preferred), under commercial CPU frequency solutions for desktop PC, the full pipeline does not require more than half-an-hour/40 min. Windows users are required to run brainArray2Flat.sh in virtual Unix environment.

2. To date, the repository from the University of Michigan represents a comprehensive and updated source of annotations for GeneChip data. For our purpose, the user should download the last release of the package based on GENCODET annotation containing *protein coding* and *non-coding* transcripts. The compressed archive available at the Michigan website (column "Zip of CDF, Seq, Map, Desc", label "Z") includes (a) mapping, (b) description, (c) probes sequence. and (d) CDF files.

   Here, exemplary, we described the procedure for the last version (v24) of the last-generation Human ClariomD arrays. However, it can be run with any other arrays upon substitution of any string referred to ClariomD with the appropriate arrays.

3. The optional parameter -n represents the *minimum* (and default) number of probes that should be considered to build the transcript expression signal (we have chosen to set 4 as default number according to previous evidences that recognize this as the minimum set to generate a reliable signal [11].

4. Transcript-level analysis enables to detect not only the level of expression but to precisely define what is expressed among coding RNA/lncRNA transcript variants, also allowing the identification and measure of low abundance transcripts or rare alternative splicing events. Transcript-centric approaches may be useful in targeted experiments where specific isoforms are expected to change. However, isoform estimation by

transcript-level analysis results more complex than gene-level analysis, due to the high degree of overlap among transcripts. Additionally, some transcripts may not be identified by irregular coverage due to possible technical biases. Even if dynamics among transcripts may not be detected with gene-level analyses, they appear more robust and accurate [12], and more easily interpretable than transcript-level approaches. Transcript profiling produces extremely large data sets that are difficult to be handled, whereas global gene expression patterns could more easily define altered molecular pathways at a lower complex level. Finally, gene-level functional investigations are more actionable than transcript ones, given the difficulty of knocking down single isoforms of genes [13].

## Acknowledgments

This work was financially supported by grants to Antonino Neri (from Associazione Italiana Ricerca sul Cancro [AIRC] [IG16722 and IG24365]).

## References

1. Kopp F, Mendell JT (2018) Functional classification and experimental dissection of long noncoding RNAs. Cell 172(3):393–407. https://doi.org/10.1016/j.cell.2018.01.011

2. Mercer TR, Dinger ME, Mattick JS (2009) Long non-coding RNAs: insights into functions. Nat Rev Genet 10(3):155–159. https://doi.org/10.1038/nrg2521

3. Slack FJ, Chinnaiyan AM (2019) The role of non-coding RNAs in oncology. Cell 179 (5):1033–1055. https://doi.org/10.1016/j. cell.2019.10.017

4. Djebali S, Davis CA, Merkel A, Dobin A, Lassmann T, Mortazavi A, Tanzer A, Lagarde J, Lin W, Schlesinger F, Xue C, Marinov GK, Khatun J, Williams BA, Zaleski C, Rozowsky J, Roder M, Kokocinski F, Abdelhamid RF, Alioto T, Antoshechkin I, Baer MT, Bar NS, Batut P, Bell K, Bell I, Chakrabortty S, Chen X, Chrast J, Curado J, Derrien T, Drenkow J, Dumais E, Dumais J, Duttagupta R, Falconnet E, Fastuca M, Fejes-Toth K, Ferreira P, Foissac S, Fullwood MJ, Gao H, Gonzalez D, Gordon A, Gunawardena H, Howald C, Jha S, Johnson R, Kapranov P, King B, Kingswood C, Luo OJ, Park E, Persaud K, Preall JB, Ribeca P, Risk B, Robyr D, Sammeth M, Schaffer L, See LH, Shahab A, Skancke J, Suzuki AM, Takahashi H, Tilgner H, Trout D, Walters N, Wang H, Wrobel J, Yu Y, Ruan X, Hayashizaki Y, Harrow J, Gerstein M, Hubbard T, Reymond A, Antonarakis SE, Hannon G, Giddings MC, Ruan Y, Wold B, Carninci P, Guigo R, Gingeras TR (2012) Landscape of transcription in human cells. Nature 489 (7414):101–108. https://doi.org/10.1038/nature11233

5. Uszczynska-Ratajczak B, Lagarde J, Frankish A, Guigo R, Johnson R (2018) Towards a complete map of the human long non-coding RNA transcriptome. Nat Rev Genet 19(9):535–548. https://doi.org/10.1038/s41576-018-0017-y

6. Kapranov P, Cheng J, Dike S, Nix DA, Duttagupta R, Willingham AT, Stadler PF, Hertel J, Hackermuller J, Hofacker IL, Bell I, Cheung E, Drenkow J, Dumais E, Patel S, Helt G, Ganesh M, Ghosh S, Piccolboni A, Sementchenko V, Tammana H, Gingeras TR (2007) RNA maps reveal new RNA classes and a possible function for pervasive transcription. Science 316(5830):1484–1488. https://doi.org/10.1126/science.1138341

7. Kapranov P, Willingham AT, Gingeras TR (2007) Genome-wide transcription and the implications for genomic organization. Nat Rev Genet 8(6):413–423. https://doi.org/10.1038/nrg2083

8. Ning Q, Li Y, Wang Z, Zhou S, Sun H, Yu G (2017) The evolution and expression pattern of human overlapping lncRNA and protein-coding gene pairs. Sci Rep 7:42775. https://doi.org/10.1038/srep42775

9. Irizarry RA, Hobbs B, Collin F, Beazer-Barclay YD, Antonellis KJ, Scherf U, Speed TP (2003) Exploration, normalization, and summaries of high density oligonucleotide array probe level data. Biostatistics 4(2):249–264. https://doi.org/10.1093/biostatistics/4.2.249

10. Frankish A, Diekhans M, Ferreira AM, Johnson R, Jungreis I, Loveland J, Mudge JM, Sisu C, Wright J, Armstrong J, Barnes I, Berry A, Bignell A, Carbonell Sala S, Chrast J, Cunningham F, Di Domenico T, Donaldson S, Fiddes IT, Garcia Giron C, Gonzalez JM, Grego T, Hardy M, Hourlier T, Hunt T, Izuogu OG, Lagarde J, Martin FJ, Martinez L, Mohanan S, Muir P, Navarro FCP, Parker A, Pei B, Pozo F, Ruffier M, Schmitt BM, Stapleton E, Suner MM, Sycheva I, Uszczynska-Ratajczak B, Xu J, Yates A, Zerbino D, Zhang Y, Aken B, Choudhary JS, Gerstein M, Guigo R, Hubbard TJP, Kellis M, Paten B, Reymond A, Tress ML, Flicek P (2019) GENCODE reference annotation for the human and mouse genomes. Nucleic Acids Res 47(D1):D766–D773. https://doi.org/10.1093/nar/gky955

11. Ferrari F, Bortoluzzi S, Coppe A, Sirota A, Safran M, Shmoish M, Ferrari S, Lancet D, Danieli GA, Bicciato S (2007) Novel definition files for human GeneChips based on GeneAnnot. BMC Bioinformatics 8:446. https://doi.org/10.1186/1471-2105-8-446

12. Soneson C, Love MI, Robinson MD (2015) Differential analyses for RNA-seq: transcript-level estimates improve gene-level inferences. F1000Res 4:1521. https://doi.org/10.12688/f1000research.7563.2

13. Kisielow M, Kleiner S, Nagasawa M, Faisal A, Nagamine Y (2002) Isoform-specific knockdown and expression of adaptor protein ShcA using small interfering RNA. Biochem J 363 (Pt 1):1–5. https://doi.org/10.1042/0264-6021:3630001

# Chapter 4

# Bioinformatic Pipelines to Analyze lncRNAs RNAseq Data

## Luca Agnelli, Stefania Bortoluzzi, and Giancarlo Pruneri

## Abstract

RNA-sequencing could be nowadays considered the gold standard to study the coding and noncoding transcriptome. The great advantage of high-throughput sequencing in the characterization and quantification of long noncoding RNA (lncRNA) resides in its capability to capture the complexity of lncRNA transcripts configuration patterns, even in the presence of several alternative isoforms, with superior accuracy and discovery power compared to other technologies such as microarrays or PCR-based methods. In this chapter, we provide a protocol for lncRNA analysis using through high-throughput sequencing, indicating the main difficulties in the annotation pipeline and showing how an accurate evaluation of the procedure can help to minimize biased observations.

**Key words** RNA sequencing, Sequencing data mapping, lncRNA quantification

## 1 Introduction

RNA sequencing (RNA-seq) is one of the methods most commonly used for high-throughput massive parallel sequencing, also called next-generation sequencing (NGS), in which several millions of sequence fragments, around 50–150 bases long, are generated from RNA samples. The RNA-seq workflows have been designed to characterize the entire transcriptome or only parts of it, such as polyadenylated RNAs. In virtue of the variety of RNA molecules (in term of length, polyadenylation, etc.), different library preparation procedures, sequencing reactions, and analysis methods should be used to capture the whole transcriptome diversity.

A nonexhaustive list of elements that should be considered for RNAseq analysis includes: (a) the source of material (standard bulk RNA analysis to analyze the whole expression from large populations of cells, single-cell sequencing to unravel critical differences between individual cells in a population); (b) the sample preparation procedures (library-based methods that imply conversion to cDNA, ligations and amplifications, or single-molecule direct sequencing to reduce manipulation artifacts at the cost of reduced

Alfons Navarro (ed.), *Long Non-Coding RNAs in Cancer*, Methods in Molecular Biology, vol. 2348,
https://doi.org/10.1007/978-1-0716-1581-2_4, © Springer Science+Business Media, LLC, part of Springer Nature 2021

resolution); (c) the expected fragment length; (d) the nature of transcripts to be captured. This last aspect is of primary importance, in light of the role that the noncoding fraction of the transcriptome is gathering during the last years in cell physiology and in pathological processes. The recent transcriptomics efforts, thanks to large-scale massive parallel sequencing procedure, have demonstrated that the large part of the genome is pervasively transcribed. However, only a minor polyadenylated fraction actually encodes known proteins, whereas more than two-thirds of human genes produce transcripts with none or with very limited coding potential, called noncoding RNAs (ncRNAs) [1].

## 2   Materials

### 2.1   Hardware Specifications

The following pipeline has been run both on an iMacPro equipped with MacOSX 10.15.6, 3.2 GHz Intel Xeon W 8-core 128GB DDRAM, through the UNIX shell (no graphical user interface is needed, unless IGV tool) and RStudio v1.3.959, and on a HPC platform running on Linux CentOS v7.7.1908 hosted by the University of Milan (https://www.indaco.unimi.it/).

## 3   Methods for lncRNA Analysis

### 3.1   Target Preparation

According to the transcript length, noncoding RNAs are stratified into small- or long-ncRNA (based on a 200 nt cutoff) [2], whose analysis by NGS requires consequently different library preparation and read-generation protocols.

The present chapter is dedicated to the basic description of lnc RNA analysis through high-throughput sequencing. Herein, we assume that the library has been prepared starting from total RNA and generated paired-end sequence data without the enrichment for polyadenylated transcripts that is normally used to focus on the coding transcriptome. TruSeq Stranded Total RNA protocol from Illumina is one of the most commonly adopted solutions, even if several competing alternatives are available.

Currently, the advantages of paired-end analysis in accuracy, cost, and effectiveness [3] have discouraged the use of single-end read sequencing, which is deprecated for long transcript analysis and remains in use only for the characterization of short RNAs, such as for miRNA sequencing. To gather appropriate coverage and results for lncRNA analysis, therefore, we suggest to use paired-end (50–150 nt) stranded preparation and reach a high sequencing dept, of at least 50–80 million reads per sample or more. This will allow to obtain a global view of gene expression, and some information on alternative splicing. This range encompasses most published RNA-seq experiments for lncRNA/whole transcriptome sequencing.

**3.2  Data Preprocessing**

Ultimately, the output generated by the sequencing pipeline (usually, the output generated from the sequencing service) is a list of paired `fastq` text files that will be used as input for the following analyses.

If the `fastq` files are generated by an in-house service, before proceeding the researchers should ensure that the data acquired have been demultiplexed and trimmed of the low-quality reads using different tools relative to the sequencing technology. With regard to Illumina-generated data processing (here taken as reference pipeline), the simplest way to process the `bcl` output is using `bcl2fastq2` tool available at the manufacturer's website (https://emea.support.illumina.com/downloads/bcl2fastq-conversion-software-v2-20.html), as well as the standard pipelines described in Bokulich et al. [4], which are extensively and clearly summarized at http://qiime.org/tutorials/processing_illumina_data.html. In principle, this pipeline should be valid to demultiplex any `fastq` file.

Then, for what concerns trimming of law-quality reads, if not yet performed by `bcl2fastq2`, the most effective and commonly used tool is represented by Trimmomatic, in virtue of its customizability [5].

After downloading the binary tool from Usadel lab web page (http://www.usadellab.org/cms/), it can be easily run under the default condition, for example, for paired-end data.

```
java -jar trimmomatic-0.39.jar PE input_forward.fq.gz input_reverse.fq.gz output_forward_paired.fq.gz output_forward_unpaired.fq.gz output_reverse_paired.fq.gz output_reverse_unpaired.fq.gz ILLUMINACLIP :TruSeq3-PE.fa:2:30:10:2:keepBothReads LEADING:N TRAILING:M MINLEN:X
```

where N and M represent the head and tail low quality bases value to be removed and X the minimal length of reads to be kept, and ILLUMINACLIP specifies: the path to a FASTA file containing all the adapters, the maximum mismatch count which still allows a full match to be performed, how accurate the match between the two "adapter ligated" reads must be for PE palindrome read alignment, how accurate the match between any adapter sequence must be against a read, the minimum length of adapter and the retention of reverse read (which may be useful if the downstream tools cannot handle a combination of paired and unpaired reads), all parameters separated by colons.

## 3.3 Alignment Pipeline

In line with the exponential growth of data produced by NGS, several bioinformatics tools have been developed to complete the several analysis steps needed, from read alignment to the reference genome to transcript sequence definition and quantification [6].

Due to both the intrinsic variability of the genome and the technical nature of NGS procedure, it is difficult to define a gold-standard bioinformatics pipeline for RNAseq analysis, and appropriate solutions could be chosen among multiple published so far, according to the experimental design. Nonetheless, even in the absence of a gold-standard procedure, anyone who faces ncRNA analysis needs to deal with the great challenge of unambiguous and reliable annotations. Based on current knowledge ncRNA genes are, in fact, usually associated with several overlapping transcripts, of different length and boundaries, which normally undergo splicing without respecting a common rule. In other words, differently from coding RNA, the same sequence from an ncRNA gene may alternatively be processed as "exonic-" or "intronic-like," thereby leading to radically different isoform (*see*, as an example, NEAT1 isoforms pattern in Fig. 1).

This implies that, independent of the alignment procedure used to map the sequenced fragments to the genome, a visual deconvolution (e.g., by IGV software) of the obtained results is often needed to depict the correct alignment and understand the meaning of the obtained count estimates. The present methodological pipeline is thus focused on describing the controversial scenario that derives from lncRNA annotation and quantification, and providing guidance on how to obtain good quality information on the noncoding transcriptome.

First, as regards the alignment procedures, it is worth summarizing briefly the differences between aligners and pseudoaligners, and highlighting their pros and cons.

The job of aligners (e.g., Bowtie, BWA, TopHat2, or STAR) is to find out where in the genome each sequencing read came from.

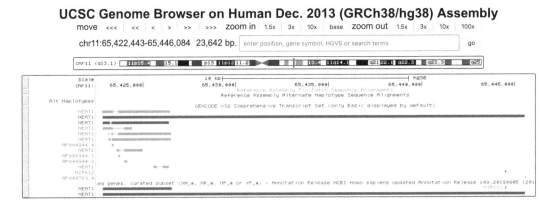

**Fig. 1** Screenshot of the pattern of NEAT1 isoforms from UCSC browser (https:/is.gd/9hGcFb)

The coordinates on the genome are included in the output, in the form of a BAM file. In the transcriptome analysis of ncRNA data, aligners like TopHat [7] and STAR [8] must be preferred since they can manage spliced reads, which is mandatory to capture differences in splicing or isoforms where unambiguous signals could be inferred.

Conversely, pseudoalignment leads simply to define the set of target sequences that the read is compatible with. The most commonly used pseudoaligners, valid for ncRNA analysis, are Kallisto [9] and Salmon [10]. Different from aligners, these are much quicker and less memory-consuming, and potentially allow to obtain transcript level expression information (whereas, e.g., STAR plus counting algorithm only give gene-level information, with some exception such as *featureCounts* [11] or *RSEM* [12]). Furthermore, pseudoaligners deal better with genes where reads map to multiple reference sequences. On the other hand, pseudoaligners usually map only reads to the reference transcriptome, rather than the genome, and their results are strictly dependent on the transcript annotation used as input; additionally, they cannot quantify transcripts or splice variants de novo, limiting the discovery power.

Although it has been reported that pseudoaligners outperform conventional alignment pipelines in lncRNA sequencing analysis [13], some issues have been recognized that limit their capability to correctly quantify lowly expressed genes and small RNAs, in particular in the presence of biological variations [14].

In reason of all these considerations, to decipher the complex scenario of ncRNA configuration, the researchers might prefer using just one of the two procedure. Here, for convenience, both are described, underlining the main difference that might be expected in the results. For sake of simplicity, Kallisto and STAR pipeline are shown together with the alignment output generated for two of the most well-characterized ncRNAs, *NEAT1* [15] and *MALAT1* [16].

The GENCODE consortium `gtf` annotation was chosen to process the data in the following example, since GENCODE represent the most commonly used annotations for conventional pipelines, whereas other more comprehensive datasets (such as https://lncipedia.org/) include a large variety of computationally inferred, nonvalidated transcripts, which are not necessarily helpful to investigators. Anyhow, the presented pipeline can be easily modified/integrated with custom annotations.

*3.3.1* Kallisto

This pipeline has been launched from system console using *kallisto* 0.46.2 (https://pachterlab.github.io/kallisto/download) on CentOS Linux release 7.7.1908 (*see* Materials section for hardware specifications).

First, to build the genome indices, download the full transcriptomes from Ensembl (files ending in `cdna.all.fa.gz`) and build the indices with *kallisto*. Namely, to build the human transcriptome index including both coding and noncoding RNA fraction, first download the coding transcriptome, which is available under cDNA on the Ensembl website, and the ncRNA one.

```
curl -O ftp://ftp.ensembl.org/pub/release-101/fasta/homo_sa
piens/cdna/Homo_sapiens.GRCh38.cdna.all.fa.gz
curl -O ftp://ftp.ensembl.org/pub/release-101/fasta/homo_sa
piens/ncrna/Homo_sapiens.GRCh38.ncrna.fa.gz
```

The two files can then be merged.

```
cat Homo_sapiens.GRCh38.cdna.all.fa.gz Homo_sapiens.GRCh38.
ncrna.fa.gz > Homo_sapiens.GRCh38.fa.gz
```

Next, run *kallisto* index. *Kallisto* works either on `.fa` and `.fa.gz` files, so there is no need to unzip the downloaded file.

```
kallisto index -i Homo_sapiens.GRCh38.idx Homo_sapiens.GRCh38.
fa.gz --make-unique
```

The following step is to obtain the pseudoalignment.

```
kallisto quant -i Homo_sapiens.GRCh38.idx -o ./OUTPUTDIR $PAT
HTOYOURFILES /YourSample_R1.fastq.gz $PATHTOYOURFILES/YourSam
ple_R2.fastq.gz --genomebam --gtf=gencode.v35.annotation.gtf
--chromosomes hg38.chrom.sizes
```

Pseudoaligners generate `.bam` files (with the corresponding `.bam.bai` index) and quantify transcript abundance, all available in the output directory.

The output of the alignment is shown in Figs. 2 and 3 (NEAT1) and Fig. 4 (MALAT1), upper panels.

The output can be easily visualized using the Integrated Genome Viewer (IGV) tool from Broad Institute (http://software.broadinstitute.org/software/igv/), where `.bam` output can be imported directly, or by other visualization tools. The easiest way to visualize the different ncRNA transcript isoforms in IGV is to convert to `bed` format the whole `gtf` file, or at least all those transcripts referred to the gene of interest.

Example:

```
grep NEAT1 gencode.v35.annotation.gtf > NEAT1.gtf
cat NEAT1.gtf | grep transcript_id | convert2bed --do-not-sort
--input=gtf - > NEAT1.bed
```

`convert2bed` is a function included in BEDOPS, a suite for high-performance genomic feature operations (v2.4.39, used herein, available at https://github.com/bedops/bedops).

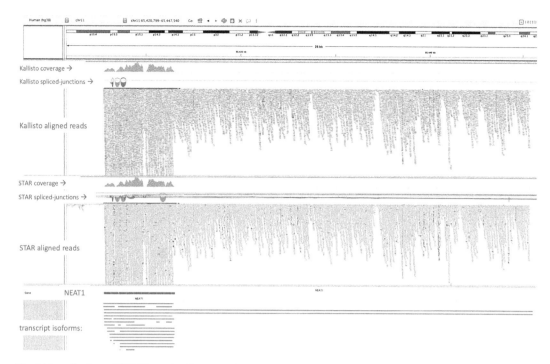

**Fig. 2** Visualization of NEAT1 reads alignment for (**a**) all transcripts, including the long-isoform and (**b**) focusing on the short 5′-isoforms, obtained either with kallisto (upper tracks) or STAR (lower tracks) procedure. The corresponding transcript GTF reference sequences are shown at the bottom

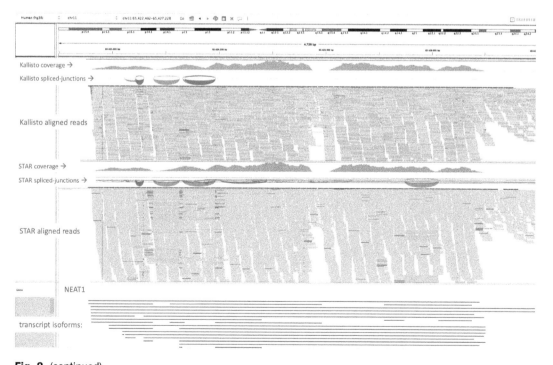

**Fig. 2** (continued)

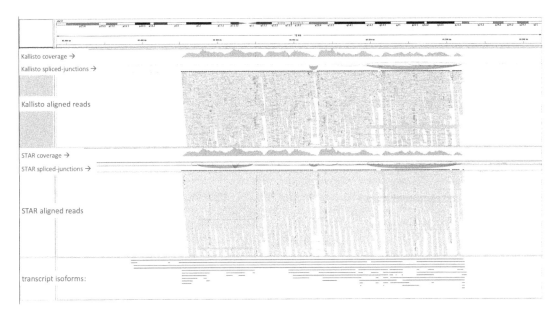

**Fig. 3** Visualization of MALAT1 reads alignment, obtained either with kallisto (upper tracks) or STAR (lower tracks) procedure. The corresponding transcript GTF reference sequences are shown at the bottom

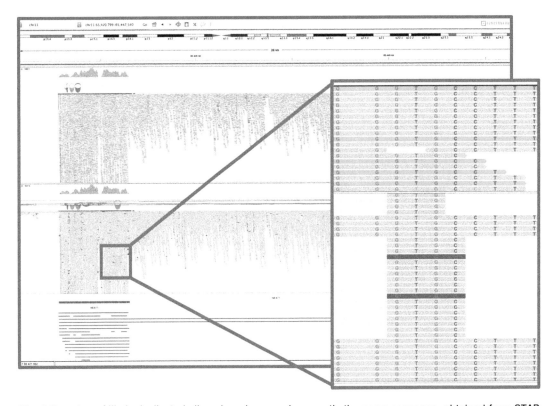

**Fig. 4** Overview of likely duplicated aligned reads, spanning exactly the same sequence, obtained from STAR analysis. The box enlarges the 3′ portion of the splitting reads (junction indicated by thin gray lines)

*3.3.2 STAR*

This pipeline has been launched from system console using *STAR* 2.7.6a (see installation instruction at https://github.com/ale xdobin/STAR) on CentOS Linux release 7.7.1908 (*see* Materials section for hardware specifications).

The first step to perform alignment with STAR is to create the genome index.

```
# download fasta
curl -O ftp://ftp.ensembl.org/pub/release-101/fasta/homo_sapiens/cdna/ Homo_sa-
piens.GRCh38.dna.primary_assembly.fa.gz


# extract archive
gunzip -c Homo_sapiens.GRCh38.dna.primary_assembly.fa.gz


# run STAR genome index generation
STAR --runThreadN 12
     --runMode genomeGenerate
     --genomeDir $PATHTOYOURFILES/Homo_sapiens.GRCh38.release.101_GENECODE.v35
     --genomeFastaFiles $PATHTOYOURFILES/Homo_sapiens.GRCh38.dna.primary_assembly.fa
     --sjdbGTFfile $PATHTOYOURFILES/gencode.v35.annotation.gtf
     --sjdbOverhang 100
```

Where `Homo_sapiens.GRCh38.dna.primary_assembly. fa` is the full `fasta` of the genome (downloaded, e.g., from Ensembl repository), the `gtf` is the transcript annotation downloaded from GENCODE consortium and 100 indicates the [number of bases – 1] of the reads.

STAR can be run with or without bedGraph generation. The first choice is less memory-consuming and might be suitable also for desktop solution with **32GB RAM** available.

Here, we report a standard instruction.

```
STAR --genomeDir
$PATHTOYOURFILES/Homo_sapiens.GRCh38.release.101_GENECODE.v35
     --genomeLoad LoadAndRemove
     --runThreadN 12
     --readFilesIn $PATHTOYOURFILES/YourSample_R1.fastq.gz
$PATHTOYOURFILES/YourSample_R2.fastq.gz
     --outFileNamePrefix YuorSample-GRCh38_
     --readFilesCommand zcat
     --outSAMunmapped Within
     --outBAMsortingThreadN 12
  --outSAMtype BAM Unsorted
  --limitBAMsortRAM 32000000000
```

To sort and index BAM files, `samtools` [17] is required (*see* installation instructions at http://www.htslib.org/). Here we use `samtools` version 1.3.1.

```
# bam files sorting
samtools sort -@ 12 -m 16G YourSample-GRCh38_Aligned.out.bam
YourSample-GRCh38_Aligned.out.sorted.bam
```

where the parameters -@ and -m represent threads and memory dedicated to the process, according to the available resources.

```
# bam file indexing
samtools index MM-055-GRCh38_Aligned.out.sorted.bam
```

STAR allows to customize several parameters, and there are many advanced options to control mapping behavior. In particular, we focus on two options that could help investigators to better analyze the occurrence of alternative splicing forms. The `--sjdbO-verhang` option tells STAR how many bases should be concatenated from donor and acceptor sides of the junctions. With 100 nt-long reads, the ideal value of `--sjdbOverhang` would be 99, which allows the 100 nt-read mapping 99 nt on one side and 1 nt on the other side. In other words, `--sjdbOverhang` represents the maximum possible overhang for your reads. On the other hand, `--alignSJDBoverhangMin` is used at the mapping step to define the minimum allowed overhang over splice junctions. For example, the default value of 3 would prohibit overhangs of only 1b or 2b. Here, for convenience, we run STAR leaving default parameters, which will produce results that might, in part, explain the difference with pseudoalignment.

The results of STAR analysis are depicted in Fig. 2a, b (NEAT1) and Fig. 3 (MALAT1), lower panels. Compared to *kallisto* output, at a first sight it is quite evident how STAR alignment depicts a more complex isoform scenario. In all likelihood, this is due to the higher capability of pseudoaligners to control duplicated reads and short overhanging between junctions. Figure 4 highlights a particular of STAR alignment output, where several likely duplicated reads with short overhangs (3–4 nt) are piled up to define a spliced junction. This does not necessarily correspond to "false positive" detection, but should anyhow be kept in consideration by the investigators before calling the occurrence of a specific transcript.

Ultimately, however, the real occurrence of a given transcript avoiding biases intrinsically associated with in silico predictions can be confirmed using direct Sanger sequencing of Q-RT-PCR with appropriate, unambiguous, primers.

*3.4  Quantification*      Next, the output of transcript quantification obtained by pseudoaligners procedure will represent the basis to obtain the quantification of detected transcripts. As stated before, `kallisto quant` procedure automatically generate two `abundance.tsv` and `abundance.h5` file in the output directory containing the transcript-per-million (TPM) bases expression value. Conversely, starting from STAR mapping, it is better to derive gene-level data (albeit, as stated before, some algorithm would offer the possibility to gather transcript information). This procedure presents limitations for investigators that are interested to capture differences at transcript-level: gene-level quantification does not account for isoforms diversification when multiple or alternatively spliced transcripts are expressed from the same gene, which is actually the most frequent situation in the lncRNA world.

Conversely, if compared with transcript-level quantification, the "meta-feature" based methods, such as *FeatureCounts* and *HTSeq* [11, 18], lead to reliable overall gene-level quantification. These algorithms are widely used in RNA-seq gene quantification in virtue of their simplicity. The "meta-feature" consists in the summarization of the singular transcriptional units considered: for example, if the features are represented by exons, all the overlapping exons from a gene are merged and the read counts per gene are obtained by considering all the reads that have been aligned to the previously generated "meta-exon."

*FeatureCounst* and *HTSeq* share quite similar procedures and lead to very similar results, with much less than 0.1% discrepancy (Fig. 5 depicts the overlapping of the raw counts obtained from a large RNA-seq proprietary dataset for almost 60,000 transcripts).

Here, exemplarily, we report *featureCounts* syntax to obtain raw expression estimation from STAR output (here we run the installed version 1.5.1). The software can be downloaded at https://bioinformaticshome.com/tools/rna-seq/descriptions/Subread.html; alternatively, R package is also available at https://www.rdocumentation.org/packages/Rsubread/versions/1.22.2/topics/featureCounts. A peculiar characteristic of this software is the capability to run on multiple samples.

```
featureCounts -p -a $ PATHTOYOURFILES /gencode.v25.annotation.
gtf -s 2 -T 5 -O -o $ PATHTOYOURFILES /NameOfYourOutputFile.
featureCounts 'cat Samples_list.featureCounts'
```

where `Sample_list.featureCounts` represents the list of all the `bam` files to be quantified. For completeness, provided the limitations described above, the procedure to extract transcript quantification can be run as such.

```
featureCounts -p -a $PATHTOYOURFILES/gencode.v25.annotation.
gtf -s 2 -T 5 -O -g "transcript_id" -f -o $ PATHTOYOURFILES /
NameOfYourOutputFile.featureCounts $ PATHTOYOURFILES /YourSam-
ple.out.sorted.bam
```

*FeatureCounts* gives raw counts. The easiest way to obtain normalized counts, if needed, is running *DESeq* function in *DESeq2* package in R environment (*see* **Note 1**).

Additionally, investigators, for some applications, may want to generate FPKM values (*see* **Note 2**).

**Fig. 5** Overlapping of the whole raw counts obtained on 40 samples for ~60,000 transcripts with HTseq (black lines) and feature counts (red dots). Each element on *x*-axis represents a transcript, *y*-axis represents the raw-counts

To this aim, we suggest using the well-known *Cufflinks* tool [19] from Cole Trapnell's lab, available at https://github.com/cole-trapnell-lab/cufflinks (here used v2.2.1). *Cufflinks* requires *samtools* being installed. The default procedure (*see* **Note 3**) can be run as such.

```
cufflinks -o
        -G $PATHTOYOURFILES /gencode.v25.annotation.gtf -p 12
        --library-type fr-secondstrand
        $PATHTOYOURFILES/YourSample.out.sorted.bam
```

***3.5  Downstream Analyses***

The methodology presented herein has been aimed at helping researchers to manage the output of high-throughput RNA-sequencing to detect lncRNA transcript, and to point out one of the most relevant issue that they should commonly face when handling for the first time the complex patterns of lncRNA annotations.

The following steps strictly depends on experimental design and investigator objectives. Typically, unsupervised (e.g., clustering or PCA) and supervised analysis (differential expression tests) are used. Specific tests must be run for alternative splicing detection, whereas interpretation of ncRNA functions, in terms of miRNA–lncRNA–gene interactions, protein–lncRNA interactions, pathway analysis, and so on, demands more complex and tailored downstream analyses that would require dedicated chapters.

We refer to the lncRNAblog container at https://www.lncrnablog.com/, where investigators can browse a wide amount of literature, tools, procedures, databases, and documentation about lncRNA world.

---

## 4   Notes

1. https://www.bioconductor.org/packages/devel/bioc/vignettes/DESeq2/inst/doc/DESeq2.html.

2. For a simple explanation of the difference between TPM and FPKM, see https://rna-seqblog.com/rpkm-fpkm-and-tpm-clearly-explained/.

3. Differently from featureCounts, cufflinks does not allow multiple sample processing. Here, for researcher's convenience, we include a short R pipeline to merge FPKM results from multiple samples at both gene and transcript level.

```
fpkm.transcripts <- c()
fpkm.genes <- c()
# create object with "Sample" dir names (replace "Sample" as opportune)
dirnames <- dir(pattern="Sample")
# loop through all directories and grab fpkm columns
for(i in 1:length(dirnames) ){
        gname <- paste(dirnames[i], "/genes.fpkm_tracking",sep="")
        tname <- paste(dirnames[i], "/isoforms.fpkm_tracking",sep="")
        x <- read.table(file=gname, sep="\t", header=T, as.is=T)
        x = x [order(x$tracking_id ),]
        y <- read.table(file=tname, sep="\t", header=T, as.is=T)
        y = y [order(y$tracking_id ),]
        if (i==1) {
            fpkm.transcripts <- y[,c("gene_id", "gene_short_name", "FPKM")]
            fpkm.genes <- x[,c("gene_id", "gene_short_name", "FPKM")]
        } else {
            fpkm.transcripts <- cbind(fpkm.transcripts, y[,"FPKM"])
            fpkm.genes <- cbind(fpkm.genes, x[,"FPKM"])
        }
}
# name the columns
colnames(fpkm.transcripts) <- c("gene.ID","gene.symbol",dirnames)
colnames(fpkm.genes) <- c("gene.ID","gene.symbol",dirnames)
# name the rows
fpkm.transcripts = fpkm.transcripts [ order(fpkm.transcripts$gene.ID ), ]
y = y[order(y$gene_id),]
all(y$gene_id == fpkm.transcripts$gene.ID)
rownames(fpkm.transcripts) <- y[,1]
rownames(fpkm.genes) <- x[,1]
```

## Acknowledgments

SB is supported by the Italian Ministry of Education, University and Research (PRIN 2017 #2017PPS2X4_003), and the Italian Association of Cancer Research, AIRC, Milan, Italy (Investigator Grant IG2017 #20052). LA is supported by the Accelerator Award #29374 through CRUK-AIRC partnership.

## References

1. Carninci P, Kasukawa T, Katayama S, Gough J, Frith MC, Maeda N, Oyama R, Ravasi T, Lenhard B, Wells C, Kodzius R, Shimokawa K, Bajic VB, Brenner SE, Batalov S, Forrest AR, Zavolan M, Davis MJ, Wilming LG, Aidinis V, Allen JE, Ambesi-Impiombato A, Apweiler R, Aturaliya RN, Bailey TL, Bansal M, Baxter L, Beisel KW, Bersano T, Bono H, Chalk AM, Chiu KP, Choudhary V, Christoffels A, Clutterbuck DR, Crowe ML, Dalla E, Dalrymple BP, de Bono B, Della Gatta G, di Bernardo D, Down T, Engstrom P, Fagiolini M, Faulkner G, Fletcher CF, Fukushima T, Furuno M, Futaki S, Gariboldi M, Georgii-Hemming P, Gingeras TR, Gojobori T, Green RE, Gustincich S, Harbers M, Hayashi Y, Hensch TK, Hirokawa N, Hill D, Huminiecki L, Iacono M, Ikeo K, Iwama A, Ishikawa T, Jakt M, Kanapin A, Katoh M, Kawasawa Y, Kelso J, Kitamura H, Kitano H, Kollias G, Krishnan SP, Kruger A, Kummerfeld SK, Kurochkin IV, Lareau LF, Lazarevic D, Lipovich L, Liu J, Liuni S, McWilliam S, Madan Babu M, Madera M, Marchionni L, Matsuda H, Matsuzawa S, Miki H, Mignone F, Miyake S, Morris K, Mottagui-Tabar S, Mulder N, Nakano N, Nakauchi H, Ng P, Nilsson R, Nishiguchi S, Nishikawa S, Nori F, Ohara O, Okazaki Y, Orlando V, Pang KC, Pavan WJ, Pavesi G, Pesole G, Petrovsky N, Piazza S, Reed J, Reid JF, Ring BZ, Ringwald M, Rost B, Ruan Y, Salzberg SL, Sandelin A, Schneider C, Schonbach C, Sekiguchi K, Semple CA, Seno S, Sessa L, Sheng Y, Shibata Y, Shimada H, Shimada K, Silva D, Sinclair B, Sperling S, Stupka E, Sugiura K, Sultana R, Takenaka Y, Taki K, Tammoja K, Tan SL, Tang S, Taylor MS, Tegner J, Teichmann SA, Ueda HR, van Nimwegen E, Verardo R, Wei CL, Yagi K, Yamanishi H, Zabarovsky E, Zhu S, Zimmer A, Hide W, Bult C, Grimmond SM, Teasdale RD, Liu ET, Brusic V, Quackenbush J, Wahlestedt C, Mattick JS, Hume DA, Kai C, Sasaki D, Tomaru Y, Fukuda S, Kanamori-Katayama M, Suzuki M, Aoki J, Arakawa T, Iida J, Imamura K, Itoh M, Kato T, Kawaji H, Kawagashira N, Kawashima T, Kojima M, Kondo S, Konno H, Nakano K, Ninomiya N, Nishio T, Okada M, Plessy C, Shibata K, Shiraki T, Suzuki S, Tagami M, Waki K, Watahiki A, Okamura-Oho Y, Suzuki H, Kawai J, Hayashizaki Y, Consortium F, Group RGER, Genome Science G (2005) The transcriptional landscape of the mammalian genome. Science 309 (5740):1559–1563. https://doi.org/10.1126/science.1112014

2. Van Roosbroeck K, Pollet J, Calin GA (2013) miRNAs and long noncoding RNAs as biomarkers in human diseases. Expert Rev Mol Diagn 13(2):183–204. https://doi.org/10.1586/erm.12.134

3. Freedman AH, Gaspar JM, Sackton TB (2020) Short paired-end reads trump long single-end reads for expression analysis. BMC Bioinformatics 21(1):149. https://doi.org/10.1186/s12859-020-3484-z

4. Bokulich NA, Subramanian S, Faith JJ, Gevers D, Gordon JI, Knight R, Mills DA, Caporaso JG (2013) Quality-filtering vastly improves diversity estimates from Illumina amplicon sequencing. Nat Methods 10 (1):57–59. https://doi.org/10.1038/nmeth.2276

5. Bolger AM, Lohse M, Usadel B (2014) Trimmomatic: a flexible trimmer for Illumina sequence data. Bioinformatics 30 (15):2114–2120. https://doi.org/10.1093/bioinformatics/btu170

6. Costa-Silva J, Domingues D, Lopes FM (2017) RNA-Seq differential expression analysis: an extended review and a software tool. PLoS One 12(12):e0190152. https://doi.org/10.1371/journal.pone.0190152

7. Kim D, Pertea G, Trapnell C, Pimentel H, Kelley R, Salzberg SL (2013) TopHat2: accurate alignment of transcriptomes in the presence of insertions, deletions and gene fusions. Genome Biol 14(4):R36. https://doi.org/10.1186/gb-2013-14-4-r36

8. Dobin A, Davis CA, Schlesinger F, Drenkow J, Zaleski C, Jha S, Batut P, Chaisson M, Gingeras TR (2013) STAR: ultrafast universal RNA-seq aligner. Bioinformatics 29(1):15–21. https://doi.org/10.1093/bioinformatics/bts635

9. Bray NL, Pimentel H, Melsted P, Pachter L (2016) Near-optimal probabilistic RNA-seq quantification. Nat Biotechnol 34 (5):525–527. https://doi.org/10.1038/nbt.3519

10. Patro R, Duggal G, Love MI, Irizarry RA, Kingsford C (2017) Salmon provides fast and bias-aware quantification of transcript expression. Nat Methods 14(4):417–419. https://doi.org/10.1038/nmeth.4197

11. Liao Y, Smyth GK, Shi W (2014) feature-Counts: an efficient general purpose program for assigning sequence reads to genomic features. Bioinformatics 30(7):923–930. https://doi.org/10.1093/bioinformatics/btt656

12. Li B, Dewey CN (2011) RSEM: accurate transcript quantification from RNA-Seq data with or without a reference genome. BMC Bioinformatics 12:323. https://doi.org/10.1186/1471-2105-12-323

13. Zheng H, Brennan K, Hernaez M, Gevaert O (2019) Benchmark of long non-coding RNA quantification for RNA sequencing of cancer samples. Gigascience 8(12):giz145. https://doi.org/10.1093/gigascience/giz145

14. Wu DC, Yao J, Ho KS, Lambowitz AM, Wilke CO (2018) Limitations of alignment-free tools in total RNA-seq quantification. BMC Genomics 19(1):510. https://doi.org/10.1186/s12864-018-4869-5

15. Dong P, Xiong Y, Yue J, Hanley SJB, Kobayashi N, Todo Y, Watari H (2018) Long non-coding RNA NEAT1: a novel target for diagnosis and therapy in human tumors. Front Genet 9:471. https://doi.org/10.3389/fgene.2018.00471

16. Arun G, Aggarwal D, Spector DL (2020) MALAT1 long non-coding RNA: functional implications. Noncoding RNA 6(2):22. https://doi.org/10.3390/ncrna6020022

17. Li H, Handsaker B, Wysoker A, Fennell T, Ruan J, Homer N, Marth G, Abecasis G, Durbin R, 1000 Genome Project Data Processing Subgroup (2009) The sequence alignment/map format and SAMtools. Bioinformatics 25(16):2078–2079. https://doi.org/10.1093/bioinformatics/btp352

18. Anders S, Pyl PT, Huber W (2015) HTSeq—a Python framework to work with high-throughput sequencing data. Bioinformatics 31(2):166–169. https://doi.org/10.1093/bioinformatics/btu638

19. Trapnell C, Williams BA, Pertea G, Mortazavi A, Kwan G, van Baren MJ, Salzberg SL, Wold BJ, Pachter L (2010) Transcript assembly and quantification by RNA-Seq reveals unannotated transcripts and isoform switching during cell differentiation. Nat Biotechnol 28(5):511–515. https://doi.org/10.1038/nbt.1621

# Chapter 5

## Single-Cell RNAseq Analysis of lncRNAs

### Stefano Cagnin, Enrico Alessio, Raphael Severino Bonadio, and Gabriele Sales

### Abstract

Mammalian genomes are pervasively transcribed and a small fraction of RNAs produced codify for proteins. The importance of noncoding RNAs for the maintenance of cell functions is well known (e.g., rRNAs, tRNAs), but only recently it was first demonstrated the involvement of microRNAs (miRNAs) in posttranscriptional regulation and then the activity of long noncoding RNAs (lncRNAs) in the regulation of miRNAs, DNA structure and protein function. LncRNAs have an expression more cell specific than other RNAs and basing on their subcellular localization exert different functions. In this book chapter we consider different protocols to evaluate the expression of lncRNAs at the single cell level using genome-wide approaches. We considered the skeletal muscle as example because the most abundant tissue in mammals involved in the regulation of metabolism and body movement. We firstly described how to isolate the smallest complete contractile system responsible for muscle metabolic and contractile traits (myofibers). We considered how to separate long and short RNAs to allow the sequencing of the full-length transcript using the SMART technique for the retrotranscription. Because of myofibers are multinucleated cells and because of it is better to perform single cell sequencing on fresh tissues we described the single-nucleus sequencing that can be applied to frozen tissues. The chapter concludes with a description of bioinformatics approaches to evaluate differential expression from single-cell or single-nucleus RNA sequencing.

**Key words** Long noncoding RNA, Myofiber, Single-nucleus RNA sequencing, Bioinformatic

## 1 Introduction

With the conclusion of the human genome project, people understood that a limited amount of DNA was involved in the synthesis of proteins. The annotated coding genes varied among 26,000 and 39,000. In 2012, it was observed that most of the human genome is transcribed and the most impressive conclusion was that the vast majority of the transcribed genome does not code for translated RNAs to synthesize proteins. Most of the human and other mammalian genomes code for noncoding RNAs [1]. Among noncoding RNAs, the most abundant are long noncoding RNAs (lncRNAs). They are described as important players in the regulation of different aspects of cellular biology. For instance, they are involved in cell

Alfons Navarro (ed.), *Long Non-Coding RNAs in Cancer*, Methods in Molecular Biology, vol. 2348,
https://doi.org/10.1007/978-1-0716-1581-2_5, © Springer Science+Business Media, LLC, part of Springer Nature 2021

differentiation [2, 3], normal functioning of differentiated cells [4–6], and also involved in the development of pathological conditions such as tumors [7–9].

Soft tissue sarcomas, fibromatoses, and hemangiomas are the most common tumors arising in muscle. Rhabdomyosarcoma is primarily a tumor that develops from skeletal muscle cells that lose their ability to fully differentiate. It is a childhood and adolescence disease and accounts for ~40% of soft tissue sarcomas [10]. Most common rhabdomyosarcomas are embryonal (60–70% of childhood cases) while alveolar type comprises for 20–25% of rhabdomyosarcoma related tumors [11]. Alveolar rhabdomyosarcomas can be also subclassified in translocated and non-translocated according to the presence of the translocations t(2;13) (q35,q14) or, t(1;13)(p36,q15) [12, 13]. These translocations involve the paired box 3 (PAX3) or paired box 7 (PAX7) and forkhead box protein O1 (FOXO1) genes. All three genes codify for transcription factors important for muscle trophism.

One of the major lineages expressing Pax3 is the skeletal muscle lineage [14]. It forms dimers with another PAX3 or with PAX7 molecules. Myogenic precursors expressing PAX3 and/or PAX7 form satellite cells that are muscle stem cells, which contribute to postnatal muscle growth and muscle regeneration. These adult satellite cells are quiescent until injury occurs, when they are activated to repair injury to form new or repair the already present myofibers.

Skeletal muscle is a complex organ and heterogenous tissue. Different cell types such as those from blood, vessels, nerves, connective tissue, and myofibers, that are the smallest complete contractile system of skeletal muscle compose this organ. Myofibers influence both muscle mechanical performance and metabolism. They are classified into different types. In mouse, type I myofibers present slow-twitch contraction and oxidative metabolism, type IIA and IIX myofibers fast-twitch contraction and oxidative metabolism, and type IIB myofibers fast-twitch contraction and glycolytic metabolism [15]. Scaling down the possibility of analyzing transcriptomic of skeletal muscle at single isolated myofiber level for mRNA, long noncoding RNA (lncRNA) and microRNA (miRNA) populations will aid in a better comprehension of the skeletal muscle pathophysiology [6, 16, 17].

This aspect is particularly true when we are talking of highly specifically expressed RNAs as lncRNAs. They show a cell-specific expression more than that evidenced for coding RNAs. For this reason, it is important to analyze lncRNAs in single cells instead of using bulk tissues or a cell population. Recently several technological improvements were done in the field of single-cell genomic and transcriptomic. Moreover, the ability of identify single molecules thorough fluorescence amplification has given a considerable boost in the comprehension of cell specificity, subcellular localization, and function of lncRNAs.

The purpose of this chapter is to describe different protocols available for the analysis of RNA expression using a single cell approach. We will elucidate important steps to consider having good results. To conclude the chapter, we will consider bioinformatics approaches have to be applied for the analysis of single cell RNA sequencing.

# 2  Materials

## 2.1  Analysis of Single Myofibers

1. 200µL tips.
2. DNA LoBind tubes.
3. Spin-X centrifuge tubes (Corning-Costar).
4. RNase/DNase-free Eppendorf microcentrifuge tube.
5. 0.2 mL PCR tube.
6. Cell culture plates: 24-well and 6-well plates.
7. Plastic Pasteur pipettes.
8. Slide-staining dishes.
9. Adult wild-type mice, weight: 33–35 g (*see* **Note 1**).
10. High-glucose Dulbecco's modified Eagle medium (DMEM).
11. 2,3-Butanedione monoxime (BDM).
12. Collagenase from *Clostridium histolyticum*, type I.
13. Fetal bovine serum (FBS).
14. Phosphate-buffered saline (PBS).
15. TRIzol Reagent.
16. Nuclease-free water.
17. Chloroform.
18. 70% v/v ethanol (dilute ethanol in nuclease-free water).
19. 75% v/v ethanol (dilute ethanol in nuclease-free water).
20. Absolute ethanol.
21. miRNeasy kit (Qiagen).
22. RNeasy micro kit (Qiagen).
23. Sodium acetate 3 M (pH 5.5).
24. Micropipette (P10, P20).
25. −80 °C freezer.
26. −20 °C freezer.
27. Forceps and scissors for microdissection.
28. 37 °C incubator.

29. Stereomicroscope.

30. Refrigerated microcentrifuge.

31. SpeedVac concentrator.

32. Thermocycler.

33. Nanodrop spectrophotometer.

34. Heat block.

35. Centrifuge.

*2.2  miRNA, lncRNA, and mRNA Sequencing Library Based on the SMART Amplification*

1. Primers for the sequencing library using the IonTorrent sequencer (Thermofisher Scientific).

   (a) SMART primer: CACACACAATTAACCCTCACTAAA ggg (uppercase deoxyribonucleotides; lower case ribonucleotides).

   (b) oligo-dT-Ion P1 Adaptor primer (primer for retrotranscription): CCTCTCTATGGGCAGTCGGTGATCCT CAGC[dT]20VN.

   (c) A Adaptor primer: CCATCTCATCCCTGCGTGTCTCC GACTCAG.

   (d) P Adaptor primer: CCTCTCTATGGGCAGTCGGTGAT .

2. Poly(A) Tailing Kit.

3. NaOAc 3 M pH 5.5.

4. Absolute ethanol.

5. 75% v/v of ethanol.

6. dNTPs.

7. RNase-free water (no DEPC treated).

8. SuperScript II (Thermo Fisher Scientific) (*see* **Note 2**).

9. Taq DNA polymerase high fidelity.

10. GenElute PCR Clean-up kit (Sigma-Aldrich).

11. E-Gel™ SizeSelect™ II Agarose Gels, 2% (Thermo Fisher Scientific).

12. E-Gel Power Snap Electrophoresis Device (Thermo Fisher Scientific).

*2.3  Single-Nucleus RNA Sequencing (snRNA-Seq)*

*See* **Note 3** for considerations about solutions.

1. 1 M Tris HCl pH 7.6 (10 mL).

2. 1 M NaCl (10 mL).

3. 1 M $MgCl_2$ (10 mL).

4. 100 mg/mL BSA (10 mL).

5. PBS 1×.

6. Igepal 10% (10 mL).

7. DAPI (10 mL).

8. Nuclei Storage Buffer: 6139µL of $H_2O$, 70µL of 1 M Tris–HCl, 70µL of 1 M NaCl, 21µL of 1 M $MgCl_2$, 700µL of 100 mg/mL BSA. Prepare fresh as needed.

9. Nuclei Lysis Buffer: 4335µL of $H_2O$, 50µL of 1 M Tris–HCl, 50µL of 1 M NaCl, 15µL of 1 M $MgCl_2$, 500µL of 100 mg/mL BSA, 50µL of 10% Igepal. Prepare fresh as needed.

10. Refrigerated swinging bucket centrifuge for microtubes.

11. 15 mL tubes.

12. 2 mL tubes.

13. Cell strainers (size 40µm).

14. Syringe and needles (size 21 G).

15. Fluorescence microscope.

16. Slides and cover slips.

## 3    Methods

### 3.1   Single-Myofiber RNA Sequencing (Single-Cell RNA-Seq)

#### 3.1.1   Myofiber Isolation

1. Collect the muscle of choice. Below, step by step procedure to collect soleus and EDL muscles (*see* **Note 4**).

   (a)  Sacrifice the mouse by performing cervical dislocation.

   (b)  Peel off the skin from one leg in order to expose the muscles.

   (c)  Carefully remove the fascia around the hindlimb muscles.

   (d)  Secure the mouse supine and start exposing the tibialis anterior (TA) and EDL tendons.

   (e)  Remove the TA muscle by cutting the distal tendon at its proximal attachment.

   (f)  Collect the EDL muscle by cutting first the distal tendon and then the proximal tendon.

   (g)  Store the EDL muscle in a well of 24 or 6 well plate containing DMEM with 3 mM BDM. Assure to cover the muscle.

   (h)  Repeat **steps 1b–g** to collect the EDL muscle of the other leg.

   (i)  Rotate the mouse and secure it in prone position.

   (j)  To expose the soleus muscle, peel off the gastrocnemius muscle by cutting its tendon.

   (k)  Collect the soleus muscle by cutting the tendon and then cutting the other end.

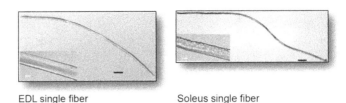

EDL single fiber                    Soleus single fiber

**Fig. 1** Images of single isolated myofibers from EDL and soleus muscles. Scale bar is for 250μm

    (l) Store the soleus muscle in a well of 24 or 6 well plate containing DMEM with 3 mM BDM.

    (m) Repeat **steps 1j–l** to collect the soleus muscle of the other leg.

    (n) Assure that there is minimal blood contamination and eventually wash muscles with new DMEM plus BDM medium.

2. Put muscles onto a well of cell culture plate (24 or 6 well plates) covered by cold DMEM with 3 mM BDM (*see* **Note 5**).

3. Incubate each muscle in 1 mL high-glucose DMEM with 3 mM BDM and 10 mg/mL of type I collagenase for 45 min at 37 °C in a well of a 24-well plate.

4. Rinse each muscle by moving it to different wells of a 6-well plate (*see* **Note 6**):

    (a) Rinse the first time using 3 mL of DMEM with 3 mM BDM.

    (b) Rinse the second time using 3 mL of DMEM with 3 mM BDM and 10% FBS.

    (c) Rinse the third time using 3 mL of DMEM with 3 mM BDM.

5. Transfer the muscles into the well of a 6-well plate containing 3 mL of DMEM with 10% FBS.

6. Separate the myofibers by gently pipetting up and down using a wide-mouth plastic Pasteur pipette (about 4 mm diameter) previously rinsed in FBS to prevent myofibers from sticking to the plastic. When about 100 myofibers have been isolated, transfer the muscle into a new well.

7. Repeat **step 6** several times until enough intact fibers have been obtained (Fig. 1).

8. Pick one by one the isolated myofibers using a micropipette (200μL tips) and a stereomicroscope, wash the myofiber first in a well containing DMEM with 3 mM BDM and 10% FBS, and second in a well containing PBS.

9. Store the myofibers in a microcentrifuge tube and proceed with the RNA extraction or nuclei isolation.

*3.1.2  Long RNA and Short RNA Separation Using RNeasy Kits (Qiagen)*

*See* **Note 7** for the optimal number of myofibers to process contemporary.

1. Each myofiber is lysed in 250μL of TRIzol Reagent pipetting up and down the solution.

2. Add 50μL of chloroform, mix by vortexing, and incubate on ice for 15 min.

3. Centrifuge the tube for 15 min at $12,000 \times g$ at 4 °C.

4. Transfer the aqueous upper phase (about 130μL) into a new tube.

5. Add 1 volume of 70% ethanol and mix.

6. Transfer the solution onto a miRNeasy column.

7. Spin for 15 s at $12,000 \times g$.

8. Long RNAs are retained by the column, whereas short RNAs are collected in the eluate (*see* **Note 8**).

9. Proceed to Long RNA purification (Subheadings 3.1.3) or miRNA purification (Subheading 3.1.4) (*see* **Note 9**).

*3.1.3  Long RNA Purification Retained in the Column*

1. Add 700μL of RWT Buffer from miRNeasy kit to the column containing long RNAs (previous section).

2. Spin for 15 s at $\geq 8000 \times g$ and discard the eluate.

3. Add 500μL of RPE Buffer from miRNeasy kit to the column.

4. Spin for 15 s at $\geq 8000 \times g$ and discard the eluate.

5. Add again 500μL of RPE Buffer from miRNeasy kit to the column.

6. Spin for 15 s at $\geq 8000 \times g$ and discard the eluate.

7. Place the column in a new collection tube.

8. Add 50μL of nuclease-free water to the center of the column and incubate at room temperature for 2 min.

9. Spin for 1 min at $\geq 8000 \times g$ to eluate long RNAs (*see* **Note 10**).

10. Use SpeedVac concentrator to reduce the volume to 14μL (*see* **Note 11**).

*3.1.4  miRNA Purification Using miRNeasy Kit*

1. Add 0.65 volumes of absolute ethanol (about 165μL) to the eluate produced after loading the aqueous phase of the TRIzol extraction into the miRNeasy columns (Subheading 3.1.2, **step 8**) and mix well.

2. Transfer the solution onto a new RNeasy micro column.

3. Spin for 15 s at $\geq 8000 \times g$ and discard the eluate.

4. Add 500μL of RPE Buffer to the column.

5. Spin for 15 s at $\geq 8000 \times g$ and discard the eluate.

6. Add 500µL of 80% ethanol to the column.

7. Spin for 2 min at ≥8000 × *g* and discard the eluate.

8. Spin again for 5 min at ≥8000 × *g* with the cap opened.

9. Transfer the column to a new collection tube.

10. Add 14µL of nuclease-free water to the center of the column and incubate at room temperature for 2 min.

11. Spin for 1 min at ≥8000 × *g* to eluate miRNAs (*see* **Note 10**).

12. Use SpeedVac concentrator to reduce the volume to 6.5µL (*see* **Note 12**).

*3.1.5 miRNA, lncRNA, and mRNA Sequencing Library Based on the SMART Amplification*

RNA processing for microarray gene expression analysis or miRNA sequencing are described in [6, 17, 18]. Remember that miRNAs and long RNAs (coding and noncoding) are separated in different Eppendorf (*see* Subheadings 3.1.2–3.1.4). Here we will fully describe the preparation of miRNA sequencing library based on the SMART protocol [19] because a first step of polyadenylation is required. In fact, mature miRNAs, purified as described in the Subheading 3.1.4, do not have a poly(A) tail that is used to bind oligo-d(T) primers for the retrotranscription reaction. Otherwise, both lncRNAs and mRNAs are polyadenylated and therefore this first step is not required for their retrotranscription and eventual amplification through the SMART protocol. The SMART amplification allows the recovery of the full-length transcripts.

*miRNA Polyadenylation*

Starting volume of purified miRNAs is 6.5µL (*see* Subheading 3.1.4, **step 12**). Using a polyA polymerase (Poly[A] Tailing Kit), add a poly(A) stretch to the 3′ end of miRNAs. Reaction should be scaled to perform it in 10µL (*see* **Note 13**).

1. Precipitate the RNA adding one-tenth of the volume of NaOAc 3 M pH 5.5.

2. Add 2.5 volumes of absolute ethanol.

3. Mix and incubate overnight at −20 °C.

4. Centrifuge at 12,000 × *g* at 4 °C for 20 min.

5. Discard the solution without disturbing the pellet.

6. Add 500µL of ethanol 75%.

7. Centrifuge at 12,000 × *g* at 4 °C for 20 min.

8. Discard the solution without disturbing the pellet.

9. Add 500µL of ethanol 75%.

10. Centrifuge at 12,000 × *g* at 4 °C for 20 min.

11. Discard the solution without disturbing the pellet.

12. Air dry the pellet for 5–10 min.

13. Resuspend the pellet in 3.2µL of RNase free water.

**Retrotranscription**

1. Perform the retrotranscription in a final volume of 10μL adding to the previous volume (*see* **Note 14**) the following reagents:

   (a)  10 pmol of oligo-dT-Ion P1 Adaptor primer.

   (b)  50 pmol of SMART primer.

2. Incubate at 72 °C for 2 min to eliminate any RNA secondary structures (*see* **Note 15**).

3. Put the solution on ice for 2 min.

4. Add First Strand Buffer to a final concentration of 1×.

5. Add DTT to a final concentration of 10 mM.

6. Add dNTPs to a final concentration of 0.5 mM.

7. Add 100 U of Superscript II.

8. Incubate at 42 °C for 2 h.

9. Inactivate the retrotranscriptase incubating the solution at 72 °C for 5 min.

**Amplification of Retrotranscribed RNA**

ssDNAs have a SMART anchor sequence (SMART primer) at the 5′-end after the end of the retrotranscription. This allows the PCR amplification to increase the cDNA content and to create a dsDNA to be sequenced. In the case of lncRNAs it has to consider the length of RNAs. In fact, if those are too long it is impossible the retrotranscription until the 5′-end. For this reason, to construct the sequencing library from long RNAs it can be necessary to fragment it and produce a 3′-end library or to consider losing the information of the 5′-end of very long transcripts.

1. A classical PCR amplification with the high fidelity Taq DNA polymerase is used to amplify cDNAs. Primers used were A Adaptor primer and P1 Adaptor primer (*see* **Note 16**).

2. As template use half volume of the previously prepared cDNA.

3. Perform a second PCR amplification using as primers A and P1. Amplification cycles of this amplification step has to be set up running the PCR amplification product on electrophoresis gel. It should appear a smear with no or a reduced number of bands that evidence the preferential amplification of specific transcripts (*see* **Note 17**). *See* the Fig. 2 for an example.

4. If necessary, bring the volume to 100μL with nuclease free water before the purification. Purify PCR products with Gen-Elute PCR Clean-up columns to eliminate primer dimers. Follow exactly the manufacturer protocol (*see* **Note 18**).

5. Size select products for sequencing using the E-Gel SizeSelect Gels (*see* **Note 19**).

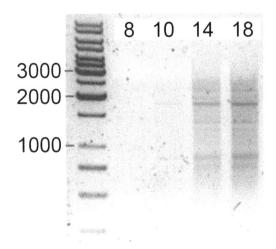

**Fig. 2** Example of PCR amplification setting. (1) The number of PCR cycles over each line are indicated. On the left of the ladder the number of nucleotides

### 3.2 Improvement with Single-Nucleus RNA Sequencing (snRNA-seq)

Previously described protocols are useful for cells that are big and manually collectable like skeletal muscle fibers or neurons. These cells cannot be analyzed with the classical high-throughput single-cell sequencing methods, based onto drop-seq for example, because too big for their separation within the water bubbles of the emulsion used to create the sequencing library (for a review of the methods for the single-cell sequencing *see* [20, 21]). An alternative for these type of cells (big dimensions, multinucleated such as myofibers) and for frozen tissues (in fact single cell sequencing is a method highly performant in fresh tissues) is the single-nucleus sequencing. Same methods used to produce RNA sequencing libraries from single cells can be used to produce RNA sequencing libraries from isolated nuclei. The main problem of this technique is to have nuclei purified from cell debris, and to have intact nuclei. It was evidenced that snRNA-seq is well suited for large-scale surveys of cellular diversity in various tissues as it provides similar resolution for cell type detection to single-cell RNA-seq [22, 23].

### 3.2.1 Single Nucleus Preparation

We recommend proceeding to the nuclei isolation with fresh tissues, but the same method can be adapted to frozen tissues. However, depending on the experimental design it is possible to freeze myofibers at −80 °C (*see* Subheading 3.1.1). If doing so, thaw myofibers on ice before starting the nuclei isolation. Keep buffers and the single-nucleus suspension always on ice to prevent clumps (*see* **Note 20**).

1. Coat 15 mL tubes by adding 1 mL of BSA stock solution in tube walls (one per each sample or pooled samples) and remove the excess volume (*see* **Note 21**).

2. Transfer the resuspension of myofibers freshly prepared (*see* Subheading 3.1.1) or thawed to the coated 15 mL tubes on ice. Recover the maximum amount of fibers by washing the vial used to recover or store myofibers (*see* Subheading 3.1.1) with 750µL of cold Nuclei Storage Buffer.

3. Centrifuge the cell suspension at $900 \times g$ for 10 min at 4 °C.

4. Discard the supernatant (leaving approximately 100µL to avoid lose cells) (*see* **Note 22**).

5. Wash the myofibers with 750µL of Nuclei Storage Buffer and repeat the centrifugation at $900 \times g$ for 10 min at 4 °C, then discard the supernatant, leaving approximately 100µL of cell suspension. Keep cells on ice between centrifugation steps.

6. Transfer the samples to 2 mL tubes.

7. Add 500µL of cold Nuclei Lysis Buffer and 1% Invitrogen™ SUPERase In™ RNase Inhibitor.

8. Perform cell lysis by doing up and down pipetting 15 times with p 1000 tips and put samples 2 min on ice.

9. Pipette 15 times with p 100 tips and wait 2 min on ice.

10. Pass samples through a needle syringe (21 G) 15 times and wait 2 min on ice.

11. Pass samples through a needle syringe (21 G) more 15 times and wait 10 min on ice.

12. Coat 50 mL tubes with 1 mL of BSA.

13. Filter samples using cell strainers (it is not necessary to put pressure) and collect the filtered fraction on 50 mL coated tubes (*see* **Note 23**).

14. Wash previous 2 mL tubes with 500µL of storage solution and pass through cell strainers to maximize nuclei recovery (*see* **Note 24**).

15. Centrifuge the filtrate at $900 \times g$ for 10 min at 4 °C.

16. Remove supernatant and leave around 100µL in the tube.

17. Wash the nuclei by adding 750µL of Nuclei Storage Buffer, centrifuging at $900 \times g$ for 10 min at 4 °C. Remove supernatant (leave approximately 100µL) and add 500µL of Nuclei Storage Buffer.

18. Separate control samples in 2 tubes for cell sorting: 200µL for the blank (1/3 volume) and 400µL for staining (2/3 volume).

19. Add 1µL of DAPI solution (final concentration 3×) to stain samples and leave them 10 min on ice.

20. Separate 10µL aliquot to check nuclei integrity and presence of cell debris on fluorescence microscope. If the nuclei are

preserved and there are no visible cell debris proceed to cell sorting.

21. Sort the cells with BD FACSAria III immediately (1× PBS + 0.1% BSA is recommended).

*3.2.2 Single-Nucleus Library Preparation for RNAseq (Bio-Rad snRNAseq)*

The following protocol is optimized for the preparation of bar-coded RNA-Seq libraries in order to be sequenced on Illumina systems. It requires a Bio-Rad ddSEQ Single-Cell Isolator and the Illumina® Bio-Rad® SureCell™ WTA 3′Library Prep Kit. Each run on the ddSSEQ system can result on 1200 single nuclei sequenced. We recommend to read the detailed protocol (Document # 1000000044178 v00, from the Bio-Rad website) before starting the experiments. Here we show the main steps and some valuable tips that should be considered. Alternative sequencing strategies can also be found in other companies (10X genomics, for example). Always proceed immediately to the next step, unless indicated a safe stop point. Delays during sample preparation can reduce data quality (*see* **Note 25**).

1. Prepare the reverse transcription enzyme mix (cell suspend buffer, DTT, RNA stabilizer, RT Enzyme and Enhancer enzyme) in a 1.7μL tube on ice, then pipette up and down 20 times and spin the solution (*see* **Note 26**).

2. Add the sorted nuclei (up to 12,000 nuclei) and keep it on ice (*see* **Note 27**).

3. In another tube, vortex and spin the Barcode buffer and 3′ Barcode mix, then prepare the Barcode mix suspension on ice.

4. In order to coencapsulate each nucleus with a unique barcode inside the droplets use the ddSEQ Single-Cell Isolator.

5. Insert the cartridge into the cartridge holder and prime the fluidics station with ddSEQ Priming Solution (*see* **Note 28**).

6. Vortex the Barcode mix suspension and homogenize the Nuclei mix suspension by pipetting (*see* **Note 29**).

7. Load the samples, barcodes and encapsulation oil in the ddSEQ cartridge and then insert the cartridge in the ddSEQ Single-Cell Isolator. The encapsulation starts automatically and takes approximately 5 min.

8. Transfer slowly the emulsion to a prechilled 96 well plate and seal the wells with an 8-tube strip cap (*see* **Note 30**).

9. Transfer the plate to a thermocycler and run the reverse transcription program (37 °C for 30 min/50 °C for 1 h/85 °C for 5 min).

10. Break the droplets adding slowly the droplet disruptor reagent, followed by adding DNase- and RNase-free water. Do not mix the aqueous and the oil layers.

11. Clean up the cDNA libraries by vortexing the magnetic beads and dispensing it into the upper aqueous layer, without mixing.

12. Homogenize carefully the upper phase without disturbing the oil layer in the bottom.

13. Place the plate on a magnetic rack.

14. After the beads attach to the tube wall, remove the supernatant and wash twice with freshly prepared 80% ethanol.

15. Seal the plate, spin down, place the plate on a magnetic rack and remove any residual ethanol.

16. Then, also using the magnetic rack, elute the samples with resuspension buffer and transfer the volume to a new plate.

17. To remove the RNA template and synthesizes a double stranded cDNA perform the reaction by combining the Second Strand Buffer and the Second Strand Enzyme in a 1.5 mL tube.

18. Add the mix into the wells, turn off the thermocycler heated lid function and run the program (16 °C for 2 h) (*see* **Note 31**).

19. After the second strand cDNA synthesis wash the samples in a similar way as the **steps 11–14** and separate a 10μL aliquot from each sample to check the library quality using a Bioanalyzer instrument. cDNA should yield more than 2 ng (400–8000 bp range). If the library construction has good quality, proceed to the tagmentation, which is a process that fragment and tag DNA with adapter sequences in a single step. These adapters are required for cluster generation during the analysis.

20. Prepare the Tagmentation Mix (Tagment Buffer and Tagment Enzyme) on ice, add it to the samples and incubate the plate at 55 °C for 5 min.

21. Immediately stop the reaction using the Tagment Stop Buffer and leave samples at room temperature for 5 min.

22. Then, add separately the DNA Adapters (a different index for each sample), Tagmentation PCR Mix and Tagment PCR Adapter and load the reaction on the thermocycler (95 °C for 30 s/15 cycles of 95 °C for 10 s 60 °C for 45 s 72 °C for 1 min/72 °C for 5 min).

23. Finally, wash twice the samples in a similar way as the **steps 11–14**.

24. Separate 1μL to assess the library quality on a Bioanalyzer instrument (typical libraries are 300–1000 bp long) and prepare the samples for sequencing according to the instrument to be used.

**Table 1**
**Algorithms to process scRNA-seq or snRNA-seq experiments**

| Algorithm | Function |
|---|---|
| Seurat<br>Scrublet | Quality check |
| HISAT2<br>STAR | Sequencing reads alignment |
| Cufflinks<br>Scripture<br>StringTie<br>Scallop | Transcript structure identification |
| CD-HIT | Redundancy reduction |
| TransDecoder<br>CPC | Identification of coding potential |
| RNAMMER | Identification of specific RNAs |
| Blast | Searching for specific categories of RNAs |
| Htseq-count<br>RSEM<br>Alevin | Transcript expression |

**3.3 Bioinformatic Analyses of Single-Cell or -Nucleus RNAseq**

The first step of the bioinformatic analysis consists in checking the quality of the sequenced reads to identify technical artifacts, including: low cell capture rates, low UMI counts per cell and mitochondrial contamination by dying cells. The Seurat software [24] is a very popular choice for implementing these filtering steps. In general, we should require at a minimum 500 distinct UMIs per cell; values between 500 and 1000, though, might suggest performing a deeper sequencing of the samples. Scrublet [25], then, is a pipeline specifically developed to identify multiplet artifacts, that is those cases in which two or more cells receive the same barcode and risk confounding downstream analyses with their hybrid transcriptome.

Reads satisfying all quality checks are aligned against the reference genome using a software specifically designed to discover de novo splice junctions such as HISAT2 [26] or STAR [27].

Individual mapping signals are clustered by genome position and summarized with the help of assemblers (such as Cufflinks [28], Scripture [29], StringTie [30] or Scallop [31]) to infer transcript structures. This likely represents the most challenging step of the entire analysis, as transcriptome assembly is negatively affected by many factors, including the ubiquity of paralogs, unevenness of read coverage and diversity of splice variants. We suggest adopting a conservative strategy, that is to focus exclusively on those transcripts that have been identified in at least two samples, or which were defined independently by two separate assemblers [32]. Moreover, single-exon transcripts and those shorter than 200 nt are usually discarded. Finally, the CD-HIT algorithm [33] is useful to further reduce redundancy: it efficiently clusters transcripts by their similarity and identifies a representative sequence for each group.

The reconstruction procedure does not discriminate between protein-coding and noncoding RNAs. If we intend to separate them into two groups, we need an appropriate annotation strategy. As a first step, we employ a program for predicting the coding potential of our newly identified sequences, such as TransDecoder (part of the Trinity platform; [34]) or the Coding Potential Calculator (CPC; [35]). Both tools evaluate the length and integrity of potential open reading frames (ORFs), and the homology with known proteins and annotated domains. Specific classes of RNAs, such as the abundant ribosomal RNAs, can be identified directly with tailored tools such as RNAMMER [36]. Lastly, annotation efforts such as RNACentral [37] provide multispecies catalogs of known noncoding RNAs which can be used as a starting point for BLAST searches.

To evaluate the level of expression of lncRNAs in different samples and conditions we have two options. We could use the same alignments computed earlier to inform transcriptome assemblers. In such a case, we would simply tally all the reads falling within each transcript body using a tool like htseq-count [38]. While this strategy is computationally cheap, it is easily confounded by multimapping reads, that is, reads that have high-scoring matches to multiple *loci* of the reference genome. Model-based approaches such as RSEM [39] or Alevin [40] explicitly track multiple alignments in a probabilistic framework and have been shown to provide more accurate estimates at a modest increase in computational times. In the Table 1 is summarized the list of algorithms cited in this paragraph that are useful for the bioinformatic processing of scRNA-seq or snRNA-seq experiments.

# 4    Notes

1. We used CD1 mouse strain.

2. IMPORTANT: use a retrotranscriptase with a terminal transferase activity. Retrotranscriptases used are MMLV (e.g., Superscript II; Thermofisher Scientific). The terminal transferase activity is important to allow the addition of three cytosines when cDNA synthesis reach 5′ end of the RNA. The three cytosines allow the binding of the SMART primer to them. Retrotranscriptase do a template switch to synthesize a sequence complementary to the SMART primer linked to the cDNA. With this method the cDNA has a tag in the 3′ (the

SMART primer) and in the 5′ (the oligo-dT-Ion P1 Adaptor primer) ends.

3. Prepare all solutions using ultrapure water (DNase and RNase free) and analytical grade reagents. Stock solutions can be prepared and stored at room temperature. When needed, measure the pH using a pH meter. We recommend using freshly prepared buffers.

4. We used EDL and soleus muscles from the hindlimb of 3 months old CD1 mice. Make sure to minimize the mechanical stress on the myofibers by handling muscles by the tendons.

5. Do not wait for more than 30 min after the muscles have been collected to avoid to alter RNA abundance.

6. Make sure to handle the muscle with care and check at the microscope that there is no loss of myofibers during these washing steps.

7. To proceed with RNA purification, it is better to avoid working with too many myofibers. We usually work with 4–6 myofibers per time.

8. Retain the eluate and process as described in Subheading 3.1.4 if you are interested in miRNA components. The binding of the RNA to the column depends on the ethanol concentration in the solution and on the length of the RNA. With a low ethanol concentration long RNAs bind to the column; increasing the ethanol concentration in the flow thorough and passing the solution through a new column, miRNAs (short RNAs) can bind to the column.

9. It is better to avoid leaving the filter to dry. The best choice is to finish to purify lncRNAs and then, if also interested to miRNAs, to follow purification steps for the eluate containing miRNAs.

10. Eventually, store the eluate at −80 °C in the eluted volume.

11. It is better to control the volume during its reduction to avoid drying the sample.

12. If you dry the solution, resuspend miRNAs in nuclease-free water and preferably use LoBind tubes for the SpeedVac step.

13. This step is not required if working with already polyadenylated RNA molecules (lncRNAs, mRNAs).

14. The retrotranscription reaction can be performed directly with purified long RNAs purified with the columns (*see* Subheading 3.1.3). In this RNA fraction long noncoding RNAs are present and can be retrotranscribed if they are polyadenylated. Using oligo-d(T) as starting primer of the retrotranscription only polyadenylated RNAs can be retrotranscribed.

15. This step is very important for long RNAs. In fact long RNAs can assume 2D structures that prevent their complete retrotranscription.

16. It was suggested to perform 10 cycles of PCR amplification to avoid reaching the plateau and lose the expression differences among transcripts. We use the following PCR cycle: 95 °C for 2 min; 10 cycles (95 °C for 25 s; 53 °C for 25 s; 72 °C for 90 s); 72 °C for 3 min; 4 °C infinite.

17. We use the following PCR cycle: 95 °C for 2 min; number of cycles to be determined experimentally (95 °C for 25 s; 62 °C for 25 s; 72 °C for 90 s); 72 °C for 3 min; 4 °C infinite.

18. To purify PCR amplicons from unincorporated primers and change the buffer you can use any kit used for this purpose. It is important to check that membranes used in the kit for the PCR purification allow the retention of the PCR amplicons discarding unincorporated primers.

19. E-Gel Power Snap Electrophoresis Device is able to run electrophoresis run with E-Gel™ SizeSelect™ II Agarose Gels. These are precast gels with two arrays of wells: the upper one for the samples loading and the lower one for the sample collection. The specific device allows to monitor continuously the electrophoresis run and therefore stop it when the desired band reached the recovery well. It is important to fill all wells with the same liquid volume to avoid differences in the electric field. The only well that can be loaded with a smallest volume is the one for the ladder. Moreover, usually external wells are not used because of having the most homogeneous electric field for all the samples run. Finally, to avoid sample contamination, if no different sequencing barcodes are used for the different samples, it is suggested not to run samples using adjacent wells.

20. Delays during nuclei preparation and handling can lead to sample failure. Make sure that you have all required consumables before you begin and keep samples and buffers on ice. Do not stop during or between steps.

21. It is important to coat the tubes to avoid nuclei to attach to the plastic.

22. Inspect the supernatant to check on the microscope for the presence of high amount of intact myofibers. If many myofibers are present in the supernatant repeat the **step 2**.

23. Chill a cell filter on ice for at least 5 min.

24. Cell strainer should allow the pass through of nuclei avoiding the contamination with cell debris.

25. Here it is described the Bio-Rad protocol for snRNAseq that can be adapted also for the scRNA-seq using the same instruments and solutions. In both cases it is important to work with

intact cells or nuclei (cell viability >95% or for nuclei <5%). If samples for nuclei analysis have a cell viability higher than 5% it means that cells are intact and therefore nuclei are not extracted from the cells. Dead or damaged cells/nuclei can release nucleic acids into the cell suspension buffer. This background signal from remains through subsequent steps and may impact the quality of the resulting analysis.

26. This enzyme mix can be used for up to 4 samples or replicates of the same sample that can be loaded in the 4 chambers of the cartridge. All chambers must be loaded.

27. Accurate nuclei and cell count is critical to achieve target nuclei throughput and to avoid multiplets. Size-based gating for automated counters or manual count may be required to avoid counting cell debris. Nuclei are typically counted on automated cell counters as dead (nonviable) cells due to their small diameter and should make up >95% of the final loaded sample (viability should be <5%). Both viable and nonviable cells should be included in total cell count. Nuclei are smaller than whole cells and are counted by automated cell counters as nonviable cells. If using an automatic cell counter, use the nonviable count to estimate the fraction of nuclei versus intact cells.

28. Take care to remove completely the ddSEQ Priming Solution because this solution can interfere with results.

29. It is important to avoid nuclei membrane ruptures. Pipet slowly and if possible use wide-bore tips.

30. Avoid disrupting the emulsion. Do not use plastic seals because it can generate static and interfere with the sample quality.

31. It is possible to store this reaction at −20 °C for up to 2 days.

## References

1. Bunch H, Lawney BP, Burkholder A, Ma D, Zheng X, Motola S, Fargo DC, Levine SS, Wang YE, Hu G (2016) RNA polymerase II promoter-proximal pausing in mammalian long non-coding genes. Genomics 108 (2):64–77. https://doi.org/10.1016/j.ygeno.2016.07.003

2. Fico A, Fiorenzano A, Pascale E, Patriarca EJ, Minchiotti G (2019) Long non-coding RNA in stem cell pluripotency and lineage commitment: functions and evolutionary conservation. Cell Mol Life Sci 76(8):1459–1471. https://doi.org/10.1007/s00018-018-3000-z

3. Chen J, Wang Y, Wang C, Hu JF, Li W (2020) LncRNA functions as a new emerging epigenetic factor in determining the fate of stem cells. Front Genet 11:277. https://doi.org/10.3389/fgene.2020.00277

4. Nobili L, Lionetti M, Neri A (2016) Long non-coding RNAs in normal and malignant hematopoiesis. Oncotarget 7 (31):50666–50681. https://doi.org/10.18632/oncotarget.9308

5. Nie JH, Li TX, Zhang XQ, Liu J (2019) Roles of non-coding RNAs in Normal human brain development, brain tumor, and neuropsychiatric disorders. Noncoding RNA 5(2):36. https://doi.org/10.3390/ncrna5020036

6. Alessio E, Buson L, Chemello F, Peggion C, Grespi F, Martini P, Massimino ML, Pacchioni B, Millino C, Romualdi C, Bertoli A, Scorrano L, Lanfranchi G, Cagnin S (2019) Single cell analysis reveals the

involvement of the long non-coding RNA Pvt1 in the modulation of muscle atrophy and mitochondrial network. Nucleic Acids Res 47 (4):1653–1670. https://doi.org/10.1093/nar/gkz007

7. Fang Y, Fullwood MJ (2016) Roles, functions, and mechanisms of long non-coding RNAs in cancer. Genomics Proteomics Bioinformatics 14(1):42–54. https://doi.org/10.1016/j.gpb.2015.09.006

8. Jiang MC, Ni JJ, Cui WY, Wang BY, Zhuo W (2019) Emerging roles of lncRNA in cancer and therapeutic opportunities. Am J Cancer Res 9(7):1354–1366

9. Martini P, Paracchini L, Caratti G, Mello-Grand M, Fruscio R, Beltrame L, Calura E, Sales G, Ravaggi A, Bignotti E, Odicino FE, Sartori E, Perego P, Katsaros D, Craparotta I, Chiorino G, Cagnin S, Mannarino L, Ceppi L, Mangioni C, Ghimenti C, D'Incalci M, Marchini S, Romualdi C (2017) lncRNAs as novel indicators of Patients' prognosis in stage I epithelial ovarian cancer: a retrospective and multicentric study. Clin Cancer Res 23 (9):2356–2366. https://doi.org/10.1158/1078-0432.CCR-16-1402

10. Arndt CA, Crist WM (1999) Common musculoskeletal tumors of childhood and adolescence. N Engl J Med 341(5):342–352. https://doi.org/10.1056/NEJM199907293410507

11. Qualman SJ, Coffin CM, Newton WA, Hojo H, Triche TJ, Parham DM, Crist WM (1998) Intergroup rhabdomyosarcoma study: update for pathologists. Pediatr Dev Pathol 1 (6):550–561. https://doi.org/10.1007/s100249900076

12. Davis RJ, D'Cruz CM, Lovell MA, Biegel JA, Barr FG (1994) Fusion of PAX7 to FKHR by the variant t(1;13)(p36;q14) translocation in alveolar rhabdomyosarcoma. Cancer Res 54 (11):2869–2872

13. Barr FG, Galili N, Holick J, Biegel JA, Rovera G, Emanuel BS (1993) Rearrangement of the PAX3 paired box gene in the paediatric solid tumour alveolar rhabdomyosarcoma. Nat Genet 3(2):113–117. https://doi.org/10.1038/ng0293-113

14. Buckingham M, Relaix F (2007) The role of Pax genes in the development of tissues and organs: Pax3 and Pax7 regulate muscle progenitor cell functions. Annu Rev Cell Dev Biol 23:645–673. https://doi.org/10.1146/annurev.cellbio.23.090506.123438

15. Schiaffino S, Reggiani C (2011) Fiber types in mammalian skeletal muscles. Physiol Rev 91 (4):1447–1531. https://doi.org/10.1152/physrev.00031.2010

16. Blackburn DM, Lazure F, Corchado AH, Perkins TJ, Najafabadi HS, Soleimani VD (2019) High-resolution genome-wide expression analysis of single myofibers using SMART-Seq. J Biol Chem 294(52):20097–20108. https://doi.org/10.1074/jbc.RA119.011506

17. Chemello F, Grespi F, Zulian A, Cancellara P, Hebert-Chatelain E, Martini P, Bean C, Alessio E, Buson L, Bazzega M, Armani A, Sandri M, Ferrazza R, Laveder P, Guella G, Reggiani C, Romualdi C, Bernardi P, Scorrano L, Cagnin S, Lanfranchi G (2019) Transcriptomic analysis of single isolated Myofibers identifies miR-27a-3p and miR-142-3p as regulators of metabolism in skeletal muscle. Cell Rep 26(13):3784–3797. e3788. https://doi.org/10.1016/j.celrep.2019.02.105

18. Chemello F, Alessio E, Buson L, Pacchioni B, Millino C, Lanfranchi G, Cagnin S (2019) Isolation and transcriptomic profiling of single Myofibers from mice. Bio-Protocol 9(19): e3378. https://doi.org/10.21769/BioProtoc.3378

19. Biscontin A, Casara S, Cagnin S, Tombolan L, Rosolen A, Lanfranchi G, De Pitta C (2010) New miRNA labeling method for bead-based quantification. BMC Mol Biol 11:44. https://doi.org/10.1186/1471-2199-11-44

20. Alessio E, Bonadio RS, Buson L, Chemello F, Cagnin S (2020) A single cell but many different transcripts: a journey into the world of long non-coding RNAs. Int J Mol Sci 21(1):302. https://doi.org/10.3390/ijms21010302

21. Hwang B, Lee JH, Bang D (2018) Single-cell RNA sequencing technologies and bioinformatics pipelines. Exp Mol Med 50(8):96. https://doi.org/10.1038/s12276-018-0071-8

22. Bakken TE, Hodge RD, Miller JA, Yao Z, Nguyen TN, Aevermann B, Barkan E, Bertagnolli D, Casper T, Dee N, Garren E, Goldy J, Graybuck LT, Kroll M, Lasken RS, Lathia K, Parry S, Rimorin C, Scheuermann RH, Schork NJ, Shehata SI, Tieu M, Phillips JW, Bernard A, Smith KA, Zeng H, Lein ES, Tasic B (2018) Single-nucleus and single-cell transcriptomes compared in matched cortical cell types. PLoS One 13(12):e0209648. https://doi.org/10.1371/journal.pone.0209648

23. Selewa A, Dohn R, Eckart H, Lozano S, Xie B, Gauchat E, Elorbany R, Rhodes K, Burnett J, Gilad Y, Pott S, Basu A (2020) Systematic comparison of high-throughput single-cell and single-nucleus transcriptomes during cardiomyocyte differentiation. Sci Rep 10 (1):1535. https://doi.org/10.1038/s41598-020-58327-6

24. Stuart T, Butler A, Hoffman P, Hafemeister C, Papalexi E, Mauck WM 3rd, Hao Y, Stoeckius M, Smibert P, Satija R (2019) Comprehensive integration of single-cell data. Cell 177(7):1888–1902. e1821. https://doi.org/10.1016/j.cell.2019.05.031

25. Wolock SL, Lopez R, Klein AM (2019) Scrublet: computational identification of cell doublets in single-cell transcriptomic data. Cell Syst 8(4):281–291. e289. https://doi.org/10.1016/j.cels.2018.11.005

26. Kim D, Langmead B, Salzberg SL (2015) HISAT: a fast spliced aligner with low memory requirements. Nat Methods 12(4):357–360. https://doi.org/10.1038/nmeth.3317

27. Dobin A, Davis CA, Schlesinger F, Drenkow J, Zaleski C, Jha S, Batut P, Chaisson M, Gingeras TR (2013) STAR: ultrafast universal RNA-seq aligner. Bioinformatics 29(1):15–21. https://doi.org/10.1093/bioinformatics/bts635

28. Trapnell C, Roberts A, Goff L, Pertea G, Kim D, Kelley DR, Pimentel H, Salzberg SL, Rinn JL, Pachter L (2012) Differential gene and transcript expression analysis of RNA-seq experiments with TopHat and cufflinks. Nat Protoc 7(3):562–578. https://doi.org/10.1038/nprot.2012.016

29. Guttman M, Garber M, Levin JZ, Donaghey J, Robinson J, Adiconis X, Fan L, Koziol MJ, Gnirke A, Nusbaum C, Rinn JL, Lander ES, Regev A (2010) Ab initio reconstruction of cell type-specific transcriptomes in mouse reveals the conserved multi-exonic structure of lincRNAs. Nat Biotechnol 28(5):503–510. https://doi.org/10.1038/nbt.1633

30. Pertea M, Pertea GM, Antonescu CM, Chang TC, Mendell JT, Salzberg SL (2015) StringTie enables improved reconstruction of a transcriptome from RNA-seq reads. Nat Biotechnol 33(3):290–295. https://doi.org/10.1038/nbt.3122

31. Shao M, Kingsford C (2017) Accurate assembly of transcripts through phase-preserving graph decomposition. Nat Biotechnol 35(12):1167–1169. https://doi.org/10.1038/nbt.4020

32. Cabili MN, Trapnell C, Goff L, Koziol M, Tazon-Vega B, Regev A, Rinn JL (2011) Integrative annotation of human large intergenic noncoding RNAs reveals global properties and specific subclasses. Genes Dev 25 (18):1915–1927. https://doi.org/10.1101/gad.17446611

33. Fu L, Niu B, Zhu Z, Wu S, Li W (2012) CD-HIT: accelerated for clustering the next-generation sequencing data. Bioinformatics 28 (23):3150–3152. https://doi.org/10.1093/bioinformatics/bts565

34. Haas BJ, Papanicolaou A, Yassour M, Grabherr M, Blood PD, Bowden J, Couger MB, Eccles D, Li B, Lieber M, MacManes MD, Ott M, Orvis J, Pochet N, Strozzi F, Weeks N, Westerman R, William T, Dewey CN, Henschel R, LeDuc RD, Friedman N, Regev A (2013) De novo transcript sequence reconstruction from RNA-seq using the trinity platform for reference generation and analysis. Nat Protoc 8(8):1494–1512. https://doi.org/10.1038/nprot.2013.084

35. Kong L, Zhang Y, Ye ZQ, Liu XQ, Zhao SQ, Wei L, Gao G (2007) CPC: assess the protein-coding potential of transcripts using sequence features and support vector machine. Nucleic Acids Res 35(Web Server issue):W345–W349. https://doi.org/10.1093/nar/gkm391

36. Lagesen K, Hallin P, Rodland EA, Staerfeldt HH, Rognes T, Ussery DW (2007) RNAmmer: consistent and rapid annotation of ribosomal RNA genes. Nucleic Acids Res 35 (9):3100–3108. https://doi.org/10.1093/nar/gkm160

37. The RNAcentral Consortium (2019) RNAcentral: a hub of information for non-coding RNA sequences. Nucleic Acids Res 47(D1): D221–D229. https://doi.org/10.1093/nar/gky1034

38. Anders S, Pyl PT, Huber W (2015) HTSeq--a python framework to work with high-throughput sequencing data. Bioinformatics 31(2):166–169. https://doi.org/10.1093/bioinformatics/btu638

39. Li B, Dewey CN (2011) RSEM: accurate transcript quantification from RNA-Seq data with or without a reference genome. BMC Bioinformatics 12:323. https://doi.org/10.1186/1471-2105-12-323

40. Srivastava A, Malik L, Smith T, Sudbery I, Patro R (2019) Alevin efficiently estimates accurate gene abundances from dscRNA-seq data. Genome Biol 20(1):65. https://doi.org/10.1186/s13059-019-1670-y

# Part III

## Validation of Identified LncRNAs

# Chapter 6

## Measuring lncRNA Expression by Real-Time PCR

### Sonam Dhamija and Manoj B. Menon

### Abstract

Long noncoding RNAs are defined as transcripts longer than 200 nt with no protein coding potential. Most lncRNAs are expressed in a tissue-specific manner and barring a few, their absolute expression is lower compared to most coding transcripts. Differential expression studies have contributed the most to the functional characterisation of the lncRNAs we know. Sensitive and specific quantification of lncRNA expression is crucial for such studies. SYBR Green dye based real time quantitative PCR is a simple and affordable method of quantitative PCR, wherein the specific binding of the dye to double stranded DNA amplicon emits fluorescence proportionate to the amount of PCR products. Here we describe a detailed protocol for successful lncRNA quantitation by reverse transcription followed by SYBR Green chemistry-based real-time PCR.

Key words Real-time PCR, lncRNA, Quantitative RT-PCR, SYBR Green, lncRNA expression

## 1 Introduction

Long noncoding RNAs (lncRNAs) are transcripts of >200 nt in length that do not encode for proteins. The advancements in high-throughput techniques in the last decade established that the genome is pervasively transcribed [1–5] and led to the discovery of not only long noncoding RNA genes but also noncoding iso-forms of the protein-coding genes [6]. Although most annotated lncRNAs are transcribed by RNA polymerase II and undergo post-transcriptional processing including 5′ capping, pre-mRNA splicing and 3′ polyadenylation [7, 8], a significant proportion of lncRNAs lack poly(A) tail [9–11] and alternative 5′ and 3′ topologies are known for few of them [12–15]. Based on the proximity of lncRNAs to the protein-coding genes, lncRNAs are classified into intergenic and intragenic. Long intergenic noncoding RNAs or lincRNAs do not overlap with any other gene, while intragenic lncRNAs completely or partially overlap with the exons or introns or both of protein-coding genes and are further classified into sense or antisense based on their orientation. In addition, bidirectional

Alfons Navarro (ed.), *Long Non-Coding RNAs in Cancer*, Methods in Molecular Biology, vol. 2348,
https://doi.org/10.1007/978-1-0716-1581-2_6, © Springer Science+Business Media, LLC, part of Springer Nature 2021

lncRNAs are those transcripts which are initiated in antisense orientation <1000 bp away from the transcriptional start site (TSS) of a protein-coding gene. These include lncRNAs overlapping with promoter regions of protein-coding genes as well as those that are divergently transcribed from the same promoter as the nearby protein-coding gene [4, 16](*see* Chapter 1).

It was established in the early phase of lncRNAs discovery that a large proportion of these transcripts are expressed at very low levels and are expressed in a cell and tissue specific manner [4, 17–19]. Moreover, it is challenging to functionally characterize lncRNAs compared to protein-coding transcripts. Most studies rely on differential expression of lncRNAs identified in a phenotypic screen, for example by microarrays or next-generation RNA sequencing [20, 21] and expression of several lncRNAs detectable in blood/urine/saliva have been shown to be of clinical relevance as diagnostic or prognostic markers [22, 23]. Therefore, it is very important to validate the expression of even the low-expressed lncRNAs identified from high-throughput data quantitatively and in a reliable way.

Quantitative real time PCR (qPCR) is considered to be the gold standard for the specific quantitation of candidate target gene expression due to simplicity and sensitivity of the technique [24]. The total RNA is extracted from the cells of interest and converted to complementary DNA (cDNA) in a reaction using reverse transcriptase and oligo-(dT) or random hexamer primer. For lncRNA transcripts, it is imperative to use random hexamer as many of them lack poly(A) tail [12]. Moreover, for lncRNA genes overlapping with other protein coding genes (e.g., antisense lncRNAs), it is advisable to use transcript specific antisense primers for reverse transcription. Quantitative real time PCR can be performed using two broad classes of chemistries. One approach depends on DNA binding fluorescent dyes like SYBR Green, a DNA minor-groove binding dye which emits strong fluorescence upon binding to double-stranded DNA (dsDNA) [25, 24]. The signals are proportionate to the amount of dsDNA present in the reaction, thus aiding in real time monitoring of PCR amplification. Alternatively, specific probe sequences labelled with a reporter and quencher dye can be used to detect the amplified products. The most commonly used probe chemistry involves the use of a Taqman probe, wherein each PCR cycle leads to the cleavage of the probe, separating quencher from the reporter dye, accumulating fluorescence signals proportionate to the number of PCR cycles. The output data generated by both probe-free and probe-based real-time PCR assays are typically represented in the form of $C_t$ (threshold cycle) value, which corresponds to the number of PCR cycles required by a particular sample to reach an arbitrary predefined threshold of fluorescence. The threshold is set in the exponential phase of PCR amplification and relative copy numbers of the template transcripts/cDNA can be calculated from the $C_t$ values using comparative CT method [26].

While SYBR Green and probe-based chemistries can achieve similar levels of sensitivities, the SYBR Green based assays require additional steps to ensure specificity. Inherently, SYBR Green chemistry is more prone to primer based nonspecificity problems as the dye binds to any double-stranded DNA in the PCR mixture, independent of whether it is the specific gene amplification product or not. The probe-based chemistries do not have this problem as the emission of fluorescence is coupled with probe-binding to the specific target DNA. While performing real-time PCR assays using SYBR Green or its alternatives, the specificity of the PCR is usually verified by a process termed as melt-curve analysis [27]. This involves slow heating of the post-PCR reaction with continuous measurement of fluorescence, usually between 65 °C and 95 °C. Upon heating, the dsDNA undergoes denaturation or melting giving rise to separate single strands. The temperature of melting ($T_m$) is defined as the temperature at which 50% of the dsDNA is converted to single strands and can be used as a signature for a specific PCR product, determined by the length and G/C content of the amplicon. As SYBR Green binding and emission of fluorescence is dependent on the presence of dsDNA, denaturation/melting can be tracked by monitoring the loss of green fluorescence and $T_m$ values can be easily determined. SYBR Green PCR followed by melt-curve analysis and $T_m$ determination is an affordable and reliable method for specific quantification of lncRNAs.

In this chapter, we will describe the steps involved in obtaining specific quantitation of long noncoding RNA expression from cell lines using SYBR Green based fluorescence detection. The successful quantitation of specific target transcripts requires accurate execution of several steps which precede the actual amplification step including primer design, RNA isolation, and reverse transcription. Basic procedures for these steps will be described in this chapter.

## 2 Materials

### 2.1 General Equipment and Facilities

1. Cell culture facility with biosafety cabinet and incubator at 37 °C with 5% $CO_2$.

2. General materials required for culturing cells (e.g., pipette boy, pipettes, flasks, and dishes), appropriate base medium with supplements depending on the cell-type, trypsin–EDTA, and phosphate buffered saline (PBS).

3. 1.5, 15, and 50 ml centrifuge tubes.

4. Tube racks and common instruments (e.g., vortex, centrifuge, dry bath, freezers) are required at different steps of the procedure.

| | |
|---|---|
| ***2.2 Primer Design*** | 1. Computer with Internet access. |

***2.3 RNA Isolation***

1. Clean RNase-free microcentrifuge tubes.

2. RNase-free 15 ml/50 ml centrifuge tubes.

3. Centrifuge with cooled microtube rotor.

4. TRI reagent (Merck).

5. Plate rocker.

6. Vortexer.

7. Chloroform.

8. Isopropanol.

9. Ethanol.

10. Nuclease-free water or DEPC-treated water.

11. DNase I and 10× incubation buffer (Roche).

12. Phenol–chloroform–isoamyl alcohol (25:24:1, pH 4.5–5).

13. Sodium acetate.

14. 10 mg/ml glycogen: Dissolve 0.1 g of glycogen in 10 ml of RNase-free water and prepare 1 ml aliquots and store in −20 °C freezer.

15. Spectrophotometer (e.g., Nanodrop™ 2000 from Thermo-Fisher Scientific).

16. Agarose.

17. 1× TBE buffer: 0.89 M Tris base, 0.89 M boric acid, 0.02 M EDTA pH 8. Weigh 108 g of Tris base and 55 g of boric acid and dissolve in 900 ml of distilled water. Add 40 ml of 0.5 M EDTA (pH 8) to it and make up to 1000 ml. Autoclave and store at RT. This constitutes 10× TBE. Dilute to 1× TBE using ultrapure water and use.

18. Agarose gel electrophoresis equipment.

19. Ethidium bromide or alternative dyes.

20. DNA loading dye.

21. UV Transilluminator.

***2.4 Reverse Transcription***

1. Random hexamer primer.

2. Gene-specific reverse primer.

3. Deoxyribonucleotides triphosphate.

4. RevertAid® reverse transcriptase (ThermoFisher Scientific).

5. Reverse transcriptase buffer (ThermoFisher Scientific).

6. RiboLock RNase inhibitor (ThermoFisher Scientific).

7. Thermocycler.

8. Nuclease-free water or DEPC-treated water.

| | |
|---|---|
| **2.5  Real-Time PCR Setup, Cycling, and Data Analysis** | 1. Forward and reverse primers. |
| | 2. SYBR Green master mix (e.g., Power SYBR Green master mix from ThermoFisher Scientific). |
| | 3. cDNA. |
| | 4. Nuclease-free water. |
| | 5. Stepper pipette. |
| | 6. Optical 96-wells PCR plate. |
| | 7. qPCR plate sealers. |
| | 8. qPCR thermocycler (e.g., StepOnePlus™ from ThermoFisher Scientific). |
| | 9. 96-well plate centrifuge. |

# 3  Methods

**3.1  Primer Design**

1. Retrieve full length sequence of the candidate lncRNA from the Nucleotide or Gene database in NCBI by providing the accession number or Gene name or Gene ID in the search box (https://www.ncbi.nlm.nih.gov/gene/) (*see* **Notes 1** and **2**).

2. In case of sense or antisense lncRNAs that overlap with protein-coding transcripts or noncoding splice-variants from protein coding genes, locate the sequence regions unique to lncRNAs of interest. This can be done either by simply viewing the genomic organization of the lncRNA–mRNA pair (e.g., when there are one or more exons unique to the lncRNA) or by aligning the sequences of the lncRNA of interest and the overlapping transcripts (e.g., in cases where only short stretches of unique sequences are present) (*see* **Note 2**).

3. Copy the complete transcript sequence or specific unique regions in plain or FASTA format and paste in Primer 3 web-server (http://bioinfo.ut.ee/primer3/) for primer design [28, 29] (*see* **Note 3**).

4. Set the following optimal parameters for real-time PCR primer design:
   (a) Product size range: 70–200. It is preferable to stay below 150 for efficient amplification.
   (b) Primer size: Minimum: 20, Optimal: 22, Maximum: 27.
   (c) Primer Tm: Minimum: 59, Optimal: 60, Maximum: 61.

5. Primer 3 output (*see* **Note 4**) is ranked for optimal performance in PCR and compatibility between primer pairs. In addition to the automated scoring by the software, select the candidate primer pairs based on the following parameters:

   (a) Select an intron-spanning primer pair or optimally an exon–exon junction spanning primer. This needs to be verified manually (*see* **Notes 5** and **6**).

   (b) Primer pairs with a G or C residue at the 3′ end, 40–60% GC content, and no self-complementarity are preferable.

   (c) Avoid nucleotide repeats in the primer sequences.

6. Analyze primers for cross-hybridization with other genes by using NCBI primer blast at https://www.ncbi.nlm.nih.gov/tools/primer-blast. A mismatch of ≥50% to other genes is acceptable (*see* **Note 7**).

**A**

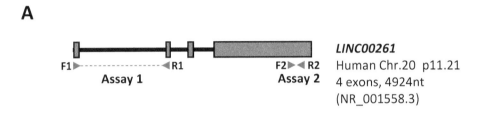

**B**

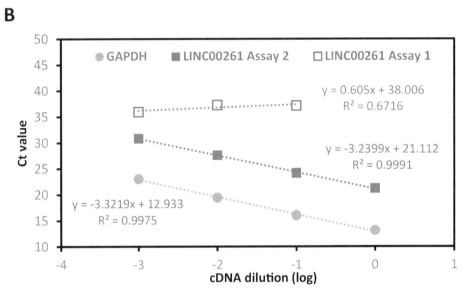

**Fig. 1** Design and efficiency analysis of primer assays for SYBR Green based lncRNA quantitation. (**a**) Genomic organization of a candidate human lncRNA (*LINC00261*) showing the four exons and localization of the two primer sets (Assay 1 and 2). Assay 1 amplicon covers 30–161 nt positions (intron-spanning) and Assay 2 amplicon covers 2943–3063 nt positions of the 4924 nt long lncRNA transcript. (**b**) The two primer assays for *LINC00261* and the control *GAPDH* mRNA primer sets were used in SYBR Green based real-time qPCR with 10-fold dilutions of human cell cDNA and $C_t$ values were plotted. While Assay 1 showed very high $C_t$ values with no dose-response, Assay 2 gave PCR efficiencies (slope $= -3.2399$, calculated PCR efficiency $= 103.5\%$) comparable to that of GAPDH (slope $= -3.3219$, calculated PCR efficiency $= 100\%$) and $R^2$ value close to the optimal value of 1

7. It is advisable to order more than 1 primer pair for a transcript and then experimentally verify for PCR efficiency and specificity with cDNA dilutions (*see* **Note 19**) (Fig. 1).

**3.2   RNA Isolation from Human Cell Lines Using TRI Reagent**

*3.2.1   Cell Lysis*

1. For adherent cells, depending on the experimental setup, ~40–100% confluent cell culture plates can be used for RNA isolation using TRI reagent (*see* **Notes 8** and **9**). Remove medium from a well or plate and wash with $1\times$ PBS. Remove the PBS completely. The recommended volumes of PBS are:
   (a)  2 ml PBS per well of a 6 well plate.
   (b)  5 ml PBS for 10 cm dish.
   (c)  10 ml PBS for 15 cm dish.

2. For suspension cells, pellet down the cells in a 15 ml centrifuge tube and discard the medium. Resuspend the pellet gently in $1\times$ PBS (5 ml buffer for ~$10^6$ cells), centrifuge and discard the supernatant.

3. Add TRI reagent to the plate or falcon under a fume-hood (*see* **Note 10**). 1 ml reagent per well is optimal for a 6 well plate, while 3–4 ml works well for 10 cm plates. For further scale-up and for suspension cells, 1 ml TRI reagent per million cells should be used.

4. Shake the dish cautiously at ~180 rpm on a plate rocker for 5–10 min. For falcon tubes, vortex for about 10–30 s until the cell pellet is suspended.

5. Transfer the cell lysate from a dish to a 1.5 ml centrifuge tube depending on the volume and vortex shortly.

6. At this stage, the lysates can be stored at $-20\,^\circ$C for short-term or $-80\,^\circ$C for long-term storage.

*3.2.2   RNA Precipitation and Extraction from 1 ml of TRI-Reagent Lysate*

1. Precool the centrifuge to 4 $^\circ$C and thaw frozen TRI reagent lysates at room temperature (RT).

2. **Hood**: Add 0.2 ml chloroform and shake vigorously for 30 s by placing the tubes in a closed microcentrifuge tubes rack and shaking in an up-and-down movement (do not vortex).

3. Leave the samples undisturbed for 2–3 min at RT and centrifuge the tubes at $12,000 \times g$ for 15–20 min at 4 $^\circ$C.

4. **Hood**: Carefully dispense the upper colorless aqueous phase to new labelled tubes, avoiding aspiration from the interphase or the organic phase.

5. Add 0.5 ml 2-propanol (IPA) to the collected upper phase and gently mix by inversion 3–4 times.

6. Incubate the samples at RT for 10 min or at $-20\,^\circ$C for 20 min for precipitation. At this stage, tubes can also be stored overnight at $-20\,^\circ$C.

7. Spin tubes at $12{,}000 \times g$ for 10 min at 4 °C.

8. Remove the supernatant completely by careful aspiration without touching the pellet (*see* **Note 11**).

9. Add 1 ml 70% ethanol to the tubes and spin at $8000 \times g$ for 5 min at 4 °C.

10. Carefully pipet the supernatant (using 1 ml tip) leaving ~50µl in the tube.

11. Spin once again at $8000 \times g$ for 1 min at 4 °C and carefully remove the remaining supernatant with a pipette (using 100µl tip).

12. Repeat the ethanol wash procedure (**steps 8–11**) twice (total three washes).

13. Preheat nuclease-free water to 65 °C for resuspension.

14. Air-dry the pellet for 5–10 min, ensuring complete removal of ethanol. Do not let the pellet to dry out completely (proceed to the next step once no droplets are visible).

15. Suspend the RNA pellet in 50µl of preheated nuclease-free water and leave on ice.

16. Determine the RNA concentration using a spectrophotometer (*see* **Note 12**).

*3.2.3 DNase Treatment, Reprecipitation, and Extraction (Optional, See **Note 13**)*

1. Precool 99% ethanol in −20 °C freezer.

2. For DNase treatment, set up the following components in a 50µl reaction: RNA (2–50µg), 10× incubation buffer—5µl, DNase-I (10 U/µl)—1µl, and water.

3. Incubate at 37 °C for 30 min in a dry-bath incubator.

4. Spin the tubes shortly to bring down the contents and add 150µl water to bring the total volume to 200µl.

5. **Hood**: Add 200µl phenol–chloroform–isoamyl alcohol (PCI, acid, pH 4–5) and shake the tubes for 15 s as in Subheading 3.2.2, **step 2**.

6. Leave the tubes undisturbed for 2 min after which centrifuge the tubes at $12{,}000 \times g$ for 2 min at RT.

7. **Hood**: Transfer the upper phase (~190µl) to a new labeled microcentrifuge tube and add 200µl chloroform to it.

8. Shake, incubate, and spin as in Subheading 3.2.3, **steps 5 and 6**.

9. **Hood**: transfer the upper phase (~170µl) to a new labeled tube.

10. Add one-tenth volume (~17µl) sodium acetate (3 M, pH 5), mix and add 1µl of 10 mg/ml glycogen if necessary (*see* **Note 14**).

11. Add 2.5 times volume (425µl) ice-cold 99% ethanol and gently mix by inverting the tubes 4–5 times.

12. Incubate the tube for at least 30–60 min at −80 °C or overnight at −20 °C for precipitation.

13. Pellet RNA by centrifugation at $16,000 \times g$ for 10 min at 4 °C and remove the supernatant.

14. Wash with 1 ml 70% ethanol twice following the **steps 9–11** from Subheading 3.2.2 for a total of two washes.

15. Air-dry the pellet for 5–10 min, ensuring complete removal of ethanol and suspend RNA in 20µl of prewarmed (65 °C) water.

16. Pipet up and down, vortex, and shortly spin at RT and leave on ice.

17. Determine RNA concentration as described previously.

*3.2.4  RNA Integrity Analysis*

1. Prepare 1% (1 g in 100 ml 1× TBE buffer) agarose gel. The volume of the gel depends on the number of samples and size of the casting tray; for example, for a medium sized-tray, weigh 0.5 g of agarose in a conical flask, add 50 ml of 1× TBE buffer to it and heat until the solution becomes clear.

2. Cool the solution to 60–70 °C, add 0.5 mg/l of ethidium bromide (*see* **Note 15**) and mix gently by swirling.

3. Pour the solution into the casting try and let it solidify for about 20–30 min.

4. Thaw the 6× DNA loading dye.

5. Take 500 ng of purified RNA and 2µl of 6× dye. Make up the volume to 12µl using water.

6. Load the samples into the gel and run at 65 V for 40 min for a medium-sized electrophoresis apparatus.

7. Remove the gel from the apparatus carefully and detect the bands under UV illuminator.

8. The presence of two major crisp bands corresponding to 28S and 18S ribosomal RNA (rRNA) at a ratio of 2:1 reflects intact total RNA isolation.

**3.3  Reverse Transcription**

Thaw all components (except the enzymes) and set up the reaction on ice. The enzymes must be brought to ice or a −20 °C cooler stand just before the addition.

1. Add total RNA (0.5 to 1µg) and Random hexamer primer—1µl (200 ng) into a nuclease-free reaction tube and make up the volume to 12.5µl (*see* **Notes 16** and **17**).

2. Incubate at 65 °C for 5 min.

3. Cool down the tubes on ice, spin down, and place it back on ice.

4. Add the following components in the order given below making the total volume of the reaction to 20μl: 5× Reaction buffer—4μl, Ribolock® RNase inhibitor (20 U/μl)—0.5μl, dNTP mix (10 mM)—2μl and Revert Aid Reverse Transcriptase (200 U/μl)—1μl.

5. Mix gently by tapping the tubes and centrifuge briefly.

6. Controls: prepare one reaction without the addition of RNA (a No Template Control or NTC) and a second reaction without the reverse transcriptase (a No RT control or NRT). During subsequent real time PCR, any amplification seen with the NTC indicates RNA/DNA contaminants in the reaction components, water or aerosol, while amplification in NRT control indicates amplicon, cDNA, or genomic DNA contamination.

7. Incubate at RT (25 °C) for 10 min, 42 °C for 60 min, 70 °C for 10 min for random hexamer primed synthesis.

8. Dilute the cDNA with nuclease-free water (*see* **Note 18**).

9. Continue with the qPCR or store the tubes at −20 °C. For long-term storage without losing RNA integrity, it is recommended to store samples at −80 °C.

**3.4 Real-Time PCR Setup, Cycling, and Data Analysis**

1. The primer pairs designed for an lncRNA should be first tested for their efficiency and specific amplification before regular use (*see* **Note 19**).

2. Add the components in the order given below to set up the reaction: Water—0.6μl, SYBR Green master mix (2×)—5μl, 10μM Forward primer—0.2μl, 10μM Reverse primer—0.2μl (*see* **Note 20**).

3. Mix gently and centrifuge briefly.

4. For multiple reactions, prepare the stock by calculating 1 extra reaction per 24 samples.

5. Dispense the reaction mixture into a PCR plate wells (6μl into each well) using a stepper pipette.

6. Add 4μl diluted cDNA (1:40) into each well (*see* **Note 21**).

7. Carefully seal the plate using optical plate seal and centrifuge briefly.

8. Run the PCR reaction in a real time PCR instrument using the following thermal program: holding stage of 95 °C for 10 min followed by a cycling stage of 95 °C for 15 s and 60 °C for 30 s repeated 40 times. For melt curve analysis: holding step of 95 °C for 15 s, 60 °C for 1 min and a subsequent heating ramp of 0.5 °C per minute until 95 °C (*see* **Note 22**). Make sure that the fluorescence signals are acquired during annealing/extension steps during cycling (60 °C for 30 s) and continuously during melt curve analysis.

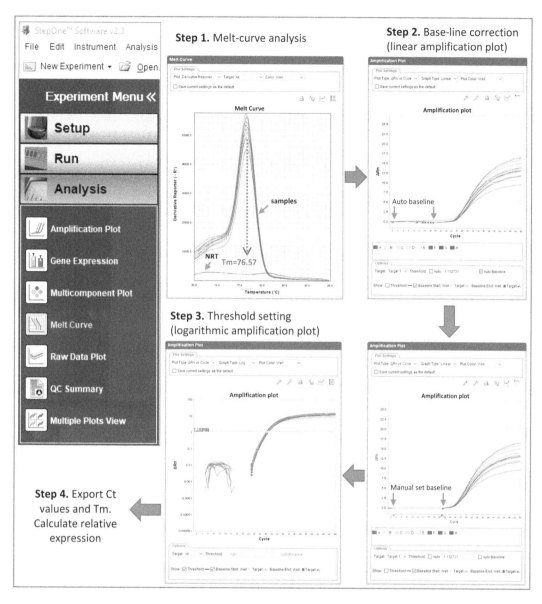

**Fig. 2** Probe-free real-time PCR data analysis. Screen captures from the StepOne software (V2.3) depicting the analysis of a qPCR run. The left panel shows the software user interface. (**Step 1**) First step is amplification specificity check by melt-curve analysis. A typical melt curve for a target is shown and the NRT (No RT control) is seen in purple as a flat line below. Every target is expected to have a unique peak and a specific Tm value across samples. (**Step 2**) Amplification plot in a linear scale with delta Rn (ΔRn, *See* **Note 24**) plotted on the y-axis and PCR cycle numbers on the x-axis with auto baseline settings (baseline start and end cycles indicated) is shown in the right top panel. To set up the baseline manually, decide the start and end cycle (*see* **Note 25**) for each target using the "Analysis Settings" on the top right side of the software screen (not shown). A manually baseline set plot is shown in the lower right panel. (**Step 3**) It shows the amplification plot in log scale (log ΔRn on y-axis) which allows the threshold to be set manually, if required. Unclick the "Auto" option below the amplification plot and move the threshold line so that it is above the background and lies in the exponential phase of the amplification curve as shown. (**Step 4**) Export the $C_t$ and $T_m$ values and calculate the relative expression levels by comparative $C_t$ method. The exported files can be analyzed in MS Excel or other alternatives

9. Once the run is completed, click the "Analysis—Melt Curve" in StepOnePlus Real-Time PCR system to view the melt curve. The presence of a prominent peak in the test reactions and absence of this peak in NTC and NRT for a selected target typically represents a specific single amplicon (*see* **Note 23** and Fig. 2).

10. View the amplification plot, which depicts the fluorescent intensity accumulated during PCR cycles (*see* **Note 24**) and set the baseline (*see* **Note 25**) and threshold as shown in Fig. 2.

11. Export the $C_t$ and $T_m$ values for each sample for both the target and reference gene into an excel spreadsheet and subtract the $C_t$ values of housekeeping (HK) gene from that of the target gene (Target $C_t$- HK $C_t$) to obtain the values for delta $C_t$ ($\Delta C_t$). The relative expression of the sample can then be obtained using the formula $1/2^{\Delta Ct}$.

12. For analysis of differential expression of lncRNA between the reference and the test sample (e.g., control and stimulated samples), the $\Delta C_t$ value of the reference sample is subtracted from $\Delta C_t$ of each sample. This gives a delta-delta $C_t$ ($\Delta\Delta C_t$) value which equals to 0 for the reference sample. Calculation using the formula $1/2^{\Delta\Delta Ct}$ then provides the fold change ($1/2^0 = 1$ for reference sample).

# 4  Notes

1. For transcripts that are not annotated by NCBI and are only part of ENSEMBL (https://www.ensembl.org) or UCSC (https://genome.ucsc.edu/cgi-bin/hgGateway) or other genome annotation servers, download the sequence from the respective server based on the gene name or other gene/transcript identifiers.

2. When designing primers for a particular transcript of a gene, obtain the sequence unique to the transcript of interest as described for overlapping lncRNAs in Subheading 3.1, **step 2**. For general quantitation of gene expression, use the regions common to all transcripts as input sequence for primer design.

3. NCBI primer design tool (https://www.ncbi.nlm.nih.gov/tools/primer-blast/) is one of the other alternative webservers for primer design. It is based on "Primer3 and BLAST" and also provides the "Intron Inclusion" option for obtaining intron-spanning primers. The primers can also be designed manually considering the specifications given in Subheading 3.1 (**steps 4** and **5**) and can be analyzed using a freely available oligo/primer analysis software like NetPrimer (http://www.premierbiosoft.com/NetPrimer/AnalyzePrimer.jsp)     that

provides the rating to each primer. A best rated primer pair is expected to give a successful amplification.

4. The primer3 output provides the reverse primer in the right 5′–3′ orientation.

5. The primer pair must be analyzed manually to ensure that the primer binding regions lie in two different exons or span the exon–exon junction. It is also important to ensure that the enclosed intron length is long enough so that no amplification occurs from the pre-mRNA or contaminating genomic DNA.

6. If the default primer output does not contain an intron-spanning primer pair, it is worthwhile to provide input sequences proximal to and encompassing the exon–exon junction. This limits the choice of primer design to this region, increasing the probability of retrieving intron-spanning primers. Primer that hybridizes partly to 3′ end of one exon and 5′ end of the adjacent exon (exon–exon junction spanning) excludes any binding to genomic DNA or unspliced transcript, thus providing high specificity.

7. In case no primer pair with required transcript selectivity is feasible with the standard design parameters, Tm range and primer length can be varied accordingly to design more primer sets. While the general guidelines must be followed for optimal amplification efficiency, successful real-time PCR primer sets have been reported with $T_m$ as low as 52–55 °C and amplicon lengths above 300 bp.

8. Total RNA including lncRNAs can also be extracted using commercial kits routinely used in most laboratories (e.g., RNeasy mini kit from Qiagen, Nucleospin RNA mini kit from Macherey-Nagel, Gene Jet RNA purification kit from Thermo-Fisher Scientific).

9. For lysis of tissue samples, add 1 ml of TRI reagent per 50–100 mg of tissue and homogenize using a homogenizer. In case the samples contain a high content of fat, polysaccharides, proteins, or extracellular materials, centrifuge the homogenate at 12,000 × $g$ for 10 min at 4 °C and use the supernatant for RNA precipitation and extraction.

10. Perform all steps involving TRI reagent, phenol, or chloroform in a chemical fume hood. Read the safety data sheets and follow the handling instructions provided with the reagent. Wear suitable protective eyewear, clothing, and gloves. Tips, tubes, gloves, and other materials contaminated with TRI reagent, phenol, or chloroform must be collected in a separate sealable container/bag. Similarly, any contaminated liquid must be collected in a separate liquid waste in a closable container.

11. Do not discard the supernatant and collect in a fresh tube when in doubt of losing the pellet. The pellet can be recovered later by centrifugation.

12. The absorbance or optical density (OD) measured at 260 nm provides the RNA concentration in ng/μl. The ratio value of ~2.0 for $OD_{260nm}/OD_{280nm}$ and >2.0 for $OD_{260nm}/OD_{230nm}$ are indicative of pure RNA. $OD_{260nm}/OD_{280nm}$ of <1.9 indicates the presence of contaminants that absorb at or near 280 nm (e.g., DNA, proteins, phenol). A ratio of <2.0 for $OD_{260nm}/OD_{230nm}$ may indicate the presence of EDTA, phenol, carbohydrates, salts or other contaminants that absorb at or near 230 nm.

13. DNase treatment is crucial for the specific detection of lncRNA transcripts and to avoid any nonspecific amplification from genomic DNA, especially when intron-spanning primers are not feasible. While using intron-spanning primer pairs of established specificity, the DNase I step can be optional.

14. Glycogen coprecipitates with RNA and facilitates pellet visibility after centrifugation, making the handling easier during subsequent washes. It is advisable to add glycogen while working with small amounts of input samples or when low RNA yields are expected.

15. Ethidium bromide is a mutagen and can be replaced with other safer alternatives for staining RNA and detection using the UV trans-illuminator.

16. LncRNAs are not necessarily poly(A)-tailed and to ensure reverse transcription of novel lncRNAs, preferably follow random hexamer primed cDNA synthesis.

17. In case of antisense lncRNAs, it is important to design primers that do not detect the overlapping transcripts on the opposite strand. In cases where this is not feasible, reverse transcription with an lncRNA-specific reverse primer ensures specific detection of the lncRNA. For reverse transcription of such transcripts, replace the random hexamer by 1μl of 20 pmol/μl of the gene-specific reverse primer (designed for the real-time PCR) in the reaction and perform reverse transcription at 50 °C for 60 min followed by 5 min enzyme inactivation at 95 °C.

18. The cDNA synthesized in a 20μl reaction is diluted 1:40 using nuclease-free water and 4μl is used for each qPCR reaction.

19. The new primer pairs should be tested using dilutions of cDNA to determine the efficiency and dynamic range of PCR primers. Use the undiluted or 1:20 diluted cDNA as the start-point (=0), serially dilute the cDNA in 10-fold dilutions (1:10 = Log value −1; 1:100 = Log value −2 and so on)

keeping a minimum of 4 dilutions. Perform the qRT-PCR with 2 or better 3 technical replicates for each cDNA dilution plus the negative controls. Plot a scatter plot with the average $C_t$ value of the technical replicates on $Y$-axis and the log dilution value $(\ldots -3, -2, -1, 0)$ on $X$-axis. Add a trend line for the graph and calculate its slope by displaying the line equation in MS Excel. The percentage efficiency of PCR is calculated using the equation: $(10^{-1/\text{slope}} - 1) \times 100$. A slope value of $-3.32$ in a standard curve indicates a primer efficiency of 100%. An efficiency between 90% and 100% is desirable $(-3.6 \geq \text{slope} \geq -3.3)$ and an assay with slope $< -3.6$ should not be used. Primer test results for a successfully used *LINC00261* primer set (Assay 2) [30] is shown in Fig. 1.

20. The PCR reaction for each sample must be done for both the target as well as a house keeping gene (GAPDH, 18S rRNA, Cyclophilin are some of the commonly used ones) to normalize for differences in the amount of input or other factors that could affect the PCR cycling. A house keeping gene, which is not affected by the study conditions or treatments has to be used.

21. While a 1:40 dilution works for most targets, for very low expressing transcripts, undiluted or 1:10 diluted cDNA can be used. A Ct value of higher than 30 should be considered cautiously.

22. For reliable detection of low abundant lncRNAs that are exclusively or predominantly localized to a specific cellular compartment, it is advisable to perform cellular fractionation (cytoplasmic, nuclear, chromatin) before RNA extraction from the fraction of interest.

23. When more than one peak is seen in the melt curve, the PCR product should be run on the gel to confirm the identity. A peak at a lower temperature may be seen due to the presence of primer dimers and a peak at a higher temperature could be indicative of the presence of intron-containing product due to the gDNA contamination or off-target amplification.

24. The SYBR master mix essentially contains a hot-start DNA polymerase, buffer, dNTPs and the SYBR Green dye (or alternatives like EvaGreen and other SYBR derivatives). The formulation varies slightly between different manufacturers. Most of them also contain the reference ROX dye, the fluorescence of which remains the same during PCR for a given reaction and is used to normalize the non–PCR-related fluctuations like optical variations due to the design of the instrument. The Rn value or the normalized fluorescence intensity for a given reaction is the SYBR Green fluorescent signal normalized to the signal of the ROX dye and delta Rn ($\Delta$Rn)

represents Rn minus the baseline value. ROX-based normalization is absolutely required for some real-time PCR equipment, while other thermocyclers do not require ROX.

25. The baseline correction is incorporated to normalize the differences in fluorescence between samples before PCR. For this purpose, a baseline range (start/end cycle) is auto-determined by the analysis software, wherein the end cycle typically falls 2–3 cycle before the start of the amplification curve. If this is not the case for any sample, the end cycle should be manually set 2–3 cycles lower to the cycle number at which the amplification first appears. The baseline correction normalizes all values in the plot to the average fluorescence from the baseline range.

## Acknowledgments

We are thankful to Prof. Dr. Sven Diederichs and Ksenia Myacheva (DKFZ, Heidelberg) for their contribution to the method.

## References

1. Okazaki Y, Furuno M, Kasukawa T, Adachi J, Bono H, Kondo S, Nikaido I, Osato N, Saito R, Suzuki H, Yamanaka I, Kiyosawa H, Yagi K, Tomaru Y, Hasegawa Y, Nogami A, Schonbach C, Gojobori T, Baldarelli R, Hill DP, Bult C, Hume DA, Quackenbush J, Schriml LM, Kanapin A, Matsuda H, Batalov S, Beisel KW, Blake JA, Bradt D, Brusic V, Chothia C, Corbani LE, Cousins S, Dalla E, Dragani TA, Fletcher CF, Forrest A, Frazer KS, Gaasterland T, Gariboldi M, Gissi C, Godzik A, Gough J, Grimmond S, Gustincich S, Hirokawa N, Jackson IJ, Jarvis ED, Kanai A, Kawaji H, Kawasawa Y, Kedzierski RM, King BL, Konagaya A, Kurochkin IV, Lee Y, Lenhard B, Lyons PA, Maglott DR, Maltais L, Marchionni L, McKenzie L, Miki H, Nagashima T, Numata K, Okido T, Pavan WJ, Pertea G, Pesole G, Petrovsky N, Pillai R, Pontius JU, Qi D, Ramachandran S, Ravasi T, Reed JC, Reed DJ, Reid J, Ring BZ, Ringwald M, Sandelin A, Schneider C, Semple CA, Setou M, Shimada K, Sultana R, Takenaka Y, Taylor MS, Teasdale RD, Tomita M, Verardo R, Wagner L, Wahlestedt C, Wang Y, Watanabe Y, Wells C, Wilming LG, Wynshaw-Boris A, Yanagisawa M, Yang I, Yang L, Yuan Z, Zavolan M, Zhu Y, Zimmer A, Carninci P, Hayatsu N, Hirozane-Kishikawa T, Konno H, Nakamura M, Sakazume N, Sato K, Shiraki T, Waki K, Kawai J, Aizawa K, Arakawa T, Fukuda S, Hara A, Hashizume W, Imotani K, Ishii Y, Itoh M, Kagawa I, Miyazaki A, Sakai K, Sasaki D, Shibata K, Shinagawa A, Yasunishi A, Yoshino M, Waterston R, Lander ES, Rogers J, Birney E, Hayashizaki Y, Consortium F, I RGERGP, Team II (2002) Analysis of the mouse transcriptome based on functional annotation of 60,770 full-length cDNAs. Nature 420(6915):563–573. https://doi.org/10.1038/nature01266

2. Bertone P, Stolc V, Royce TE, Rozowsky JS, Urban AE, Zhu X, Rinn JL, Tongprasit W, Samanta M, Weissman S, Gerstein M, Snyder M (2004) Global identification of human transcribed sequences with genome tiling arrays. Science 306(5705):2242–2246. https://doi.org/10.1126/science.1103388

3. Carninci P, Kasukawa T, Katayama S, Gough J, Frith MC, Maeda N, Oyama R, Ravasi T, Lenhard B, Wells C, Kodzius R, Shimokawa K, Bajic VB, Brenner SE, Batalov S, Forrest AR, Zavolan M, Davis MJ, Wilming LG, Aidinis V, Allen JE, Ambesi-Impiombato A, Apweiler R, Aturaliya RN, Bailey TL, Bansal M, Baxter L, Beisel KW, Bersano T, Bono H, Chalk AM, Chiu KP, Choudhary V, Christoffels A, Clutterbuck DR, Crowe ML, Dalla E, Dalrymple BP, de Bono B, Della Gatta G, di Bernardo D, Down T, Engstrom P, Fagiolini M, Faulkner G, Fletcher CF, Fukushima T,

Furuno M, Futaki S, Gariboldi M, Georgii-Hemming P, Gingeras TR, Gojobori T, Green RE, Gustincich S, Harbers M, Hayashi Y, Hensch TK, Hirokawa N, Hill D, Huminiecki L, Iacono M, Ikeo K, Iwama A, Ishikawa T, Jakt M, Kanapin A, Katoh M, Kawasawa Y, Kelso J, Kitamura H, Kitano H, Kollias G, Krishnan SP, Kruger A, Kummerfeld SK, Kurochkin IV, Lareau LF, Lazarevic D, Lipovich L, Liu J, Liuni S, McWilliam S, Madan Babu M, Madera M, Marchionni L, Matsuda H, Matsuzawa S, Miki H, Mignone F, Miyake S, Morris K, Mottagui-Tabar S, Mulder N, Nakano N, Nakauchi H, Ng P, Nilsson R, Nishiguchi S, Nishikawa S, Nori F, Ohara O, Okazaki Y, Orlando V, Pang KC, Pavan WJ, Pavesi G, Pesole G, Petrovsky N, Piazza S, Reed J, Reid JF, Ring BZ, Ringwald M, Rost B, Ruan Y, Salzberg SL, Sandelin A, Schneider C, Schonbach C, Sekiguchi K, Semple CA, Seno S, Sessa L, Sheng Y, Shibata Y, Shimada H, Shimada K, Silva D, Sinclair B, Sperling S, Stupka E, Sugiura K, Sultana R, Takenaka Y, Taki K, Tammoja K, Tan SL, Tang S, Taylor MS, Tegner J, Teichmann SA, Ueda HR, van Nimwegen E, Verardo R, Wei CL, Yagi K, Yamanishi H, Zabarovsky E, Zhu S, Zimmer A, Hide W, Bult C, Grimmond SM, Teasdale RD, Liu ET, Brusic V, Quackenbush J, Wahlestedt C, Mattick JS, Hume DA, Kai C, Sasaki D, Tomaru Y, Fukuda S, Kanamori-Katayama M, Suzuki M, Aoki J, Arakawa T, Iida J, Imamura K, Itoh M, Kato T, Kawaji H, Kawagashira N, Kawashima T, Kojima M, Kondo S, Konno H, Nakano K, Ninomiya N, Nishio T, Okada M, Plessy C, Shibata K, Shiraki T, Suzuki S, Tagami M, Waki K, Watahiki A, Okamura-Oho Y, Suzuki H, Kawai J, Hayashizaki Y, Consortium F, Group RGER, Genome Science G (2005) The transcriptional landscape of the mammalian genome. Science 309 (5740):1559–1563. https://doi.org/10.1126/science.1112014

4. Derrien T, Johnson R, Bussotti G, Tanzer A, Djebali S, Tilgner H, Guernec G, Martin D, Merkel A, Knowles DG, Lagarde J, Veeravalli L, Ruan X, Ruan Y, Lassmann T, Carninci P, Brown JB, Lipovich L, Gonzalez JM, Thomas M, Davis CA, Shiekhattar R, Gingeras TR, Hubbard TJ, Notredame C, Harrow J, Guigo R (2012) The GENCODE v7 catalog of human long noncoding RNAs: analysis of their gene structure, evolution, and expression. Genome Res 22(9):1775–1789. https://doi.org/10.1101/gr.132159.111

5. Trapnell C, Williams BA, Pertea G, Mortazavi A, Kwan G, van Baren MJ, Salzberg SL, Wold BJ, Pachter L (2010) Transcript assembly and quantification by RNA-Seq reveals unannotated transcripts and isoform switching during cell differentiation. Nat Biotechnol 28(5):511–515. https://doi.org/10.1038/nbt.1621

6. Dhamija S, Menon MB (2018) Non-coding transcript variants of protein-coding genes - what are they good for? RNA Biol 15 (8):1025–1031. https://doi.org/10.1080/15476286.2018.1511675

7. Guttman M, Amit I, Garber M, French C, Lin MF, Feldser D, Huarte M, Zuk O, Carey BW, Cassady JP, Cabili MN, Jaenisch R, Mikkelsen TS, Jacks T, Hacohen N, Bernstein BE, Kellis M, Regev A, Rinn JL, Lander ES (2009) Chromatin signature reveals over a thousand highly conserved large non-coding RNAs in mammals. Nature 458 (7235):223–227. https://doi.org/10.1038/nature07672

8. Djebali S, Davis CA, Merkel A, Dobin A, Lassmann T, Mortazavi A, Tanzer A, Lagarde J, Lin W, Schlesinger F, Xue C, Marinov GK, Khatun J, Williams BA, Zaleski C, Rozowsky J, Roder M, Kokocinski F, Abdelhamid RF, Alioto T, Antoshechkin I, Baer MT, Bar NS, Batut P, Bell K, Bell I, Chakrabortty S, Chen X, Chrast J, Curado J, Derrien T, Drenkow J, Dumais E, Dumais J, Duttagupta R, Falconnet E, Fastuca M, Fejes-Toth K, Ferreira P, Foissac S, Fullwood MJ, Gao H, Gonzalez D, Gordon A, Gunawardena H, Howald C, Jha S, Johnson R, Kapranov P, King B, Kingswood C, Luo OJ, Park E, Persaud K, Preall JB, Ribeca P, Risk B, Robyr D, Sammeth M, Schaffer L, See LH, Shahab A, Skancke J, Suzuki AM, Takahashi H, Tilgner H, Trout D, Walters N, Wang H, Wrobel J, Yu Y, Ruan X, Hayashizaki Y, Harrow J, Gerstein M, Hubbard T, Reymond A, Antonarakis SE, Hannon G, Giddings MC, Ruan Y, Wold B, Carninci P, Guigo R, Gingeras TR (2012) Landscape of transcription in human cells. Nature 489 (7414):101–108. https://doi.org/10.1038/nature11233

9. Sun Q, Hao Q, Prasanth KV (2018) Nuclear long noncoding RNAs: key regulators of gene expression. Trends Genet 34(2):142–157. https://doi.org/10.1016/j.tig.2017.11.005

10. Yang L, Duff MO, Graveley BR, Carmichael GG, Chen LL (2011) Genomewide characterization of non-polyadenylated RNAs. Genome Biol 12(2):R16. https://doi.org/10.1186/gb-2011-12-2-r16

11. Kim TK, Hemberg M, Gray JM, Costa AM, Bear DM, Wu J, Harmin DA, Laptewicz M, Barbara-Haley K, Kuersten S, Markenscoff-Papadimitriou E, Kuhl D, Bito H, Worley PF, Kreiman G, Greenberg ME (2010) Widespread transcription at neuronal activity-regulated enhancers. Nature 465(7295):182–187. https://doi.org/10.1038/nature09033

12. Wilusz JE, JnBaptiste CK, Lu LY, Kuhn CD, Joshua-Tor L, Sharp PA (2012) A triple helix stabilizes the 3′ ends of long noncoding RNAs that lack poly(A) tails. Genes Dev 26 (21):2392–2407. https://doi.org/10.1101/gad.204438.112

13. Brown JA, Valenstein ML, Yario TA, Tycowski KT, Steitz JA (2012) Formation of triple-helical structures by the 3′-end sequences of MALAT1 and MENbeta noncoding RNAs. Proc Natl Acad Sci U S A 109 (47):19202–19207. https://doi.org/10.1073/pnas.1217338109

14. Yin QF, Yang L, Zhang Y, Xiang JF, Wu YW, Carmichael GG, Chen LL (2012) Long non-coding RNAs with snoRNA ends. Mol Cell 48 (2):219–230. https://doi.org/10.1016/j.molcel.2012.07.033

15. Memczak S, Jens M, Elefsinioti A, Torti F, Krueger J, Rybak A, Maier L, Mackowiak SD, Gregersen LH, Munschauer M, Loewer A, Ziebold U, Landthaler M, Kocks C, le Noble F, Rajewsky N (2013) Circular RNAs are a large class of animal RNAs with regulatory potency. Nature 495(7441):333–338. https://doi.org/10.1038/nature11928

16. Sigova AA, Mullen AC, Molinie B, Gupta S, Orlando DA, Guenther MG, Almada AE, Lin C, Sharp PA, Giallourakis CC, Young RA (2013) Divergent transcription of long non-coding RNA/mRNA gene pairs in embryonic stem cells. Proc Natl Acad Sci U S A 110 (8):2876–2881. https://doi.org/10.1073/pnas.1221904110

17. Cabili MN, Trapnell C, Goff L, Koziol M, Tazon-Vega B, Regev A, Rinn JL (2011) Integrative annotation of human large intergenic noncoding RNAs reveals global properties and specific subclasses. Genes Dev 25 (18):1915–1927. https://doi.org/10.1101/gad.17446611

18. Zhou Q, Wan Q, Jiang Y, Liu J, Qiang L, Sun L (2020) A landscape of murine long non-coding RNAs reveals the leading transcriptome alterations in adipose tissue during aging. Cell Rep 31(8):107694. https://doi.org/10.1016/j.celrep.2020.107694

19. Ransohoff JD, Wei Y, Khavari PA (2018) The functions and unique features of long intergenic non-coding RNA. Nat Rev Mol Cell Biol 19(3):143–157. https://doi.org/10.1038/nrm.2017.104

20. Yuan JH, Yang F, Wang F, Ma JZ, Guo YJ, Tao QF, Liu F, Pan W, Wang TT, Zhou CC, Wang SB, Wang YZ, Yang Y, Yang N, Zhou WP, Yang GS, Sun SH (2014) A long noncoding RNA activated by TGF-beta promotes the invasion-metastasis cascade in hepatocellular carcinoma. Cancer Cell 25(5):666–681. https://doi.org/10.1016/j.ccr.2014.03.010

21. Kawasaki Y, Miyamoto M, Oda T, Matsumura K, Negishi L, Nakato R, Suda S, Yokota N, Shirahige K, Akiyama T (2019) The novel lncRNA CALIC upregulates AXL to promote colon cancer metastasis. EMBO Rep 20 (8):e47052. https://doi.org/10.15252/embr.201847052

22. Hessels D, Schalken JA (2009) The use of PCA3 in the diagnosis of prostate cancer. Nat Rev Urol 6(5):255–261. https://doi.org/10.1038/nrurol.2009.40

23. Yang Z, Li X, Yang Y, He Z, Qu X, Zhang Y (2016) Long noncoding RNAs in the progression, metastasis, and prognosis of osteosarcoma. Cell Death Dis 7(9):e2389. https://doi.org/10.1038/cddis.2016.272

24. Schmittgen TD, Zakrajsek BA, Mills AG, Gorn V, Singer MJ, Reed MW (2000) Quantitative reverse transcription-polymerase chain reaction to study mRNA decay: comparison of endpoint and real-time methods. Anal Biochem 285(2):194–204. https://doi.org/10.1006/abio.2000.4753

25. Morrison TB, Weis JJ, Wittwer CT (1998) Quantification of low-copy transcripts by continuous SYBR Green I monitoring during amplification. BioTechniques 24(6):954–958, 960, 962

26. Schmittgen TD, Livak KJ (2008) Analyzing real-time PCR data by the comparative C (T) method. Nat Protoc 3(6):1101–1108. https://doi.org/10.1038/nprot.2008.73

27. Ririe KM, Rasmussen RP, Wittwer CT (1997) Product differentiation by analysis of DNA melting curves during the polymerase chain reaction. Anal Biochem 245(2):154–160. https://doi.org/10.1006/abio.1996.9916

28. Untergasser A, Cutcutache I, Koressaar T, Ye J, Faircloth BC, Remm M, Rozen SG (2012) Primer3--new capabilities and interfaces. Nucleic Acids Res 40(15):e115. https://doi.org/10.1093/nar/gks596

29. Koressaar T, Remm M (2007) Enhancements and modifications of primer design program Primer3. Bioinformatics 23(10):1289–1291. https://doi.org/10.1093/bioinformatics/btm091

30. Dhamija S, Becker AC, Sharma Y, Myacheva K, Seiler J, Diederichs S (2018) LINC00261 and the adjacent gene FOXA2 are epithelial markers and are suppressed during lung cancer tumorigenesis and progression. Noncoding RNA 5(1). https://doi.org/10.3390/ncrna5010002

# Chapter 7

# Quantitation of Long Noncoding RNA Using Digital PCR

## Yu Ota, Irene K. Yan, and Tushar Patel

## Abstract

Long noncoding RNAs (lncRNAs) are implicated in many physiological or disease processes and alterations in their expression may contribute to the development of various diseases. Accurate quantitation of lncRNA can be useful in measuring changes in expression in different settings such as in the circulation where the measurement of lncRNA may be useful as a biomarker of disease. However, the low levels of lncRNA expression require the use of highly sensitive detection technologies for accurate quantitation. Digital polymerase chain reaction (dPCR) is a sensitive method for absolute quantification of lncRNA and can be useful for measurement of gene expression when transcript levels are low. By providing a direct measurement without normalization, the use of dPCR may provide advantages for quantitation of low-abundance targets.

**Key words** Long noncoding RNA, Digital PCR, Gene expression

## 1 Introduction

Long noncoding RNAs (lncRNAs) are defined as gene transcripts of more than 200 nucleotides that are not translated into proteins. Many lncRNAs have been implicated in disease processes [1]. Alterations in lncRNA expression between normal and diseased tissue provides the basis for their use as biomarkers of disease [2]. However, the levels of lncRNA may be very low, making it difficult to detect or to quantitate their expression. Although quantitative polymerase chain reaction (qPCR) is a well-established tool for quantifying gene expression, it is not well-suited for detecting low abundance targets such as most lncRNA. Furthermore, there is a lack of a consistent reference for normalizing lncRNA, especially in body fluids [3]. Digital polymerase chain reaction (dPCR) has a greater sensitivity that qPCR and can detect smaller fold change differences. Furthermore, unlike qPCR, dPCR allows for absolute quantification without the need for standard curves or reference [3–5]. Thus, ddPCR provides the ability to quantify lncRNAs with high precision and sensitivity [6].

Alfons Navarro (ed.), *Long Non-Coding RNAs in Cancer*, Methods in Molecular Biology, vol. 2348,
https://doi.org/10.1007/978-1-0716-1581-2_7, © Springer Science+Business Media, LLC, part of Springer Nature 2021

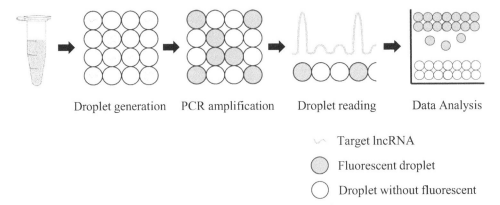

Droplet generation    PCR amplification    Droplet reading    Data Analysis

⌣ Target lncRNA

◉ Fluorescent droplet

○ Droplet without fluorescent

**Fig. 1** Schematic showing the droplet digital PCR workflow. RNA is isolated and cDNA generated. Samples are randomly partitioned across discrete droplets and the droplets are amplified to end-point through thermal cycling. After amplification, fluorescence amplitudes for droplets are read as either positive or negative. Finally, positive droplets are counted and Poisson statistics are applied to estimate the average target concentration

Herein we describe the workflow and methods for quantitation of lncRNA using droplet digital PCR (ddPCR). With this technique, sample DNA is randomly partitioned across discrete droplets using microfluidic circuits and surfactant chemistry. The template DNA efficiently is encapsulated in its own droplet and counted separately. PCR amplification is then performed using fluorescence-based detection technology to allow detection of positive droplets. Positive droplets are counted and Poisson statistics are then applied to derive the mean number of target sequences within each droplet and used to estimate the average target concentration (Fig. 1) [7–12]. These protocols should be valuable to researchers interested in the role and contribution of lncRNAs to disease biomarkers.

## 2    Materials

### 2.1    Equipment

1. Thermal cycler (*see* **Note 1**).
2. Heat sealer (*see* **Note 2**).
3. Droplet generator (Bio-Rad QX200, 186-4002) (*see* **Note 3**).
4. Droplet Reader (Bio-Rad QX200, 186-4003) (*see* **Note 4**).
5. QuantaSoft Software (Bio-Rad) (*see* **Note 5**).

### 2.2    cDNA Synthesis

1. Total RNA (*see* **Note 6**).
2. cDNA synthesis kit. cDNA synthesis can be performed using iScript cDNA Synthesis Kit (Bio-Rad) or an alternative cDNA synthesis kit.

**2.3 ddPCR Reaction Setup**

1. ddPCR master mix (*see* **Note 7**).

2. cDNA template (*see* **Note 8**).

3. Primers (*see* **Note 9**).

4. Probe (*see* **Note 10**).

5. 96-well PCR plate.

**2.4 Droplet Generation and PCR Amplification**

1. Droplet generator oil (*see* **Note 11**):
   (a)  For TaqMan experiments, use Bio-Rad, 186-3005.
   (b)  For EvaGreen experiments, use Bio-Rad 186-4005.

2. DG8 Cartridge (Bio-Rad, 186-4008) (*see* **Note 12**).

3. DG8 Gasket (Bio-Rad, 186-3009).

4. Cartridge Holder (Bio-Rad, 186-3051).

5. ddPCR supermix:
   (a)  For TaqMan experiments, use the supermix for probes (Bio-Rad, 186-3023).
   (b)  For EvaGreen experiments, use EvaGreen supermix (Bio-Rad, 186-4034 and custom primers).

6. Multichannel pipettes (*see* **Note 13**).

7. Reagent trough (*see* **Note 14**).

8. Pierceable Foil Heat Seal (Bio-Rad, 181-4040).

9. Eppendorf 96-well twin.tec PCR plates (Eppendorf, 951020346).

10. Plate sealer (*see* **Note 15**).

# 3    Methods

Use standard lab precautions to avoid contamination of the reaction mix and sample. Work in an RNase-free work area, and use filtered pipette tips and nuclease-free water.

**3.1 Sample Preparation**

1. Prepare DNase treated RNA in 10 µl of nuclease-free water. The recommended concentration of RNA template is 100 fg to 1 µg.

2. If using iScript cDNA Synthesis Kit, mix 4 µl 5× iScript Buffer, 1 µl iScript RT, 0.2 µl RNase inhibitor (20 units/µl), and 4.8 µl water in PCR tubes. Add 10 µl RNA from previous step to the 10 µl reaction.

3. Incubate using the following reaction protocol: 5 min at 25 °C, 30 min at 42 °C, 5 min at 85 °C, and hold at 4 °C.

4. Template cDNA should be diluted to avoid saturating the droplet reader (*see* **Note 16**).

**3.2 ddPCR Reaction Setup for TaqMan**

1. Prepare the reaction master mix: 20 μl of master mix will contain 5 μl nuclease free water, 10 μl ddPCR Master mix for TaqMan FAM/VIC probes, 1 μl of ddPCR assay mix (20×), and 4 μl of template cDNA (*see* **Note 17**).

2. Plate samples into a 96-well PCR plate in preparation for droplet generation. A multichannel pipette can then be used to load the samples into the Droplet Generator cartridge (*see* **Note 18**).

**3.3 ddPCR Reaction Setup for EvaGreen**

1. Prepare the reaction master mix: 20 μl of master mix will contain 4 μl nuclease free water, 2 μl Primer Pairs 5 μM, 10 μl of ddPCR master mix for EvaGreen, and 4 μl of template cDNA (*see* **Note 17**).

2. Plate samples into a 96-well PCR plate in preparation for droplet generation. A multichannel pipette can then be used to load the samples into the Droplet Generator cartridge (*see* **Note 18**).

**3.4 Droplet Generation**

1. Insert the DG8 cartridge into the cartridge holder and lock in to place.

2. Transfer 20 μl samples to the sample wells (middle row) of the DG8 cartridge using a multichannel pipette (*see* **Note 19**).

3. Fill the oil wells (bottom row) of the DG8 cartridge with 70 μl droplet generation oil using a multichannel pipette.

4. Hook the gasket over the cartridge holder.

5. Press the button of the droplet generator to open the door and place the cartridge holder into the instrument.

6. Press the button again to close the door and droplets will automatically generate (*see* **Note 20**).

7. When droplet generation is complete, open the door, remove the cartridge holder from the unit, and carefully remove and discard the gasket.

8. The top wells of the cartridge contain droplets. Pipet slowly 35 μl of droplets into column of Eppendorf twin.tec. 96-well plate (*see* **Note 21**).

9. Repeat **steps 3–7**. Generate the droplets of all samples and transfer to the 96-well plate.

10. Place foil heat seal on top of the 96-well plate and set the plate onto the plate sealer, and then depress for 5 s.

11. Rotate plate and depress again for 5 s (*see* **Note 22**).

**Table 1**
**TaqMan Assay**

| Segment | Cycles | Temperature (°C) | Time (s) |
|---------|--------|------------------|----------|
| 1 | 1 | 95 | 600 |
| 2 | 40 | 94 | 30 |
|   |   | 60 | 60 |
| 3 | 1 | 98 | 600 |

**Table 2**
**EvaGreen Assay**

| Segment | Cycles | Temperature (°C) | Time (s) |
|---------|--------|------------------|----------|
| 1 | 1 | 95 | 300 |
| 2 | 40 | 95 | 30 |
|   |   | 60 | 60 |
| 3 | 1 | 4 | 300 |
|   | 1 | 90 | 300 |

**3.5 PCR Amplification**

1. Once the 96-well plate containing the droplets is sealed, load it plate into the thermal cycler and run the protocol for endpoint PCR. Refer to Tables 1 or 2 for cycling conditions (*see* **Note 23**).

2. When PCR amplification is complete, read the droplets using the droplet reader immediately after or store at 4 °C overnight.

**3.6 Droplet Reading**

1. Following PCR amplification in the droplets, insert 96-well plate into the droplet reader plate holder.

2. Place the plate and holder in the droplet reader.

3. Set up the experiment details in QuantaSoft software including sample ID and target, and designate which assays correspond to which channels, such as FAM and HEX.

4. Make sure there is enough the droplet reader oil in the instrument and the waste is empty.

5. Once the plate layout is complete, start the droplet reading process (*see* **Note 24**).

**3.7 Data Analysis**

1. After the droplet reader has finished sample run, the QuantaSoft software begins to analyze the data in each well.

2. If experiment type was set up for absolute quantification (ABS) analysis, automatic thresholding determines target concentrations. Positive and negative droplets in fluorescence amplitude are viewed on the scatter-plot.

3. The threshold may be manually adjusted on scatter plots. The histograms can assist in setting the threshold (*see* **Note 25**) (Fig. 2).

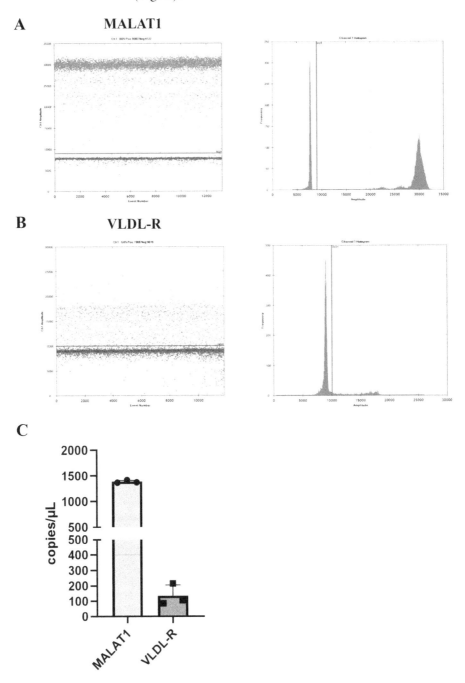

**Fig. 2** Quantitation of lncRNA using droplet digital PCR. Quantification of MALAT1 (**a**) and VLDL-R (**b**) in HepG2 cells by ddPCR. The scatter-plot (left) shows positive droplets and negative droplets, and the histogram (right) can assist in setting the threshold. MALAT1 (**a**) There is a better separation between positive droplets and negative droplets in MALAT1 compared with that in VLDL-R (**b**). (**c**) Quantitation of MALAT1 and VLDL-R expression in HepG2 cells. Data are expressed as mean and standard error from technical triplicates

4. After set threshold manually, the software will complete the calculations. The concentration reported is copies/µl of the final ddPCR reaction (*see* **Note 26**).

# 4   Notes

1. cDNA synthesis and ddPCR amplification will be carried out using thermal cycler.

2. The sample plate should be sealed using heat sealer prior to amplification.

3. The droplet generator will partition each sample into approximately 20,000 nanoliter-sized droplets by water-oil emulsion droplet technology with microfluidics.

4. The droplet reader will analyze each droplet individually using a two color detection system.

5. The number of positive and negative droplets will be measured for data analysis.

6. RNA should be DNase treated to avoid genomic DNA contamination. The concentration and purity of RNA should be evaluated to ensure quality of the preparation.

7. Either EvaGreen chemistry with custom primers or TaqMan hydrolysis probes labeled with FAM and HEX or VIC reporter fluorophores can be used.

8. Serial dilutions can be used to determine the optimal starting concentration. The cDNA template should be diluted to prevent saturation of target copy number.

9. When primers are designed and synthesized, follow same guidelines as qRT-PCR primers. They should be validated by qRT-PCR prior to use in dPCR. The recommended concentration of primer is 900 nM each, but this might need to be optimized based on the specific gene.

10. The QX200 Droplet Digital PCR system is compatible with TaqMan hydrolysis probe or EvaGreen dsDNA binding dye chemistries. The probe sequence should be chosen between the two primers of the amplicon. Primer sequence should not overlap with the probe. The probe should have melting temperature 3–10 °C higher than the primer. The probe must be <30 nucleotides length and not have a G at the 5′ end. The recommended concentration of probe is 250 nM, but might require optimization.

11. Droplet generator oil has a limited shelf life. It is important to use fresh oil to avoid lower droplet counts. There is separate oil depending on TaqMan experiments or EvaGreen experiments.

12. This cartridge generates eight samples each.

13. The advantage of using a p20 and p200 multichannel pipette is that samples can be loaded efficiently.

14. The use of a reagent trough will make it easier to distribute the samples.

15. The sample plate should be sealed prior to PCR. The plate sealer should be warmed up at least 15 min before using.

16. If the target copy number is known to be high, plan to reduce the starting sample accordingly. If the target copy number is unknown, the optimal starting concentration should be determined. The user can be done by using different range of dilutions.

17. It is important to prepare Sample wells as well as No Template Control (NTC) wells. NTC wells can be used to help set threshold during analysis.

18. It is recommended to prepare a little extra volume so as to ensure that 20 μl of mixture is transferred to the cartridge.

19. Air bubbles can cover the bottom of the well and affect the droplet counts and data quality. To avoid creating air bubbles, make sure the tip reaches the bottom of the wells.

20. The flashing green light indicates indicate droplet generation is in progress. When droplet generation is complete, indicator light is solid green. If the cartridge is accidentally removed prior to completion, droplet counts will be affected.

21. It is important to draw and pipet slowly and uniformly to avoid shearing or coalescing the droplets.

22. Confirm that all the wells in the plate are sealed properly to prevent evaporation.

23. A 2.5 °C/s ramp rate is essential to ensure each droplet reaches proper temperature.

24. Priming the system should be required to clean the dead volume of old reagents, if the instrument has been idle for over 1 month. Perform this prior to running assay acquisition.

25. Set the threshold for No Template Control (NTC) wells and apply the same threshold to Sample wells.

26. For more information about reporting results, follow the MIQE guidelines [13, 14].

## References

1. Kopp F, Mendell JT (2018) Functional classification and experimental dissection of long noncoding RNAs. Cell 172(3):393–407. https://doi.org/10.1016/j.cell.2018.01.011

2. Kazimierczyk M, Kasprowicz MK, Kasprzyk ME, Wrzesinski J (2020) Human long noncoding RNA Interactome: detection, characterization and function. Int J Mol Sci 21

(3):1027. https://doi.org/10.3390/ijms21031027

3. Mohankumar S, Patel T (2016) Extracellular vesicle long noncoding RNA as potential biomarkers of liver cancer. Brief Funct Genomics 15(3):249–256. https://doi.org/10.1093/bfgp/elv058

4. Hindson CM, Chevillet JR, Briggs HA, Gallichotte EN, Ruf IK, Hindson BJ, Vessella RL, Tewari M (2013) Absolute quantification by droplet digital PCR versus analog real-time PCR. Nat Methods 10(10):1003–1005. https://doi.org/10.1038/nmeth.2633

5. Wang C, Ding Q, Plant P, Basheer M, Yang C, Tawedrous E, Krizova A, Boulos C, Farag M, Cheng Y, Yousef GM (2019) Droplet digital PCR improves urinary exosomal miRNA detection compared to real-time PCR. Clin Biochem 67:54–59. https://doi.org/10.1016/j.clinbiochem.2019.03.008

6. Dodd DW, Gagnon KT, Corey DR (2013) Digital quantitation of potential therapeutic target RNAs. Nucleic Acid Ther 23(3):188–194. https://doi.org/10.1089/nat.2013.0427

7. Yan IK, Lohray R, Patel T (2018) Droplet digital PCR for quantitation of extracellular RNA. Methods Mol Biol 1740:155–162. https://doi.org/10.1007/978-1-4939-7652-2_12

8. Takahashi K, Yan IK, Kim C, Kim J, Patel T (2014) Analysis of extracellular RNA by digital PCR. Front Oncol 4:129. https://doi.org/10.3389/fonc.2014.00129

9. Valpione S, Campana L (2019) Detection of circulating tumor DNA (ctDNA) by digital droplet polymerase chain reaction (dd-PCR) in liquid biopsies. Methods Enzymol 629:1–15. https://doi.org/10.1016/bs.mie.2019.08.002

10. Pinheiro LB, Coleman VA, Hindson CM, Herrmann J, Hindson BJ, Bhat S, Emslie KR (2012) Evaluation of a droplet digital polymerase chain reaction format for DNA copy number quantification. Anal Chem 84(2):1003–1011. https://doi.org/10.1021/ac202578x

11. Nyaruaba R, Mwaliko C, Kering KK, Wei H (2019) Droplet digital PCR applications in the tuberculosis world. Tuberculosis (Edinb) 117:85–92. https://doi.org/10.1016/j.tube.2019.07.001

12. Wang P, Jing F, Li G, Wu Z, Cheng Z, Zhang J, Zhang H, Jia C, Jin Q, Mao H, Zhao J (2015) Absolute quantification of lung cancer related microRNA by droplet digital PCR. Biosens Bioelectron 74:836–842. https://doi.org/10.1016/j.bios.2015.07.048

13. Huggett JF, Cowen S, Foy CA (2015) Considerations for digital PCR as an accurate molecular diagnostic tool. Clin Chem 61(1):79–88. https://doi.org/10.1373/clinchem.2014.221366

14. Huggett JF, Foy CA, Benes V, Emslie K, Garson JA, Haynes R, Hellemans J, Kubista M, Mueller RD, Nolan T, Pfaffl MW, Shipley GL, Vandesompele J, Wittwer CT, Bustin SA (2013) The digital MIQE guidelines: minimum information for publication of quantitative digital PCR experiments. Clin Chem 59(6):892–902. https://doi.org/10.1373/clinchem.2013.206375

# Chapter 8

# Detection of lncRNA by LNA-Based In Situ Hybridization in Paraffin-Embedded Cancer Cell Spheroids

Boye Schnack Nielsen, Jesper Larsen, Jakob Høffding, Son Ly Nhat, Natasha Helleberg Madsen, Trine Møller, Bjørn Holst, and Kim Holmstrøm

## Abstract

Cancer cell spheroids are considered important preclinical tools to evaluate the efficacy of new drugs. In cancer cell spheroids, the cells assemble and grow in 3D structures with cell contact interactions that are partly impermeable, which leads to central hypoxia and necrosis. The cell spheroids thus possess several features identified in clinical tumors. Not only will the effect and behavior of therapeutic drugs in 3D cell spheroids be affected more similarly than in cells grown on culture plates, but molecular interactions and signaling pathways in cells are also more likely to mimic the in vivo situation. The monitoring of various biomarkers including lncRNAs in 3D cell spheroids is important to assess a potentially induced phenotype in the cells and the effects of drugs. Specifically, for lncRNAs, in situ localization can be done using locked nucleic acid (LNA) probe technology. Here we present a protocol for preparation of cell spheroids for use in LNA probe–based in situ hybridization to study lncRNA expression in paraffin embedded 3D cancer cell spheroids.

**Key words** lncRNA, Spheroid, LNA, In situ hybridization, MALAT1, UCA1

## 1 Introduction

In three-dimensional (3D) cell cultures, the cells have the capacity to interact and grow as organized cell clusters different from cells grown as monolayers on plastic surfaces (2D). 3D cancer cell cultures form spheroid-like structures if grown in low-attachment vials and, after extended growth, form necrotic cores reflecting that the semi-impermeable cell-cell interactions are preventing sufficient oxygen and nutrients access to the cells located in the center [1]. Cancer cells in adenocarcinoma-type tumors typically grow in organized clusters mimicking the gland-like structures that they derived from and may form central or luminal necrosis. Therefore, 3D cancer cell cultures are more similar to the in vivo tissue structures than cells grown in monolayers, and are found to be an attractive replacement of intervention studies of cancer cell growth

Alfons Navarro (ed.), *Long Non-Coding RNAs in Cancer*, Methods in Molecular Biology, vol. 2348,
https://doi.org/10.1007/978-1-0716-1581-2_8, © Springer Science+Business Media, LLC, part of Springer Nature 2021

in mice, strongly advocated by legal ethical authorities for reducing use of experimental animals. In this method paper, we describe how to culture 3D cell spheroids and how to embed them in paraffin for morphological and biomarker analyses.

For 3D cell cultures to be ideal models for drug efficacy testing, the 3D cell models must also mimic cancer cell characteristics at the molecular level, including general regulatory and signaling pathways in response to the external factors. In addition, the microenvironment, as composed of the extracellular space and the normal nonmalignant cells, surrounding cancer cells are providing a growth support constituting growth factors, matrix proteases, and signaling molecules. Mixing normal epithelial cells or cancerous epithelial cells with fibroblastic cells facilitates branching morphogenesis [2] or with immune cells [3] enables studies on immunotherapeutic targets. Thus, mixed-cell-culture models also allow for drug testing, targeting and intercellular signaling. Also 3D pancreas cancer models, where mixing was done with monocytes [4], suggested that M2-like macrophages developed as a result of intercellular signaling.

Key regulatory pathways are controlled at the RNA level and involve control of translation by mRNA splicing or binding of microRNAs. Long noncoding RNAs (lncRNAs) take part in this regulatory machinery. The group of lncRNAs constitutes at least 60,000 genes, which is 3- to 4-fold higher than the number of protein-encoding genes [5, 6]. Most LncRNAs functions are only partly characterized, but many are deregulated in cancer. In this work, we have included expression analyses of Metastasis associated in lung adenocarcinoma transcript 1 (MALAT1 lncRNA) and Urothelial carcinoma associated 1 (UCA1 lncRNA) as examples.

Although functions attributed to lncRNAs include regulation of transcription and translation, and mRNA splicing, their functions have only sporadically been identified and characterized. LncRNAs are known as intergenic RNA, intronic RNA, antisense transcripts, or pseudogenes. Many lncRNAs execute their function in the nuclei where they bind to chromosomal structures and affect RNA transcription [7]. Cabili et al. [8] showed by in situ hybridization (ISH) on cultured cells that the majority of lncRNAs are located in the nuclei in contrast to mRNAs that almost all are in the cytoplasm. Some lncRNAs are found in the cytoplasm that can lead to their presence in exosomes, which can act as messengers between cells [9].

MALAT1 is, in its mature spliced form, an 8–9000 nucleotides long lncRNA and is one of the most abundant lncRNA. Elevated levels of MALAT1 is associated with poor prognosis in several cancer types, including breast and colon cancer [10, 11]. MALAT1 was found, in a genetic breast tumor model, to be essential for tumor cell differentiation and to promote metastasis [12]. However, the function of MALAT1 in tumor growth and dissemination is debated [13]. MALAT1 localizes to nuclear speckles where it may have several functions, including contributing to transcription and RNA splicing [14].

UCA1 is a lncRNA of almost 3000 nucleotides that was originally found in bladder transitional cell carcinoma [15], and has since been reported to be upregulated in several cancer types, including colorectal and breast cancer [16–18], where increased expression of UCA1 is indicating poor prognosis. UCA1 is reported to be involved in tumor growth, apoptosis and invasion, probably through binding (sponging) or regulating expression of microRNAs [19].

We have previously explored methods to detect lncRNAs in cultured cells on glass slides using ISH methods, including locked nucleic acid (LNA) probe technology, multiple DNA oligonucleotide probe principle, and branched DNA probe technology [20], and found that LNA probes were useful at least for the detection of relatively abundant targets, including MALAT1. In addition, we have reported ISH methods for detection of microRNA in paraffin embedded cultured cells [21], and frozen and paraffin embedded tissue samples using LNA probes [22–24]. Here we present how to prepare paraffin embedded cell spheroids (PECS) and how to perform LNA-based ISH on the PECS.

## 2   Materials

### 2.1   Reagents and Buffers

1. Human cancer cell lines: HT29 (from colorectal adenocarcinoma), MCF7 (from breast cancer), HT1080 (from fibrosarcoma), LS174T (from colorectal adenocarcinoma). Normal human skin fibroblast: 1BR.3.G (*see* **Note 1**).

2. DMEM medium for HT-29 and 1BR.3.G: DMEM (Dulbecco's Modified Eagle's Medium), 10% FBS (heat-inactivated, 30 min at +56°), 1% pen/strep, 1% GlutaMAX.

3. EMEM medium for LS-174T, MCF7 and HT-1080: EMEM (Eagle's minimum essential medium), 10% FBS (heat-inactivated, 30 min at +56°), 1% Pen/Strep, 1% GlutaMAX, 1% MEM NEAA (Minimum essential medium, nonessential amino acids), 1% sodium pyruvate.

4. Human formalin-fixed paraffin embedded (FFPE) samples. FFPE tissue samples from human colon and breast cancer (BioIVT).

5. HEPES.

6. Ultralow-attachment round-bottom 96-well plates.

7. TrypLE express (Gibco).

8. 10% Neutral-buffered formalin (NBF).

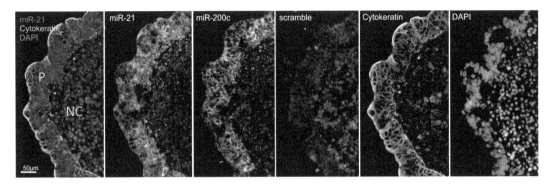

**Fig. 1** LNA-based ISH for microRNA detection in PECS. Sections from PECS (here LS174T cells) were hybridized with LNA probes to miR-21, miR-200c and a scramble probe on three serial sections. The LNA probes were stained with Cy3 (red), and followed by immunohistochemical staining of cytokeratin using Alexa 488 (green). The image segment of the spheroid in the individual figures, shows the periphery (P) with live cells and a necrotic core (NC) mostly with dead cells with loss of cytokeratin. Images were obtained using epifluorescence microscopy, here showing black-and-white (channel) images as presented to facilitate comparison and interpretation. Both miR-21 and miR-200 ISH signals are located in the cytoplasm of live cells in the periphery, whereas the necrotic core area mainly shows autofluorescence

9. HistoGel™ (Thermo Fisher Scientific).

10. LNA™ probe (QIAGEN). In this study we used double-DIG-labeled LNA™ probes specific for MALAT1 and UCA1 designed using Qiagen's design tools (*see* **Note 2**). Other LNA probes tested include miR-21, miR-200c as well as the negative control probe, scramble, *see* [21]. We initially evaluated basal experimental parameters with the LNA probes to miR-21 and miR-200 (Fig. 1) in a variety of PECS.

11. In situ hybridization buffer (microRNA ISH buffer set, QIAGEN).

12. PBS 1×, RNase-free quality.

13. Tween-20 and a 10% solution in RNase-depleted water.

14. RNase-depleted water, for example, RNase-free Milli-Q water (Millipore).

15. 20× SSC buffer, RNase-free quality.

16. Sheep anti-DIG-POD: Diluted 1:400 times in blocking solution.

17. Primary antibody: mouse monoclonal antibody against cytokeratin (Dako-Agilent).

18. Secondary antibody: Alexa 488–conjugated goat anti-mouse (Jackson ImmunoResearch).

19. Tyramine signal amplification (TSA) reagent: for example, TSA–Cy3 (PerkinElmer).

20. Antifade Prolong Gold with DAPI (Invitrogen).

21. SuperFrost® Plus (Thermo Fisher Scientific).

22. For RNase-depleting solution: RNaseZAP, RNase Away, or similar.

23. Proteinase-K buffer: To 900 mL Milli-Q water, add 5 mL of 1 M Tris–HCl (pH 7.4), 2 mL 0.5 M EDTA, and 0.2 mL 5 M NaCl. Adjust volume to 1000 mL.

24. 15 μg/mL Proteinase-K reagent: To 10 mL of 1× proteinase-K buffer, add 7.5 μL proteinase-K stock of 20 mg/mL.

25. 0.1× SSC buffer: To 995 mL Milli-Q water, add 5 mL 20× SSC. The SSC buffer should be autoclaved.

26. 0.1% PBST: to 1 L of PBS (pH 7.4), add 1 mL Tween-20.

27. Blocking solution: To 37.5 mL of Milli-Q water, add 5 mL 1 M Tris–HCl (pH 7.5), 1.5 mL 5 M NaCl, 5 mL fetal bovine serum (FBS), and 100 μL diluted Tween 20 (10% solution).

28. 3% hydrogen peroxide: Add 3 mL of $H_2O_2$ to 80 mL of PBS and make up to 100 mL with PBS.

### 2.2 Equipment

1. Cell culture hood and 37 °C Incubator.

2. Centrifuge for cell culture plates (ROTANTA 460R).

3. Biopsy cassettes.

4. Parafilm.

5. Plastic cryo molds or similar.

6. Microtome.

7. Ethanol and water-resistant marking pen.

8. Hybridizer (Dako).

9. Shandon Sequenza Slide racks (Thermo Scientific).

10. Horizontal humidifying chamber.

11. Glassware: All glassware, including Coplin jars, glass-staining racks, and stacks of cover glass and bottles for buffers, were heat-treated in an oven at 180 °C for 8 h. The items were covered by aluminum foil before being placed in the oven in order to prevent contamination when removing the items afterward.

## 3   Methods

### 3.1   HT29 Cell Spheroid Preparation and Embedding of Cells

1. Culture cell lines at standard conditions (37 °C, 5% $CO_2$, 20% $O_2$), for example in 75 mL culture flasks, in a growth medium recommended by the manufacturer for 7 days. Growth medium used here: DMEM medium for HT-29 and 1BR.3.G and EMEM medium for LS-174T, MCF7, and HT-1080 (*see* Subheading 2.1 for medium composition).

2. Remove the culture medium and wash with PBS. Detach the cells in the culture flask by adding 2 mL of TrypLE to a T75 tissue culture flask for 5–10 min at 37 °C until detached. Add 8 mL culture medium to stop the reactions.

3. Transfer cells to 15 mL tubes and centrifuge for 5 min at 500 × *g*.

4. Resuspend cells in 1 mL culture medium and remove 100µL for cell counting. Count cells manually or use a cell counter.

5. Prepare cell spheroids by seeding 10,000 tumor cells in monoculture or 1:1 coculture with fibroblasts (*see* **Note 1**) in 200µL culture medium per well in ultralow-attachment round-bottom 96-well plates.

6. Spin the well plates at 500 RPM, for 10 min, at 25 °C, and incubate for 7–14 days at standard conditions.

7. Change spheroid culture medium twice a week. When changing media, aspirate 100µL of old media with a multichannel pipette while holding the plate tilted. Add new media slowly on the side of the wells to not disturb the spheroids.

8. Carefully isolate spheroids one-by-one from the wells using a pipette with large opening into a 1.5 mL Eppendorf tube.

9. Wash gently with PBS one time and add 1 mL of 10% NBF for fixation 24–72 h at room temperature.

10. Next day, place the HistoGel (stored at 4 °C) at 60 °C for 30 min until melted.

11. Gently remove the formalin and add PBS for gentle washing.

12. Transfer the spheroids to a piece of parafilm and cover with 100–150µL prewarmed HistoGel. Leave to cool down to room temperature.

**Table 1**
**Steps to follow during dehydration and paraffin embedding of PECS**

| Step | # cycles | Time (min) | Reagent | Temperature |
|------|----------|------------|---------|-------------|
| 1 | 2 | 30 | 70% ethanol | RT |
| 2 | 2 | 30 | 96% ethanol | RT |
| 3 | 2 | 30 | 99% ethanol | RT |
| 4 | 1 | 30 | Xylene | RT |
| 5 | 1 | 60 | Xylene | RT |
| 6 | 1 | 60 | Paraffin | 60 °C |
| 7 | 1 | Over night | Paraffin | 60 °C |

13. Transfer the HistoGel-embedded spheroids using a scalpel to prelabeled paraffin embedding cassettes and run dehydration and paraffin embedding steps (see **Note 3**) as indicated in Table 1.

14. Remove the paraffin embedded spheroids from the cassette and use traditional paraffin embedding molds to obtain the paraffin blocks.

*3.2 Tissue Sections*

1. Prepare the working area for RNA work using RNaseZAP, including bench top, microtome, blade holder, brushes, tweezers, cooling plate, and water bath.

2. Set the cooling plate to $-15\ °C$ and then place the FFPE block on the plate.

3. Fill the warm water bath with RNase-free Milli-Q water and set the temperature to $40–50\ °C$ depending on the type of paraffin used for embedding.

4. Prepare another water bath in an RNase-free Coplin jar containing RNase–free Milli–Q water at room temperature.

5. Insert a new disposable blade in the knife carrier, and place the block in the cassette clamp. Carefully cut sections off the block until spheroids and HistoGel become visible in the sections (see **Note 4**).

6. Cut 6µm sections (see **Note 4**) and place them into a jar with RNase-free Milli-Q water at room temperature, in order to prevent folding. Sections from human cancer FFPE blocks were cut at 5µm thickness.

7. Transfer the slide to a heated water bath of about $40–50\ °C$, in order to avoid folding, then carefully place sections uniformly on separate SuperFrost® Plus glass slides. Allow water to slide away from in between the paraffin section and the glass slide to avoid sections falling off during deparaffinization.

8. Let the slides dry for 2 h at room temperature, draw an outline around of the HistoGel if visible using an ethanol-resistant pen on the back of the slide (see **Note 4**), and store at $4\ °C$ in a dry box containing silica gel.

9. Melt paraffin at $60\ °C$ on the day prior to the ISH experiment and store dry at room temperature.

*3.3 In Situ Hybridization*

1. Deparaffinize slides in xylene and ethanol solutions in Coplin jars ending up in PBS. Place slides in xylene for 15 min (via 2–3 Coplin jars) and then hydrate through ethanol solutions 99% (three Coplin jars), 96% (two Coplin jars), and 70% (two Coplin jars) to PBS (two Coplin jars), 5 min in each jar. In parallel, prepare a water bath and SSC buffer to be heated to $55\ °C$ (or the hybridization temperature).

2. Predigestion of tissue sections is done by applying 300μL/slide of the proteinase-K reagent at 15μg/mL directly on the tissue and incubating for 10–30 min at 37 °C (*see* **Note 5**) in a horizontal humidifying chamber or in a hybridizer.

3. Prepare LNA probes. The LNA™ probe needed is first denatured and then diluted in Qiagen ISH buffer. Example for 1 mL probe solution containing 25 nM LNA™ probe (*see*

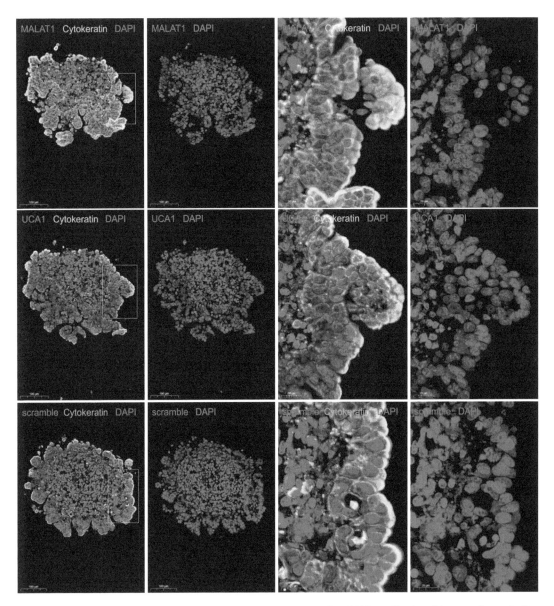

**Fig. 2** Expression of MALAT1 and UCA1 in MCF7 cell spheroids. The MCF7 cell spheroids were formed after 7 days of coculture with fibroblasts. After paraffin embedding, tissue sections were prepared for LNA ISH. The tissue sections were incubated with LNA probes to MALAT1 (10 nM), UCA1 (20 nM) and scramble (20 nM) all at 57 °C, and subsequently for cytokeratin (CK) by immunofluorescence. (Images were obtained using a confocal slide scanner as also described elsewhere [25])

**Note 6**): From a 25µM probe stock, transfer 1µL into a 1.5-mL nonstick Eppendorf tube and place the tube at 90 °C in a block heater for 4 min. Spin down shortly, and immediately add 1 mL ISH buffer into the tube. In the examples in Fig. 2, the MALAT1 probe was prepared at 10 nM, the UCA1 probe at 20 nM, and the scramble probe at 20 nM.

4. Discard the proteinase-K reagent and wash twice with PBS.

5. Remove excess PBS and immediately apply 50µL DIG probe solution and gently shield with cover glass.

6. Place the slides in the hybridizer and start a preset hybridization program for 1 h at 55–57 °C (*see* **Note 7**). The MALAT1 probe is hybridized at 57 °C and the UCA1 probe at 54 °C (Fig. 2).

7. Place slides into 54–57 °C prewarmed 0.1× SSC in a Coplin jar. The cover slides will easily detach. Then transfer slides to another casket with 55 °C prewarmed 0.1× SSC. Wash slides thrice using 55 °C prewarmed 0.1× SSC.

8. Discard the SSC washing buffer and wash twice with PBS in a Coplin jar.

9. Remove PBS and add freshly prepared 3% hydrogen peroxide and incubate at room temperature for 15 min.

10. Transfer slides to PBS-T and mount the slides into Shandon Sequenza® slide racks. Avoid air bubbles during mounting.

11. Incubate 300µL blocking solution for 15 min at room temperature.

12. Detect DIG probes by applying sheep anti-DIG-POD diluted 1:400 in blocking solution and incubate for 30 min at room temperature.

13. Wash each slide with 300µL PBS twice for 2 min.

14. Incubate 150µL freshly prepared TSA–Cy3 reagent for 5–15 min at RT. Protect from light during development.

15. Wash each slide with 300µL PBS once for 2 min.

16. Detection of protein markers is then done by incubating 200µL primary antibody diluted in PBS containing 1% BSA for 30 min at room temperature.

17. Wash each slide thrice with 300µL of PBS.

18. The protein marker antibodies are detected by incubating Alexa 488–conjugated detecting antibody (e.g., anti-mouse) diluted 1:400 in PBS and incubate 150µL on each slide for 30–60 min at room temperature.

19. Wash each slide twice with 300µL of PBS.

20. Mount slides with antifade ProLong Gold containing DAPI. Store slides in dark and at 4 °C. Evaluate staining result after 24 h. Avoid wiping off the circular outline placed on back of the slide.

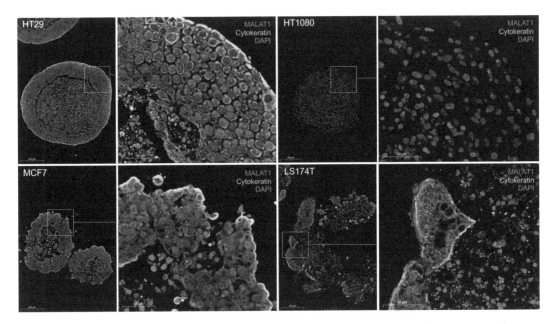

**Fig. 3** Expression of MALAT1 in HT29, MCF7, HT1080, and LS174T cell spheroids. The cell spheroids were formed after 7 days of coculture with fibroblasts, except for the HT29 that were cultured alone. After paraffin embedding, tissue sections were prepared for LNA ISH, and subsequently for cytokeratin (CK) by immunofluorescence. The tissue sections were incubated with LNA probes to MALAT1 (10 nM) at 57 °C. MALAT1 ISH signal is evident in nuclear structures of the cancer cells in all 4 cell spheroids. Cytokeratin is not expressed in the HT1080 fibrosarcoma cell line. (Images were obtained using a confocal slide scanner as also described elsewhere [25])

21. Evaluate slides using epifluorescence microscopy (Fig. 1) or a slide scanner (Figs. 2, 3, 4) with filters allowing detection of Alexa 488, Cy3, and DAPI emission (*see* **Note 8**). Standardize the exposure time according to the optimized intensity for the target probe signal (e.g., MALAT1), and use the same for comparison with staining intensities in the other control sections, including scramble. The spheroid sections are often small and may be difficult to identify or detect, even with the preview camera on the slide scanner. This is facilitated by carefully cleaning the slide surface to remove dust fragments on the slide and by drawing helper points or lines with a pen. For scanning at 20×, we used a Pannoramic Confocal slide scanner (3D-HisTech) equipped with DAPI, FITC, and TRITC filters [25]. Six focal planes were used to provide the projected images in Figs. 2 and 3, where MALAT1 in nuclear speckles are easily detected. In Fig. 4, MALAT1 and UCA probe were applied to human colon and breast cancer, respectively, to allow comparison of expression and localization in genuine human tumors.

22. Considerations on the specificity of the signal are required for the evaluation of ISH results (*see* **Note 6**).

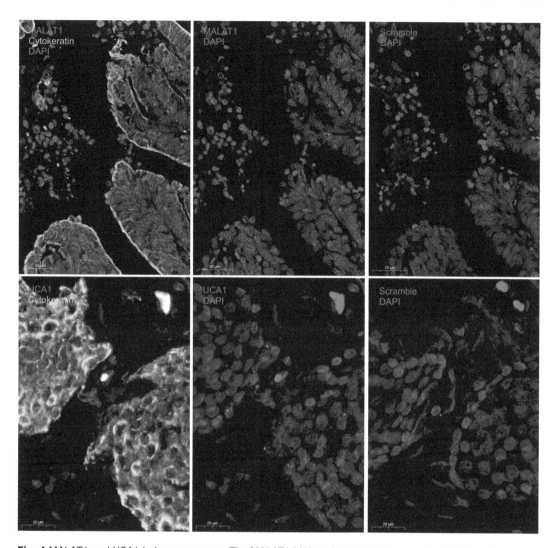

**Fig. 4** MALAT1 and UCA1 in human cancer. The MALAT1 LNA probe (at 5 nM) was submitted to colon cancer FFPE samples and UCA1 LNA probe (at 20 nM) to human breast cancer FFPE samples. After ISH, sections were stained for cytokeratin (CK) by immunofluorescence. The MALAT1 ISH signal is seen in nuclear structures in the cancer cells. The UCA1 ISH signal is seen as a more diffuse nuclear stain in the cancer cells. The scramble probe was added to serial sections using similar experimental conditions, and the images processed identically to the MALAT1 and UCA1 probes, respectively. Thus, the HT29 cancer cell spheroids and MCF7 cancer cell spheroids (Figs. 2 and 3) represent well the expression in genuine human tumors. The exposure time for the MALAT1 ISH signal was significantly shorter than that for UCA1, suggesting that UCA1 expression levels are magnitudes lower than that of MALAT1. The yellow spots (Af) are tissue embedded autofluorescence

## 4    Notes

1. Mixed Cell cultures. We mixed cultured cancer cell lines with normal transformed human skin fibroblasts to facilitate the development of compact and round cancer spheroids

[4]. Between 5000 and 10,000 fibroblasts were added on the first day of spheroid growth. Cells have been tested to be viable after up to 4 weeks of coculture in ULA plates. The effect of adding normal skin fibroblasts into mixed cultures on the growth rate and molecular processes still remains to be characterized.

2. LNA probe design. For a target lncRNA of interest, identify and acquire the FASTA sequence, for example, from GenBank (https://www.ncbi.nlm.nih.gov/genbank/). Go to Qiagen's website to design ISH LNA probes (https://geneglobe. qiagen.com/dk/customize/detection-ish/). Follow the indications on the website, and the design algorithm will suggest a list of LNA probes that subsequently can be ordered with DIG labels or FAM labels. With our experience, it is recommended to obtain at least two different LNA probes to the same target to evaluate which one will perform best. In addition, mixing two (nonoverlapping) LNA probes to the same target transcript may improve sensitivity of the assay.

3. Paraffin Embedding. We present here a manual method for paraffin embedding the cell spheroids. Handling of the small spheroids is facilitated by the HistoGel compound that is not replaced by paraffin during the embedding process, but remain and can be visualized in the embedded sample as a slight orange-colored area.

4. Spheroid sections. We tested both 5 and 6μm thick sections. The spheroids cut at 5μm were often damaged and we therefore set the microtome at 6μm. Place the paraffin sections systematically in the same region of the glass slide to facilitate the identification of the small spheroids in a fluorescence microscope. It can be hard to see the small cell spheroids directly on the glass slides. Here, we suggest to draw an outline on the back of the slide before starting the staining procedure. We have worked around this challenge also in other ways by (1) placing a hematoxylin-stained spheroid together with the unstained during embedding, (2) getting adjacent sections for hematoxylin staining and identify the presence in a bright field microscope, and (3) cutting sections throughout the spheroid and stain every 5th (e.g., sections number 1, 6, 11, and 16) with hematoxylin and retain the remaining for molecular staining, ISH or immunohistochemistry. Discard slides without content of spheroid.

5. Pretreatment with proteinase-K. We tested Proteinase-K treatment at a fixed concentration (15μg/mL) and varied the duration from 0 to 30 min. No ISH signal was seen without pretreatment. The signal intensity was highest after 10 min showing slight decrease at longer duration. Prolonged

Proteinase-K did not deteriorate morphology, which may be beneficial for some target sequences. We did not see any effect of the duration of Proteinase-K treatment on the background staining.

6. LNA probe concentration. It is recommended to test LNA probes in the range from 5 to 50 nM when diluted in the Qiagen hybridization buffer. The probe concentration and the hybridization temperature are strongly inter-related, thus, decreasing the hybridization temperature may be associated with a decreased probe concentration to obtain the best signal-to-background ratio. The background signal is both derived from the probe and from the detection system. This can be clarified using a no-probe (or hybridization buffer only) reference slide.

7. Hybridization temperature. The standard hybridization temperature for LNA probes with $T_m$ of 83–85 °C is 57 °C. For different probes, we test a hybridization temperature range from 52 to 58 °C using the hybridizer/heating plates.

8. Fluorescence assay. The basic double fluorescence assay using green (e.g., FITC, FAM, Cy2, or Alexa Fluor 488) and red (e.g., TRITC, Cy3, Alexa Fluor 555) fluorophores is presented here. Using the TSA technology for DIG-probe detection, the typical green substrate is TSA-FITC and the red substrate is TSA-Cy3. Additional antibody markers can be added, see for example [23].

## Acknowledgments

This study was supported by The Danish Agency for Science and Higher Education.

## References

1. Simiantonaki N, Kurzik-Dumke U, Karyofylli G, Jayasinghe C, Kirkpatrick CJ (2007) Loss of E-cadherin in the vicinity of necrosis in colorectal carcinomas: association with NFkappaB expression. Int J Oncol 31 (2):269–275

2. Koledova Z (2017) 3D Coculture of mammary organoids with fibrospheres: a model for studying epithelial-stromal interactions during mammary branching morphogenesis. Methods Mol Biol 1612:107–124. https://doi.org/10.1007/978-1-4939-7021-6_8

3. Osswald A, Hedrich V, Sommergruber W (2019) 3D-3 tumor models in drug discovery for analysis of immune cell infiltration.

Methods Mol Biol 1953:151–162. https://doi.org/10.1007/978-1-4939-9145-7_10

4. Kuen J, Darowski D, Kluge T, Majety M (2017) Pancreatic cancer cell/fibroblast co-culture induces M2 like macrophages that influence therapeutic response in a 3D model. PLoS One 12(7):e0182039. https://doi.org/10.1371/journal.pone.0182039

5. Kapranov P, Cheng J, Dike S, Nix DA, Duttagupta R, Willingham AT, Stadler PF, Hertel J, Hackermuller J, Hofacker IL, Bell I, Cheung E, Drenkow J, Dumais E, Patel S, Helt G, Ganesh M, Ghosh S, Piccolboni A, Sementchenko V, Tammana H, Gingeras TR (2007) RNA maps reveal new RNA classes and

a possible function for pervasive transcription. Science 316(5830):1484–1488. https://doi.org/10.1126/science.1138341

6. Iyer MK, Niknafs YS, Malik R, Singhal U, Sahu A, Hosono Y, Barrette TR, Prensner JR, Evans JR, Zhao S, Poliakov A, Cao X, Dhanasekaran SM, Wu YM, Robinson DR, Beer DG, Feng FY, Iyer HK, Chinnaiyan AM (2015) The landscape of long noncoding RNAs in the human transcriptome. Nat Genet 47 (3):199–208. https://doi.org/10.1038/ng.3192

7. Khalil AM, Guttman M, Huarte M, Garber M, Raj A, Rivea Morales D, Thomas K, Presser A, Bernstein BE, van Oudenaarden A, Regev A, Lander ES, Rinn JL (2009) Many human large intergenic noncoding RNAs associate with chromatin-modifying complexes and affect gene expression. Proc Natl Acad Sci U S A 106(28):11667–11672. https://doi.org/10.1073/pnas.0904715106

8. Cabili MN, Dunagin MC, McClanahan PD, Biaesch A, Padovan-Merhar O, Regev A, Rinn JL, Raj A (2015) Localization and abundance analysis of human lncRNAs at single-cell and single-molecule resolution. Genome Biol 16:20. https://doi.org/10.1186/s13059-015-0586-4

9. Poulet C, Njock MS, Moermans C, Louis E, Louis R, Malaise M, Guiot J (2020) Exosomal long non-coding RNAs in lung diseases. Int J Mol Sci 21(10):ix76. https://doi.org/10.3390/ijms21103580

10. Meseure D, Vacher S, Lallemand F, Alsibai KD, Hatem R, Chemlali W, Nicolas A, De Koning L, Pasmant E, Callens C, Lidereau R, Morillon A, Bieche I (2016) Prognostic value of a newly identified MALAT1 alternatively spliced transcript in breast cancer. Br J Cancer 114(12):1395–1404. https://doi.org/10.1038/bjc.2016.123

11. Wang C, Zhang Q, Hu Y, Zhu J, Yang J (2019) Emerging role of long non-coding RNA MALAT1 in predicting clinical outcomes of patients with digestive system malignancies: a meta-analysis. Oncol Lett 17(2):2159–2170. https://doi.org/10.3892/ol.2018.9875

12. Arun G, Diermeier S, Akerman M, Chang KC, Wilkinson JE, Hearn S, Kim Y, MacLeod AR, Krainer AR, Norton L, Brogi E, Egeblad M, Spector DL (2016) Differentiation of mammary tumors and reduction in metastasis upon Malat1 lncRNA loss. Genes Dev 30(1):34–51. https://doi.org/10.1101/gad.270959.115

13. Chen Q, Zhu C, Jin Y (2020) The oncogenic and tumor suppressive functions of the long noncoding RNA MALAT1: an emerging controversy. Front Genet 11:93. https://doi.org/10.3389/fgene.2020.00093

14. Arun G, Aggarwal D, Spector DL (2020) MALAT1 long non-coding RNA: functional implications. Noncoding RNA 6(2):22. https://doi.org/10.3390/ncrna6020022

15. Wang XS, Zhang Z, Wang HC, Cai JL, Xu QW, Li MQ, Chen YC, Qian XP, Lu TJ, Yu LZ, Zhang Y, Xin DQ, Na YQ, Chen WF (2006) Rapid identification of UCA1 as a very sensitive and specific unique marker for human bladder carcinoma. Clin Cancer Res 12 (16):4851–4858. https://doi.org/10.1158/1078-0432.CCR-06-0134

16. Han Y, Yang YN, Yuan HH, Zhang TT, Sui H, Wei XL, Liu L, Huang P, Zhang WJ, Bai YX (2014) UCA1, a long non-coding RNA up-regulated in colorectal cancer influences cell proliferation, apoptosis and cell cycle distribution. Pathology 46(5):396–401. https://doi.org/10.1097/PAT.0000000000000125

17. Jiang Y, Du F, Chen F, Qin N, Jiang Z, Zhou J, Jiang T, Pu Z, Cheng Y, Chen J, Dai J, Ma H, Jin G, Hu Z, Yu H, Shen H (2017) Potentially functional variants in lncRNAs are associated with breast cancer risk in a Chinese population. Mol Carcinog 56(9):2048–2057. https://doi.org/10.1002/mc.22659

18. Kalmar A, Nagy ZB, Galamb O, Csabai I, Bodor A, Wichmann B, Valcz G, Bartak BK, Tulassay Z, Igaz P, Molnar B (2019) Genome-wide expression profiling in colorectal cancer focusing on lncRNAs in the adenoma-carcinoma transition. BMC Cancer 19 (1):1059. https://doi.org/10.1186/s12885-019-6180-5

19. Xuan W, Yu H, Zhang X, Song D (2019) Crosstalk between the lncRNA UCA1 and microRNAs in cancer. FEBS Lett 593 (15):1901–1914. https://doi.org/10.1002/1873-3468.13470

20. Soares RJ, Maglieri G, Gutschner T, Diederichs S, Lund AH, Nielsen BS, Holmstrom K (2018) Evaluation of fluorescence in situ hybridization techniques to study long non-coding RNA expression in cultured cells. Nucleic Acids Res 46(1):e4. https://doi.org/10.1093/nar/gkx946

21. James JP, Johnsen L, Moller T, Nielsen BS (2020) MicroRNA in situ hybridization in paraffin-embedded cultured cells. Methods Mol Biol 2148:99–110. https://doi.org/10.1007/978-1-0716-0623-0_6

22. Moller T, James JP, Holmstrom K, Sorensen FB, Lindebjerg J, Nielsen BS (2019) Co-detection of miR-21 and TNF-alpha mRNA in budding cancer cells in colorectal

cancer. Int J Mol Sci 20(8):1907. https://doi.org/10.3390/ijms20081907

23. Nielsen BS, Holmstrom K (2019) Combined MicroRNA in situ hybridization and Immunohistochemical detection of protein markers. Methods Mol Biol 1953:271–286. https://doi.org/10.1007/978-1-4939-9145-7_17

24. Nielsen BS, Moller T, Holmstrom K (2014) Chromogen detection of microRNA in frozen clinical tissue samples using LNA probe technology. Methods Mol Biol 1211:77–84. https://doi.org/10.1007/978-1-4939-1459-3_7

25. Knudsen KN, Lindebjerg J, Kalmar A, Molnar B, Sorensen FB, Hansen TF, Nielsen BS (2018) miR-21 expression analysis in budding colon cancer cells by confocal slide scanning microscopy. Clin Exp Metastasis 35 (8):819–830. https://doi.org/10.1007/s10585-018-9945-3

# Part IV

**Functional Studies To Decipher the Role of Identified LncRNAs**

# Chapter 9

# In Vitro Silencing of lncRNA Expression Using siRNAs

## Meike S. Thijssen, Jennifer Bintz, and Luis Arnes

## Abstract

Recent advances in sequencing technologies have uncovered the existence of thousands of long noncoding RNAs (lncRNAs) with dysregulated expression in cancer. As a result, there is burgeoning interest in understanding their function and biological significance in both homeostasis and disease. RNA interference (RNAi) enables sequence-specific gene silencing and can, in principle, be employed to silence virtually any gene. However, when applied to lncRNAs, it is important to consider current limitations in their annotation and current principles regarding lncRNA regulation and function when assessing their phenotype in cancer cell lines. In this chapter we describe the analysis of lncRNA splicing variant expression, including subcellular localization, transfection of siRNAs in cancer cell lines, and validation of gene silencing by quantitative PCR and single molecule in situ hybridization. All protocols can be performed in a laboratory with essential equipment for cell culture, molecular biology, and imaging.

**Key words** Small interfering RNAs, Long noncoding RNAs, Alternative splicing, Subcellular localization, In situ hybridization, Cancer

## 1 Introduction

A large fraction of the noncoding genome generates various species of noncoding RNAs with largely unknown functions [1]. Among them, lncRNAs have been described as tissue- and cell-type specific, with dysregulated expression during cancer progression [2, 3]. Furthermore, a subset of them overlap with single nucleotide polymorphisms associated with cancer risk, and as more cancer genomes are sequenced, it is to be expected that additional lncRNAs will emerge in genomic regions associated with cancer traits [3–5]. Recent years have seen an explosion of functional studies investigating lncRNA function in a multitude of cellular systems. These studies have highlighted the functional significance of specific lncRNAs in human health and disease [6]. However, as a whole, lncRNAs remain an underexplored set of potential cancer-driving genes, guaranteeing that they will continue to attract attention and form the focus of functional studies for the foreseeable future.

Alfons Navarro (ed.), *Long Non-Coding RNAs in Cancer*, Methods in Molecular Biology, vol. 2348,
https://doi.org/10.1007/978-1-0716-1581-2_9, © Springer Science+Business Media, LLC, part of Springer Nature 2021

There are several genetic tools available to interrogate gene function that can be classified according to the targeted molecule: DNA, RNA or protein (e.g., CRISPR-Cas9, RNAi and the auxin-inducible degron system, respectively) [7, 8]. Amongst existing RNA-targeting methods, RNAi is particularly suitable for silencing lncRNAs, as in principle, it directly exposes the RNA-mediated function(s) of the targeted lncRNA locus, revealing their physiological relevance. This is particularly important if the interrogated lncRNA is located in a locus harboring DNA regulatory elements such as enhancers or boundaries of chromatin domains [9, 10]. However, one should always consider the caveat that interpretation of phenotypes resulting from the use of small interfering RNAs (siRNAs) can be confounded by off-target effects and, as such, parallel analyses using several distinct target-specific siRNAs are crucial [11]. Nevertheless, the technology is evolving rapidly and RNAi-based therapies have recently been approved by the relevant authorities in the clinical setting [12]. These important advances open a window of opportunity to translate the findings in cell lines into preclinical models of cancer and may represent a novel toolset with which to target human malignancies. As we learn more about lncRNAs, it is important to consider relevant characteristics of their regulation and function that may affect the outcome of their silencing with siRNAs.

The starting point of any expression-function analysis for a specific lncRNA is the identification of a locus of interest containing an annotated lncRNA. At present, the lncRNA sequence from most current annotation efforts is reliant upon transcriptome reconstruction of short sequenced reads, which is inherently challenging and typically yields incomplete gene structures (*see* [13] for review). Such challenges are exacerbated when studying lncRNAs, which in general, are expressed in low abundance in a cell-type specific manner and are alternatively spliced compared to coding genes, leading to low coverage and poor gene annotation [14–16]. Furthermore, the exons of lncRNAs tend to be weakly conserved through evolution [17, 18] and the DNA sequence of the lncRNA is not yet informative regarding functional domains within the mature transcript, such as Pfam domains or the open reading frame in protein-coding genes. Recently, the field has seen promising developments in the prediction of lncRNA 3D structure that might inform the presence of functional domains. However, this is still challenging due to the flexible nature of long RNA molecules compared to proteins [19]. Hence, an initial characterization of the lncRNA sequence is key to designing siRNAs targeting the mature transcript in the cell line of interest.

Another important consideration is that lncRNAs can localize to distinct subcellular domains to exert their function (s) [20, 21]. Hence, it is crucial to consider the accessibility of the cellular compartments where the lncRNA is expressed to the RNAi machinery. Moreover, to interpret the phenotype resulting from loss-of-function, it is important that the cellular localization of the lncRNA is consistent with the cellular function(s) perturbed following knockdown. If this is not the case, then observed phenotypes may be attributed to indirect effects of the loss of lncRNA expression, or perhaps off-target effects of the siRNAs.

Overall, many factors can contribute to the efficiency of RNA silencing. Design algorithms are continuously optimizing predicted target efficiency as we continue to acquire insight into RNA structure and RNA–protein interactions. However, when silencing lncRNAs, we should consider that alternative transcripts diverging from the reference annotation may be expressed in the cell line of interest and that their expression is cell-type-specific and restricted to subcellular compartments. In this chapter, we describe a routine analysis to assess the transcript model, the localization of the lncRNA by cellular fractionation, and knockdown validation by two orthogonal methods in our cell line of interest. Here, we compile well-established protocols to conduct a loss-of-function analysis of a candidate lncRNA in a eukaryotic cell line.

## 2    Materials

### 2.1  Manual Annotation of the lncRNA of Interest

1. RNA of appropriate cells/tissue as starting material.
2. SuperScript™ III First-Strand Synthesis System (Thermo Fisher Scientific).
3. DNA oligonucleotides for screening alternative exons.
4. GoTaq DNA polymerase (Promega).
5. QIAquick PCR & Gel Cleanup Kit (QIAGEN).
6. TOPO® TA Cloning® Kit with pCR™II-TOPO® vector (Thermo Fisher Scientific).
7. One Shot chemically competent TOP10 cells (Thermo Fisher Scientific).
8. QIAprep Spin Miniprep Kit (QIAGEN).
9. Nuclease-free water.

### 2.2  Analysis of Cellular Localization in the Relevant Cell Line

1. Cell culture media (DMEM or other, depending on cell type).
2. Phosphatase-buffered saline (PBS): 150 mM NaCl, 10 mM Tris–HCl, pH 7.4.
3. Accutase®.
4. 1 M NaCl solution: add 58.44 g sodium chloride into a 1 L glass bottle. Make up to 1 L with RNase-free water and sterile-filter.

5. 10% Igepal CA-630/NP-40 solution: add 20 mL Igepal CA-630/NP-40 to 150 mL RNase-free water in a 200 mL glass bottle and dissolve using a magnetic stirrer. Make up to 200 mL with RNase-free water and sterile-filter.

6. Cell lysis buffer: 10 mM Tris pH 7.4, 150 mM NaCl, 0.15% Igepal CA-630/NP-40. Fill about 100 mL RNase-free water into a 200 mL glass bottle. Add 30 mL 1 M NaCl solution, 2 mL 1 M Tris pH 7.4 and 3 mL 10% Igepal CA-630/NP-40 solution. Fill up to 200 mL with RNase-free water and sterile-filter.

7. Sucrose buffer: 10 mM Tris pH 7.4, 150 mM NaCl, 24% sucrose. Add 48 g sucrose into a glass bottle. Add 30 mL 1 M NaCl solution and 2 mL 1 M Tris pH 7.4. Add RNase-free water to a volume of around 180 mL and dissolve the sucrose using a magnetic stirrer. Make up to 200 mL with RNase-free water and sterile-filter.

8. TRIzol™ Reagent (Thermo Fisher Scientific).

9. Chloroform.

10. Isopropanol.

11. Nuclease-free water.

12. SuperScript™ III First-Strand Synthesis System (Thermo Fisher Scientific).

13. iQ SYBR Green Supermix (Bio-Rad).

### 2.3 Tissue Culture and Transfection of siRNAs

1. Cell culture media (DMEM or other, depending on cell type).

2. Synthetic siRNA oligonucleotides targeting the lncRNA of interest and positive and negative controls.

3. Lipofectamine 3000 Transfection Reagent (Invitrogen™, Thermofisher Scientific #L3000-015).

4. Refrigerated centrifuge.

### 2.4 Validation of lncRNA Silencing by Quantitative PCR and Single-Molecule In Situ Hybridization

1. TRIzol™ Reagent (Thermo Fisher Scientific).

2. SuperScript™ III First-Strand Synthesis System (Thermo Fisher Scientific).

3. iQ SYBR Green Supermix (Bio-Rad).

## 3  Methods

### 3.1 Manual Annotation of the lncRNA of Interest

1. Obtain the RNA sequence of the lncRNA via your own transcriptome analysis or an updated genome annotation (e.g., GENECODE, NONCODE, RefSeq) (see Note 1). Identify the regions shared between all splice variants (Fig. 1).

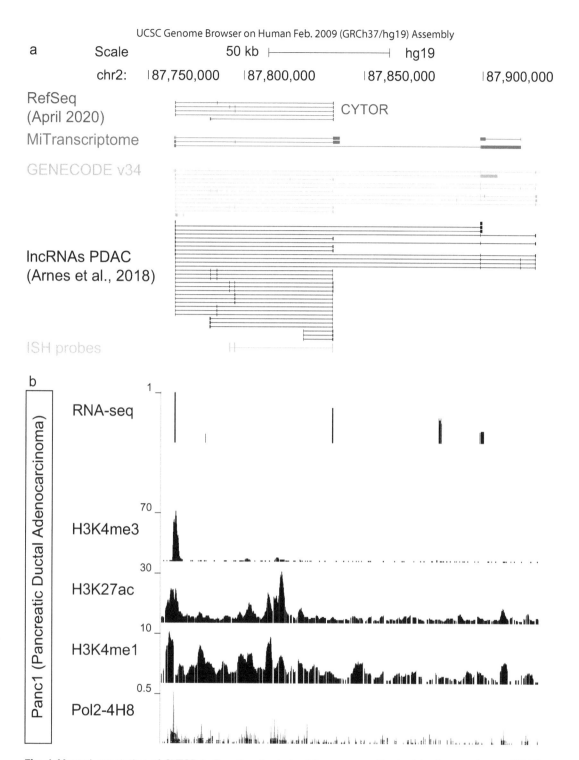

**Fig. 1** Manual annotation of CYTOR in Panc1 cells derived from pancreatic ductal adenocarcinoma (PDAC). (**a**) Snapshot of the CYTOR locus (chr2:87,753,243-87,907,544, GRCh37/hg19), also know as LINC00152, using the UCSC genome browser (*see* **Note 2**) depicting alternative transcript models from RefSeq, MiTranscriptome, GENECODE, and our own transcriptome analysis in PDAC. Besides, the transcript model used to design in situ hybridization probes is depicted as ISH probes. (**b**) Integrative analysis using sequencing datasets in public repositories (ENCODE) in Panc1 cells. The presence of H3K4me3 and pol2-4h8 binding in the first expressed exon (defined by RNA-seq) suggest that this genomic location corresponds to the transcription start site. Besides, the presence of H3K4me1 and H3K27ac could indicate the presence of an enhancer or an enhancer RNA (eRNA). We find that these chromatin modifications are common in lncRNAs

2. Design primers to validate the expression of the lncRNA and identify alternative splicing within the RNA sequence using Primer3. Use flanking PCR with oligonucleotides mapping to the first and last exons of the lncRNA.

3. Isolate RNA from the appropriate cells/tissue and perform first strand cDNA synthesis with 1 μg of RNA (*see* **Note 3**). Dilute the cDNA 1:5 with nuclease-free water.

4. Carry out PCR amplification using flanking primers to identify cell-type-specific alternative splicing (*see* **Note 4**). Run the PCR products with DNA dye on a 2% agarose gel at 90 V to visualize alternative transcripts (if different sizes) amplified with the primers (Fig. 2).

5. To check the sequence of the isoforms, excise the bands from the gel and extract the different products separately from the gel using the QIAquick gel extraction kit following the manufacturer's instructions (*see* **Note 5**).

6. Clone the amplicons into a vector for bacterial amplification using the TOPO® TA Cloning® Kit. Select three colonies from each amplicon and isolate the plasmid using the QIAprep Spin Miniprep Kit following the manufacturer's instructions.

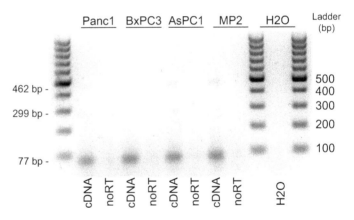

**Fig. 2** Analysis of transcripts model by flanking PCR in relevant cancer cell lines. Here we isolated RNA from a panel of PDAC cell lines and performed RT-PCR using primers to the first (GATCTTCACAGCACAGTTCCT) and last exon (AGCTTC CTGTTTCATCTCCCA ) of the RefSeq splicing variant (chr2:87,754,946-87,821,037; GRCh37/hg19; *see* **Note 4**). The analysis reveals the expression of CYTOR in PDAC cell lines and at least three splicing variants. The amplicons were corroborated to correspond to CYTOR or the paralog MIR4435-2HG by sanger sequencing, consistent with previous analysis in HeLa cells [32]. The analysis is not intended as an exhaustive characterization of CYTOR mature transcript in PDAC cell lines, and additional experiments would be required to determine the presence of the long isoform. noRT: cDNA reaction without reverse transcriptase. $H_2O$: PCR reaction without cDNA. MP2: MiaPaCa2

7. Sequence the obtained plasmid using Sanger sequencing with the M13 reverse primer to obtain the sequence of the inserted fragment.

8. Use an alignment tool (e.g., BLAST) to identify splicing variants expressed by the cell line of interest and supply the sequence to an siRNA-designing tool (*see* **Note 6**).

9. Select several potential siRNAs targeting an exon common to all the splice variants, ensuring no overlap with a coding gene. Occasionally, predesigned and validated siRNAs might be available targeting the gene of interest. In this case, validate that the target sequence is expressed in all potential forms of the lncRNA in the cell line of interest using flanking PCR (*see* **Note 7**).

10. Consider using at least two siRNAs per lncRNA target as well as positive and negative controls (nontargeting [NT] or scrambled siRNAs). If the siRNA contains chemical modifications, the same modifications should apply to the control. For the initial characterization of lncRNA function in cancer cell lines, the smallest size of siRNA (2–5 nmol) will provide sufficient material to assess knockdown efficiency and preliminary phenotypic analysis.

***3.2  Analysis of Cellular Localization in the Relevant Cell Line (Adapted from [22])***

1. All buffers should be chilled on ice, centrifugation steps carried out at 4 °C and samples kept on ice throughout the protocol. It is crucial to maintain RNase-free working conditions throughout.

2. Plate cells in 10 cm culture dishes with the appropriate growth medium (e.g., DMEM) and grow them to 70–90% confluency (Fig. 3a).

3. Prepare the buffers needed for the fractionation protocol. Each sample from a 10 cm dish requires 400 μL cell lysis buffer and 1 mL sucrose buffer (*see* **Note 8**).

4. Aspirate the medium from the cultured cells, wash them with PBS and aspirate the liquid again.

5. Add 2 mL Accutase to the cells and incubate at 37 °C for 5 min in a 5% $CO_2$ incubator (*see* **Note 9**).

6. Add 10 mL culture medium (e.g., DMEM) and transfer the sample to a 15 mL Falcon tube.

7. Centrifuge the tube at $200 \times g$ for 5 min and aspirate the supernatant.

8. Resuspend the cell pellet in 5 mL PBS and centrifuge again at $200 \times g$ for 5 min. Aspirate the supernatant.

9. Resuspend the cell pellet in 1 mL PBS. Transfer the sample to a 1.5 mL Eppendorf tube.

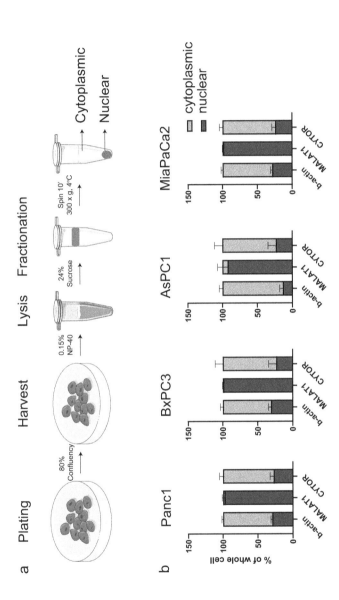

**Fig. 3** Analysis of cellular localization of CYTOR in PDAC cell lines. (**a**) Cellular fractionation protocol: cells were plated and grown to 80% confluency (time was different per cell line), after which cells were harvested. NP-40/Igepal buffer was used for the specific lysis of plasma membranes, but not nuclear membranes. The sucrose buffer enabled separation of the fractions after centrifugation: the pellet is the nuclear fraction and the supernatant is the cytoplasmic fraction. (**b**) The expression of CYTOR (LINC00152), β-actin (cytoplasmic control) and MALAT1 (nuclear control) in both fractions was measured by qPCR. The nuclear-cytoplasmic localization profile of CYTOR resembles that of β-actin, which means that its transcripts are mostly located in the cytoplasm, but around 25% is nuclear. Transcript localization is similar for all PDAC cell lines studied. $n = 3$ for all conditions and all cell lines

10. Centrifuge the sample at $200 \times g$ for 2 min. Carefully pipet off the supernatant and discard.

11. Resuspend the cell pellet in 400 µL cell lysis buffer by gently pipetting up and down five times (*see* **Note 10**). Incubate the samples on ice for 5 min.

12. Prepare 1.5 mL Eppendorf tubes containing 1 mL chilled sucrose buffer and keep them on ice.

13. Transfer the cell lysate to the Eppendorf tube containing 1 mL sucrose buffer by carefully adding it on top of the sucrose buffer (*see* **Note 11**).

14. Centrifuge the sample for 10 min at $3500 \times g$. Following centrifugation, the pellet comprises the nuclear fraction and the supernatant is the cytoplasmic fraction.

15. Collect all supernatant (cytoplasmic fraction) in a new Eppendorf tube and centrifuge for 1 min at $14,000 \times g$ (*see* **Note 12**). Transfer the supernatant to a new Eppendorf tube.

16. Transfer 200 µL of the cytoplasmic fraction to a new Eppendorf tube and add 1 mL TRIzol for RNA extraction. The remaining cytoplasmic fraction can be stored at $-80\ °C$.

17. Resuspend the nuclear pellet (from **step 14**) also in 1 mL TRIzol for RNA extraction and store the samples at $-80\ °C$ until RNA extraction.

18. To extract the RNA, add 200 µL of chloroform to the TRIzol sample, mix and centrifuge for 15 min at $12,000 \times g$. Transfer the aqueous upper phase to an Eppendorf tube with 500 µL isopropanol, mix and centrifuge for 10 min at $12,000 \times g$. Mix 300 µL 70% ethanol with the RNA pellet and centrifuge for 5 min at $12,000 \times g$. After air-drying the pellet, resuspend it in 20 µL RNase-free water and measure RNA concentration.

19. Use 1 µg of RNA to perform first strand cDNA synthesis. Dilute the cDNA (1:5) with nuclease-free water.

20. These cDNA samples are used to measure the expression of the RNA of interest in both nuclear and cytoplasmic fractions by qPCR. Use beta-actin and MALAT1 as cytoplasmic and nuclear controls, respectively (*see* **Note 13**). Localization can be expressed as the percentage of total RNA expression within the nuclear and cytoplasmic fractions (Fig. 3b).

21. The efficiency of siRNA-mediated knockdown may be compromised when silencing lncRNAs enriched in the nucleus (*see* **Note 14**). For such lncRNAs, consider using antisense oligonucleotides (ASOs) as a superior alternative (*see* **Note 15**) [23].

*3.3 Tissue Culture and Transfection of siRNAs*

1. Plate cells in 12-well plates with 100,000 cells per well with the appropriate growth medium (e.g., DMEM) and allow them to attach to the plate for at least 12 (but optimally 24) hours (h).

2. Prepare a transfection mix for a final concentration of 5 nM siRNA per well. Per 100 μL MEM medium, add 0.5μL siRNA, vortex and incubate for 5 min at room temperature (RT). Subsequently, add 1–3 μL Lipofectamine, vortex, and incubate for 15 min at RT (*see* **Note 16**).

3. For a 12-well plate, ensure that there is 400 μL appropriate culture medium (e.g., DMEM) per well. Add 100 μL siRNA mastermix to each well without vortexing before use so as not to disrupt the formed lipofectamine-siRNA complexes.

4. When using the siRNA for knockdown for the first time, harvest the cells at various timepoints to study the knockdown efficiency. 12 h, 24 h, 36 h, 48 h, and 72 h post-transfection are suitable timepoints for analysis (*see* **Note 17**).

5. For harvesting, wash the cells with PBS, add 500 μL PBS per well and scrape the cells from the plate. Transfer the samples to Eppendorf tubes and centrifuge at $200 \times g$ for 5 min. Aspirate the supernatant and add 300 μL TRIzol per sample/tube.

*3.4 Confirmation of lncRNA Knockdown by Quantitative RT-PCR and Single-Molecule In Situ Hybridization*

1. Use 1 μg of RNA to perform first strand cDNA synthesis. Dilute the cDNA (1:5) with nuclease-free water.

2. Measure the expression of the lncRNA of interest with appropriate primers using qPCR (Fig. 4a).

3. Normalize the lncRNA expression to that of the housekeeping gene and compare expression in the presence of the siRNA to that in the NT-siRNA condition as control. One should aim for a decrease in expression of the lncRNA of at least 70% compared to NT control cells.

4. The timepoint showing the lowest lncRNA expression in the siRNA-targeted cells compared to the NT control cells serves as the best timepoint for further functional experiments. NT siRNA conditions should be consistently incorporated as controls for all analyses.

5. In addition to qPCR, siRNA-mediated knockdown efficiency can also be determined through orthogonal methods such as single molecule RNA fluorescence in situ hybridization (Fig. 4b; *see* **Note 18**). The visualization of lncRNAs using RNA-FISH is extensively covered in other chapters in this volume (*see* Chapter 8).

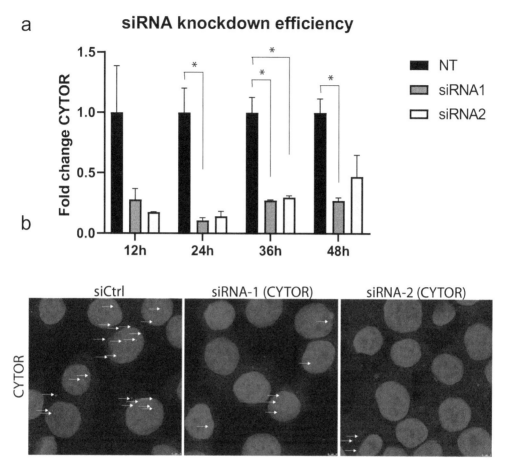

**Fig. 4** Confirmation of lncRNA knockdown by qPCR and single molecule in situ hybridization. (**a**) PANC1 cells are transfected with 5 nM NT siRNA, siRNA1 or siRNA2 targeting the last exon of CYTOR (predesigned silencer select siRNA). After 12 h, 24 h, 36 h, and 48 h, cells of all conditions are harvested, after which RNA extraction, cDNA synthesis and qPCR are carried out. CYTOR expression seems reduced at all timepoints, but knockdown seems most efficient after 24 h. CYTOR siRNA results are compared to NT siRNA as negative control. Data are represented as mean ± SEM with $n = 2$ and expression levels are normalized by housekeeping gene TBP. Statistical significance is determined with an unpaired multiple $t$-test, where $p < 0.05 =$ *. (**b**) In situ hybridization for CYTOR visualizes punctae (white arrows) in both nucleus and cytoplasm. This suggests that the protocol is able to visualize CYTOR transcripts; however, in low amounts meaning that localization of the transcript cannot be confidently confirmed. CYTOR expression is downregulated after knockdown with siRNA1 or siRNA2 respectively. Probes are stained with OPAL™ 570 (red) and nuclei are counterstained with DAPI (blue). Images are captured with ×63 objective

# 4    Notes

1. To manually annotate the mature sequence of the lncRNA of interest, integrate experimental evidence from independent sources preferably relating to the cell line of interest. There is a wealth of data available in public repositories such as ENCODE (https://www.encodeproject.org) and FANTOM

(http://fantom.gsc.riken.jp). Map the transcriptional start site with ChIP-seq data from epigenetic modifications associated with promoters (e.g., H3K4me3) or Cap analysis of gene expression (CAGE-seq). The polyadenylation site can be used to map the $3'$ end cleavage of polyadenylated lncRNAs [24]. If available, long read sequencing will provide the splicing variants [25, 26].

2. There are several human genome reference assemblies (or builds). The genome coordinates differ between assemblies; therefore, it is crucial that all dataset used in the analysis are from the same reference genome. For experienced users, it is possible to switch between reference genomes (e.g., LiftOver tool or remapping the data from raw files). In the example, we used GRCh37/hg19 assembly as the reference genome to be able to integrate ChIP-seq data from ENCODE in Panc1 cells, our cell line of interest.

3. To capture both polyadenylated and nonpolyadenylated lncRNAs, perform first strand cDNA synthesis using an equal mixture of random hexamers and poly-dT oligonucleotides. In addition, for low-abundance targets, lncRNA-specific primers might help to enrich the transcripts of interest and splicing variants.

4. To exclude possible DNA contamination of the RNA isolation, include a control with no reverse transcriptase in the first strand cDNA synthesis (a "noRT" control).

5. To increase the yield of the gel extraction, run several PCR reactions in parallel then combine the corresponding products from the replicate PCR reactions on one column.

6. There are several siRNA design websites available from both commercial and noncommercial sources (www.thermofisher.com; www.idtdna.com; www.horizondiscovery.com). Targeting intronic sequences is rarely effective, typically resulting in poor gene silencing.

7. If available for the specific lncRNA of interest, predesigned siRNAs have been validated and screened using off-target prediction algorithms. Use at least two independent siRNAs targeting the lncRNA of interest.

8. Prepare volumes of buffers in excess of those required for the number of samples processed. Buffers can be stored at 4 °C for a prolonged period, but protocol performance is optimal and most consistent with freshly prepared buffers.

9. The trypsin alternative Accutase is used to detach the cells in this protocol. Alternatively, or when cells are not fully detached after incubation, the cells can be scraped from the plates.

10. Incubation with cell lysis buffer containing Igepal CA-630/NP-40 disrupts the plasma membrane while leaving the nuclear membrane intact.

11. The sucrose buffer is used to separate and clean the nuclei and cytoplasmic fraction of the cells. This buffer has a higher density than the cell lysate, so the cell lysate should form a visible layer on top of the sucrose buffer.

12. This additional high-speed centrifugation step is incorporated in the protocol to separate the cytoplasmic fraction from remaining contamination sometimes evident as floating material.

13. Beta-actin is used as cytoplasmic control and MALAT1 as nuclear control to verify the efficiency of the fractionation. The fraction of beta-actin in the nucleus should not be higher than 35% and the fraction of MALAT1 in the cytoplasm should only be around 1%.

14. Although siRNA silencing is more efficient with cytoplasmic lncRNAs, silencing of nuclear lncRNAs with siRNAs is possible and is consistent with the localization of the RNAi machinery in the nucleus [27, 28].

15. Nuclear lncRNAs are preferentially silenced with ASOs that utilize cellular ribonuclease H (RNaseH) to cleave target RNAs. However, ASOs can induce premature transcription termination, and thus this should always be considered when interpreting a phenotype resulting from their use [29]. This is particularly relevant if silencing of the lncRNA affects the expression of neighboring genes. Ultimately, validation of any phenotype will require multiple and independent approaches (*see* [30] for review).

16. Transfection of high concentrations of siRNA can potentially result in off-target effects mediated by overloading the endogenous RNAi machinery. As a rule of thumb, we avoid using more than 10 nM, preferably 5 nM, of Silencer Select siRNAs (Thermo Fisher Scientific) [31].

17. Upon first working with siRNAs or a cell line, it is recommended to optimize transfection conditions using fluorescently labeled siRNAs acquired from commercial vendors. Using this approach, one can ascertain the lowest effective Lipofectamine 3000 concentration to use by determining the lowest amount of Lipofectamine 3000 reagent at which the majority of cells incorporate the siRNA based upon a positive fluorescent signal.

18. We have used probes from Stellaris and Advanced Cell Diagnostics (ACD), who provide all the materials and reagents and assist with the design of the probes for the RNA of interest. They also have detailed protocol manuals and excellent technical support.

## Acknowledgments

We thank Philip Allan Seymour and Mohamed Osman, members of the Arnes laboratory, for technical assistance and critical reading of the manuscript. The Novo Nordisk Foundation Center for Stem Cell Biology is supported by grant number NNF17CC0027852.

## References

1. Djebali S, Davis CA, Merkel A, Dobin A, Lassmann T, Mortazavi A, Tanzer A, Lagarde J, Lin W, Schlesinger F, Xue C, Marinov GK, Khatun J, Williams BA, Zaleski C, Rozowsky J, Roder M, Kokocinski F, Abdelhamid RF, Alioto T, Antoshechkin I, Baer MT, Bar NS, Batut P, Bell K, Bell I, Chakrabortty S, Chen X, Chrast J, Curado J, Derrien T, Drenkow J, Dumais E, Dumais J, Duttagupta R, Falconnet E, Fastuca M, Fejes-Toth K, Ferreira P, Foissac S, Fullwood MJ, Gao H, Gonzalez D, Gordon A, Gunawardena H, Howald C, Jha S, Johnson R, Kapranov P, King B, Kingswood C, Luo OJ, Park E, Persaud K, Preall JB, Ribeca P, Risk B, Robyr D, Sammeth M, Schaffer L, See LH, Shahab A, Skancke J, Suzuki AM, Takahashi H, Tilgner H, Trout D, Walters N, Wang H, Wrobel J, Yu Y, Ruan X, Hayashizaki Y, Harrow J, Gerstein M, Hubbard T, Reymond A, Antonarakis SE, Hannon G, Giddings MC, Ruan Y, Wold B, Carninci P, Guigo R, Gingeras TR (2012) Landscape of transcription in human cells. Nature 489 (7414):101–108. https://doi.org/10.1038/nature11233

2. Cabili MN, Trapnell C, Goff L, Koziol M, Tazon-Vega B, Regev A, Rinn JL (2011) Integrative annotation of human large intergenic noncoding RNAs reveals global properties and specific subclasses. Genes Dev 25 (18):1915–1927. https://doi.org/10.1101/gad.17446611

3. Iyer MK, Niknafs YS, Malik R, Singhal U, Sahu A, Hosono Y, Barrette TR, Prensner JR, Evans JR, Zhao S, Poliakov A, Cao X, Dhanasekaran SM, Wu YM, Robinson DR, Beer DG, Feng FY, Iyer HK, Chinnaiyan AM (2015) The landscape of long noncoding RNAs in the human transcriptome. Nat Genet 47 (3):199–208. https://doi.org/10.1038/ng. 3192

4. Hon CC, Ramilowski JA, Harshbarger J, Bertin N, Rackham OJ, Gough J, Denisenko E, Schmeier S, Poulsen TM, Severin J, Lizio M, Kawaji H, Kasukawa T,

Itoh M, Burroughs AM, Noma S, Djebali S, Alam T, Medvedeva YA, Testa AC, Lipovich L, Yip CW, Abugessaisa I, Mendez M, Hasegawa A, Tang D, Lassmann T, Heutink P, Babina M, Wells CA, Kojima S, Nakamura Y, Suzuki H, Daub CO, de Hoon MJ, Arner E, Hayashizaki Y, Carninci P, Forrest AR (2017) An atlas of human long non-coding RNAs with accurate 5′ ends. Nature 543(7644):199–204. https://doi.org/10.1038/nature21374

5. Rheinbay E, Nielsen MM, Abascal F, Wala JA, Shapira O, Tiao G, Hornshoj H, Hess JM, Juul RI, Lin Z, Feuerbach L, Sabarinathan R, Madsen T, Kim J, Mularoni L, Shuai S, Lanzos A, Herrmann C, Maruvka YE, Shen C, Amin SB, Bandopadhayay P, Bertl J, Boroevich KA, Busanovich J, Carlevaro-Fita J, Chakravarty D, Chan CWY, Craft D, Dhingra P, Diamanti K, Fonseca NA, Gonzalez-Perez A, Guo Q, Hamilton MP, Haradhvala NJ, Hong C, Isaev K, Johnson TA, Juul M, Kahles A, Kahraman A, Kim Y, Komorowski J, Kumar K, Kumar S, Lee D, Lehmann KV, Li Y, Liu EM, Lochovsky L, Park K, Pich O, Roberts ND, Saksena G, Schumacher SE, Sidiropoulos N, Sieverling L, Sinnott-Armstrong N, Stewart C, Tamborero D, Tubio JMC, Umer HM, Uuskula-Reimand L, Wadelius C, Wadi L, Yao X, Zhang CZ, Zhang J, Haber JE, Hobolth A, Imielinski M, Kellis M, Lawrence MS, von Mering C, Nakagawa H, Raphael BJ, Rubin MA, Sander C, Stein LD, Stuart JM, Tsunoda T, Wheeler DA, Johnson R, Reimand J, Gerstein M, Khurana E, Campbell PJ, Lopez-Bigas N, Weischenfeldt J, Beroukhim R, Martincorena I, Pedersen JS, Getz G, Drivers P, Functional Interpretation Working G, Group PSVW, Consortium P (2020) Analyses of non-coding somatic drivers in 2,658 cancer whole genomes. Nature 578 (7793):102–111. https://doi.org/10.1038/s41586-020-1965-x

6. Quek XC, Thomson DW, Maag JL, Bartonicek N, Signal B, Clark MB, Gloss BS, Dinger ME (2015) lncRNAdb v2.0: expanding the reference database for functional long

noncoding RNAs. Nucleic Acids Res 43(Database issue):D168–D173. https://doi.org/10.1093/nar/gku988

7. Housden BE, Muhar M, Gemberling M, Gersbach CA, Stainier DY, Seydoux G, Mohr SE, Zuber J, Perrimon N (2017) Loss-of-function genetic tools for animal models: cross-species and cross-platform differences. Nat Rev Genet 18(1):24–40. https://doi.org/10.1038/nrg.2016.118

8. Lin A, Sheltzer JM (2020) Discovering and validating cancer genetic dependencies: approaches and pitfalls. Nat Rev Genet 21(11):671–682. https://doi.org/10.1038/s41576-020-0247-7

9. Gil N, Ulitsky I (2019) Regulation of gene expression by cis-acting long non-coding RNAs. Nat Rev Genet 21:102–117. https://doi.org/10.1038/s41576-019-0184-5

10. Amaral PP, Leonardi T, Han N, Vire E, Gascoigne DK, Arias-Carrasco R, Buscher M, Pandolfini L, Zhang A, Pluchino S, Maracaja-Coutinho V, Nakaya HI, Hemberg M, Shiekhattar R, Enright AJ, Kouzarides T (2018) Genomic positional conservation identifies topological anchor point RNAs linked to developmental loci. Genome Biol 19(1):32. https://doi.org/10.1186/s13059-018-1405-5

11. Stojic L, Lun ATL, Mangei J, Mascalchi P, Quarantotti V, Barr AR, Bakal C, Marioni JC, Gergely F, Odom DT (2018) Specificity of RNAi, LNA and CRISPRi as loss-of-function methods in transcriptional analysis. Nucleic Acids Res 46(12):5950–5966. https://doi.org/10.1093/nar/gky437

12. Adams D, Gonzalez-Duarte A, O'Riordan WD, Yang CC, Ueda M, Kristen AV, Tournev I, Schmidt HH, Coelho T, Berk JL, Lin KP, Vita G, Attarian S, Plante-Bordeneuve-V, Mezei MM, Campistol JM, Buades J, Brannagan TH 3rd, Kim BJ, Oh J, Parman Y, Sekijima Y, Hawkins PN, Solomon SD, Polydefkis M, Dyck PJ, Gandhi PJ, Goyal S, Chen J, Strahs AL, Nochur SV, Sweetser MT, Garg PP, Vaishnaw AK, Gollob JA, Suhr OB (2018) Patisiran, an RNAi therapeutic, for hereditary transthyretin amyloidosis. New England J Med 379(1):11–21. https://doi.org/10.1056/NEJMoa1716153

13. Uszczynska-Ratajczak B, Lagarde J, Frankish A, Guigo R, Johnson R (2018) Towards a complete map of the human long non-coding RNA transcriptome. Nat Rev Genet 19(9):535–548. https://doi.org/10.1038/s41576-018-0017-y

14. Mele M, Mattioli K, Mallard W, Shechner DM, Gerhardinger C, Rinn JL (2017) Chromatin environment, transcriptional regulation, and splicing distinguish lincRNAs and mRNAs. Genome Res 27(1):27–37. https://doi.org/10.1101/gr.214205.116

15. Deveson IW, Brunck ME, Blackburn J, Tseng E, Hon T, Clark TA, Clark MB, Crawford J, Dinger ME, Nielsen LK, Mattick JS, Mercer TR (2018) Universal alternative splicing of noncoding exons. Cell Syst 6(2):245–255. e245. https://doi.org/10.1016/j.cels.2017.12.005

16. Mattioli K, Volders PJ, Gerhardinger C, Lee JC, Maass PG, Mele M, Rinn JL (2019) High-throughput functional analysis of lncRNA core promoters elucidates rules governing tissue specificity. Genome Res 29(3):344–355. https://doi.org/10.1101/gr.242222.118

17. Nitsche A, Rose D, Fasold M, Reiche K, Stadler PF (2015) Comparison of splice sites reveals that long noncoding RNAs are evolutionarily well conserved. RNA 21(5):801–812. https://doi.org/10.1261/rna.046342.114

18. Hezroni H, Koppstein D, Schwartz MG, Avrutin A, Bartel DP, Ulitsky I (2015) Principles of long noncoding RNA evolution derived from direct comparison of transcriptomes in 17 species. Cell Rep 11(7):1110–1122. https://doi.org/10.1016/j.celrep.2015.04.023

19. Kim DN, Thiel BC, Mrozowich T, Hennelly SP, Hofacker IL, Patel TR, Sanbonmatsu KY (2020) Zinc-finger protein CNBP alters the 3-D structure of lncRNA Braveheart in solution. Nat Commun 11(1):148. https://doi.org/10.1038/s41467-019-13942-4

20. Mas-Ponte D, Carlevaro-Fita J, Palumbo E, Hermoso Pulido T, Guigo R, Johnson R (2017) LncATLAS database for subcellular localization of long noncoding RNAs. RNA 23(7):1080–1087. https://doi.org/10.1261/rna.060814.117

21. Cabili MN, Dunagin MC, McClanahan PD, Biaesch A, Padovan-Merhar O, Regev A, Rinn JL, Raj A (2015) Localization and abundance analysis of human lncRNAs at single-cell and single-molecule resolution. Genome Biol 16:20. https://doi.org/10.1186/s13059-015-0586-4

22. Conrad T, Orom UA (2017) Cellular fractionation and isolation of chromatin-associated RNA. Methods Mol Biol 1468:1–9. https://doi.org/10.1007/978-1-4939-4035-6_1

23. Lennox KA, Behlke MA (2016) Cellular localization of long non-coding RNAs affects silencing by RNAi more than by antisense oligonucleotides. Nucleic Acids Res 44

(2):863–877. https://doi.org/10.1093/nar/gkv1206

24. Herrmann CJ, Schmidt R, Kanitz A, Artimo P, Gruber AJ, Zavolan M (2020) PolyASite 2.0: a consolidated atlas of polyadenylation sites from 3′ end sequencing. Nucleic Acids Res 48(D1): D174–D179. https://doi.org/10.1093/nar/gkz918

25. Lagarde J, Uszczynska-Ratajczak B, Carbonell S, Perez-Lluch S, Abad A, Davis C, Gingeras TR, Frankish A, Harrow J, Guigo R, Johnson R (2017) High-throughput annotation of full-length long noncoding RNAs with capture long-read sequencing. Nat Genet 49 (12):1731–1740. https://doi.org/10.1038/ng.3988

26. Sharon D, Tilgner H, Grubert F, Snyder M (2013) A single-molecule long-read survey of the human transcriptome. Nat Biotechnol 31 (11):1009–1014. https://doi.org/10.1038/nbt.2705

27. Ntini E, Louloupi A, Liz J, Muino JM, Marsico A, Orom UAV (2018) Long ncRNA A-ROD activates its target gene DKK1 at its release from chromatin. Nat Commun 9 (1):1636. https://doi.org/10.1038/s41467-018-04100-3

28. Gagnon KT, Li L, Chu Y, Janowski BA, Corey DR (2014) RNAi factors are present and active

in human cell nuclei. Cell Rep 6(1):211–221. https://doi.org/10.1016/j.celrep.2013.12.013

29. Lee JS, Mendell JT (2020) Antisense-mediated transcript knockdown triggers premature transcription termination. Mol Cell 77 (5):1044–1054. e1043. https://doi.org/10.1016/j.molcel.2019.12.011

30. Kopp F, Mendell JT (2018) Functional classification and experimental dissection of long noncoding RNAs. Cell 172(3):393–407. https://doi.org/10.1016/j.cell.2018.01.011

31. Grimm D, Streetz KL, Jopling CL, Storm TA, Pandey K, Davis CR, Marion P, Salazar F, Kay MA (2006) Fatality in mice due to oversaturation of cellular microRNA/short hairpin RNA pathways. Nature 441(7092):537–541. https://doi.org/10.1038/nature04791

32. Notzold L, Frank L, Gandhi M, Polycarpou-Schwarz M, Gross M, Gunkel M, Beil N, Erfle H, Harder N, Rohr K, Trendel J, Krijgsveld J, Longerich T, Schirmacher P, Boutros M, Erhardt S, Diederichs S (2017) The long non-coding RNA LINC00152 is essential for cell cycle progression through mitosis in HeLa cells. Sci Rep 7(1):2265. https://doi.org/10.1038/s41598-017-02357-0

# Chapter 10

# In Vitro Silencing of lncRNAs Using LNA GapmeRs

**Elisa Taiana, Vanessa Favasuli, Domenica Ronchetti, Eugenio Morelli, Pierfrancesco Tassone, Giuseppe Viglietto, Nikhil C. Munshi, Antonino Neri, and Nicola Amodio**

## Abstract

Despite substantial advancements have been achieved in the identification of long noncoding RNA (lncRNA) molecules, many challenges still remain into their functional characterization. Loss-of-function approaches are needed to study oncogenic lncRNAs, which appear more difficult to knock down by RNA interference as compared to mRNAs. In this chapter, we present a protocol based on the use of a novel class of antisense oligonucleotides, named locked nucleic acid (LNA) GapmeRs, to inhibit the oncogenic lncRNA NEAT1 in multiple myeloma cells. Overall, this approach holds many advantages, including its possible independence from delivery reagents as well as the capability to knock down lncRNAs even in hard-to-transfect suspension cells, like hematopoietic cells.

**Key words** ncRNA, lncRNA, ASO, LNA-GapmeR, Electroporation, Gymnosis, Multiple myeloma cells

## 1 Introduction

Since they cover the 98.5% of the whole human transcriptome, it is not surprising that non-coding RNAs (ncRNAs) are critically involved in any physiologic and pathologic process [1]. These molecules can be roughly divided in two major classes, that is, short (<200 nucleotides) noncoding (sncRNAs) and long (>200 nucleotides) noncoding RNAs (lncRNAs). The latter comprise a heterogeneous and pleiotropic group of molecules devoid of protein-coding capacity, exerting diverse functions, including in *cis* or in *trans* transcriptional regulation, organization of nuclear domains as well as physical and functional partnering with proteins or RNAs [2, 3].

LncRNAs have been linked to all the hallmarks of cancer, acting either as oncogenes, which are often overexpressed, or tumor suppressors, which are instead downregulated in human neoplasias [4].

Alfons Navarro (ed.), *Long Non-Coding RNAs in Cancer*, Methods in Molecular Biology, vol. 2348,
https://doi.org/10.1007/978-1-0716-1581-2_10, © Springer Science+Business Media, LLC, part of Springer Nature 2021

Tissue specificity of lncRNAs has prompted the development of selective approaches for their therapeutic targeting [5]. In this regard, RNA interference has represented the first strategy to inhibit lncRNAs through a RISC-mediated degradation. However, due to the extensive secondary structure or the possible nuclear localization, lncRNAs may become inaccessible to siRNAs, making antisense oligonucleotides (ASOs) the most valuable strategy for targeting [6].

ASOs are small RNA/DNA-based oligonucleotides capable to cross the cell membrane, selectively capable of binding to RNA through the Watson–Crick hybridization criteria [6]. Most of ASOs are double-stranded oligonucleotides that use the RISC complex to induce RNA degradation, or single-stranded oligonucleotides inhibiting RNA function through different mechanisms, such as alteration of RNA splicing, degradation by RNase H, inhibition of $5'$ cap formation and steric blockade of protein translation. Advantages of ASOs over siRNAs include their independence on the RISC machinery, higher specificity and reduced off-target effects. Chemical modifications have been introduced to overcome some constraints, like off-target or toxic effects, high vulnerability to degradation by exo- and endonucleases, low affinity for the target, and poor tissue uptake. These ASO modifications are referred to as first generation, and include a change in the phosphodiester with a phosphorothioate bond, that protects the oligonucleotide from degradation and increases the binding to receptor sites or plasma proteins [7]; conversely, second-generation modifications refer to changes in the sugar moiety of the nucleobase which increases the binding affinity to the target [8]. The most relevant second-generation modification is the LNA (locked nucleic acid) [9], a class of nucleic acid analogs with Watson–Crick base-pairing rules toward complementary DNA and RNA, and having unprecedented binding affinity. LNA oligonucleotides contain modified RNA nucleotides with an extra bridge linking the $2'$-O and $4'$-C atoms thus "locking" the ribose ring. This leads to an increased affinity for complementary RNA targets, without loss of sequence specificity [10]. The superior performance of single-stranded LNA-ASOs, especially for in vivo applications, is becoming widely recognized in various diseases including cancer [11]. Notably, some of these LNA-ASOs have been tested in clinical trials with encouraging results for future clinical [12]. LNA GapmeRs are single-stranded ASOs to the targeted RNA, normally around 15 nucleotides in length, with the most $5'$ and $3'$ stretch of nucleotides "locked," leaving the middle stretch as unmodified DNA nucleotides. Upon binding of the LNA GapmeR to RNA, the central unmodified nucleotides form a DNA/RNA duplex that is recognized and cleaved by RNase H, effectively degrading the target RNA [13, 14]. Given that RNase H is ubiquitously expressed both in the nucleus and the cytoplasm, LNA GapmeRs are able to target any RNA molecule regardless of intracellular location.

One significant advantage of LNA GapmeR compared to other ASOs is also the passive uptake at low micromolar concentrations, through a process, named gymnosis, which does not require any delivery system, but rather takes advantage of the normal growth properties of tissue cultured cells in order to elicit a productive oligonucleotide uptake. At the abovementioned doses, this silencing can be continuously maintained up to 6 months, with little or no toxicity [15], and even in hard to transfect suspension cells [16–19]. Importantly, the pattern of gene silencing of in vitro gymnotically treated cells well correlates with in vivo silencing, making in vitro findings closer to the real scenario [20]. Although unmodified LNA may stimulate an immune response in cells, LNA GapmeRs are less likely to be immunogenic, while toxicity seems highly sequence-dependent. Both these issues can be reduced by careful screening of LNA GapmeRs, while the use of the lowest effective concentration and the inclusion of appropriate nontargeting negative control could prevent false-positive effects [21]. At the same time, we would recommend verifying, through quantitative real time analysis of specific target, that LNA GapmeR sequences do not induce activation of the interferon pathway.

Here, we report, as a part of previous publications of our group, the use of LNA GapmeRs to successfully target the oncogenic lncRNA NEAT1 in multiple myeloma cells [19]. This approach looks promising in the context of the ncRNA-based therapy of human malignancies.

## 2  Materials

1. Cells.
2. Antibiotic-free growth medium.
3. Complete growth medium.
4. Multiwell tissue culture plates.
5. Phosphate buffered saline (PBS) without $Ca^{2+}$ and $Mg^{2+}$.
6. Antisense LNA GapmeRs (*see* **Note 1**).
7. Nuclease-free water.
8. DNase-free microcentrifuge tubes.
9. 15 mL conical centrifuge tube.
10. Neon Transfection System and Neon Transfection Kit.
11. Fluorescence microscope.
12. Quantitative PCR reagents and instrument.

## 3    Methods

### 3.1    LNA GapmeR Electroporation for Suspension Cells Using the Neon Transfection System

Neon Transfection System is a benchtop electroporation device that employs an electroporation technology by using the pipette tip as an electroporation chamber to efficiently transfect mammalian cells.

1. 48 h before transfection, split cells to $4 \times 10^5$ cells/mL.

2. On the day of transfection, prewarm an aliquot of antibiotic-free growth medium, containing serum.

3. Resuspend and take an aliquot of cell culture, count the cells to determine the cell density.

4. Transfer the required number of cells to a microcentrifuge tube or 15 mL conical tube and pellet the cells by centrifugation at $900 \times g$ for 5 min at room temperature (RT) (*see* **Notes 2** and **3**).

5. Wash the cells with PBS and pellet the cells by centrifugation at $900 \times g$ for 5 min at RT.

6. Aspirate the PBS and suspend the cell pellet in Resuspension Buffer T, suggested for suspension blood cells instead of Buffer R, at a final density of $5 \times 10^6$ cells/mL. Gently suspend the cells to obtain a single cell suspension, without creating air bubbles in the solution.

7. Prepare 12-well plates by adding to the wells 0.9 mL of pre-warmed antibiotic-free culture medium containing serum and preincubate plates in a humidified 37 °C and 5% $CO_2$ incubator.

8. Pipet the desire amount of LNA GapmeR into a sterile, 1.5 mL microcentrifuge tube (*see* **Note 4**).

9. Add 100 μL (500,000 cells) of cells suspended in Buffer T to the tube containing LNA-GapmeR and gently mix.

10. Aspirate the cell-LNA GapmeR mixture into the 100 μL Neon Tip (*see* **Note 5**).

11. Insert the Neon Pipette with the sample mixture into the right allocation within the Neon device, ensure to have selected the appropriate electroporation protocol (for some specific HMCLs, namely, RPMI-8226, NCI-H929, and AMO-1, we have optimized the protocol using the following instrument setting: 1100 V, 30 width, and 2 Pulse) and proceed with the electroporation reaction.

12. At the end of the electroporation reaction, slowly remove the Neon Pipette from the Neon device and immediately release the sample from the Neon Tip into the prepared culture plate containing prewarmed antibiotic-free medium (*see* **Note 6**).

13. Gently rock the plate to assure adequate distribution of the cells within the well.

14. Repeat the same procedure for all samples (*see* **Note 7**).

15. Incubate the plate in a humidified 37 °C and 5% $CO_2$ incubator for 24–48 h and, at the end, process samples to evaluate electroporation and silencing efficiency (fluorescence microscopy for positive fluorescent control and quantitative RT-PCR for all samples) (*see* **Note 8**).

*3.2 LNA GapmeR Gymnotic Delivery for Suspension Cells*

At micromolar concentration, naked LNA GapmeRs are able to passively cross the plasma cell membrane through a cellular passive uptake mechanism previously referred as gymnosis [15].

1. Forty-eight hours before transfection, split cells to $4 \times 10^5$ cells/mL.

2. On the day of transfection, prewarm an aliquot of complete culture medium (*see* **Note 9**).

3. Resuspend and take an aliquot of cell culture, count the cells to determine the cell density.

4. Transfer the required number of cells to a microcentrifuge tube or 15 mL conical tube and pellet the cells by centrifugation at $900 \times g$ for 5 min at RT (*see* **Note 10**).

5. Suspend the cell pellet in complete culture medium and transfer the cell suspension in the multiwell plate.

6. Add directly the desired amount of LNA GapmeR from the stock solution to cell suspension (*see* **Notes 11** and **12**).

7. Gently rock the plate to ensure adequate distribution of cells and LNA GapmeR.

8. Incubate the plate in a humidified 37 °C and 5% $CO_2$ incubator for the desired time and, at the end, process samples to evaluate electroporation and silencing efficiency (fluorescence microscopy for positive fluorescent control and quantitative RT-PCR for all samples) (*see* **Note 8**).

# 4    Notes

1. LNA GapmeRs were reconstituted with nuclease-free water at 50 μM (for electroporation) or 25 mg/mL (for gymnotic delivery) and stored at −80 °C. Because LNA GapmeRs are susceptible to degradation by exonucleases, it is highly recommended to wear powder-free gloves while handling, as well as to use DNase-free reagents and filter pipette tips. Furthermore, to minimize the risk of degradation and/or contamination, it is preferable to work under a tissue culture hood.

2. For Human Multiple Myeloma Cell Lines (HMCLs) we consider to electroporate $0.5 \times 10^6$ cells each sample and to seed samples in 1 mL final of fresh growth medium.

   The optimal combination of cell density and electroporation conditions must be determined. Optimizing electroporation efficiencies is crucial for maximizing lncRNA inhibition while minimizing secondary effects. Optimal electroporation conditions can be reached by adjusting the following.

   (a) Cell density at time of electroporation.

   (b) Amount of LNA GapmeR.

   (c) Electroporation parameters (voltage, pulse and width).

3. We recommend to consider taking a sufficient number of cells to set up the following adequate experimental control conditions to ensure that the resulting phenotype is due to antisense inhibition of the targeted RNA.

   (a) Negative control.
   - Unelectroporated cells.
   - Electroporated cells (without LNA GapmeR addiction).
   - Cells in the presence of LNA GapmeR alone (without electroporation procedure).
   - Electroporated cells with scrambled LNA GapmeR (to be used at the same concentration of the targeting LNA GapmeR).

   (b) Positive control.
   - Electroporated cells with a positive (possibly fluorescent) control LNA GapmeR known to efficiently silence a target gene within cells. It allows confirmation that the LNA GapmeR delivery process in each experiment is successful.

4. Generally, LNA GapmeRs delivered by electroporation or by the use of transfection reagents display potent activity at final concentrations of 1–50 nM, but a more extensive range of 1–100 nM can be used in optimization experiments. Considering a final volume (for each sample) of 1 mL, in order to electroporate using 50 nM of LNA GapmeR, you need to move in a microcentrifuge tube 1 μL of LNA GapmeR stock solution.

5. Avoid air bubbles during pipetting as air bubbles lead to lowered or failed transfection efficiency. If you notice air bubbles in the tip, discard the sample and carefully aspirate the fresh sample into the tip again without any air bubbles. If you are using 10 μL Neon Tip consider to adjust the cell concentration, LNA GapmeR volume and final growth medium amount appropriately (take care that the amount of LNA GapmeRs

should not exceed 1/10 of the final buffer volume used to suspend cells for Neon electroporation).

6. We strongly recommend seeding electroporated cells into growth medium without antibiotics that can greatly affect cells viability after transfection.

7. Take care to use the same Neon Tip for a maximum of two samples (in case of the same experimental condition), then discard the Neon Tip and use a new one. If the Neon Tips are used more than two times, the electrode function of the piston will decrease, thus affecting the reproducibility of the transfection conditions within or between experiments.

8. From our experience, to evaluate LNA GapmeRs silencing efficiency in order to select the best LNA GapmeR to use for functional approaches, we recommend starting to analyze the target knockdown (KD) efficiency from 48 h postelectroporation (Fig. 1a) or 48–72 h post–gymnotic delivery (Fig. 1b).

9. In contrast with electroporation, the gymnotic delivery of LNA GapmeRs does not rely on pores formation in the plasma cell membrane, allowing, if required, the use of antibiotics-supplemented growth medium without affecting cell viability.

10. It is important to seed cells at low plating density to reach confluence on the final day of the experiment. Based on our experience, in the case of HMCLs, in order to end the experiment on day 6, the cell number at plating ranged from $0.5 \times 10^3$ to $2.5 \times 10^3$ in 96-well plates, from $2.5 \times 10^4$ to

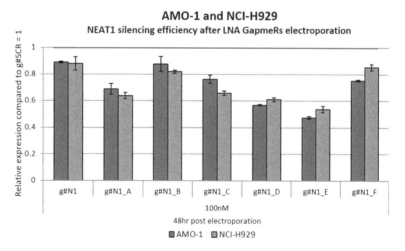

**Fig. 1** Quantitative real-time PCR (qRT-PCR) evaluation of target knockdown (KD) efficiency; (**a**) qRT-PCR of NEAT1 in AMO-1 and NCI-H929 after 48 h from electroporation of a panel of LNA GapmeR sequences. (**b**) qRT-PCR of NEAT1 in AMO-1 and NCI-H929 at the reported time point upon LNA GapmeR gymnotic delivery; NEAT1 expression was expressed as $2^{-\Delta\Delta Ct}$ relative to the scramble LNA GapmeR at the same time point

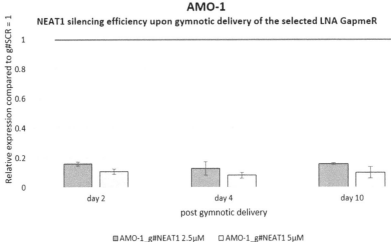

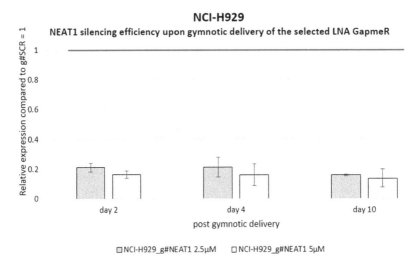

**Fig. 1** (continued)

$10 \times 10^4$ in 12-well plates, and from $1 \times 10^5$ to $3 \times 10^5$ in 6-well plates.

11. Appropriate LNA GapmeR solution should be added at a final concentration ranging from 1 to 50 μM.

12. Always remember to set up the experiment with the adequate control conditions to ensure that the phenotype is due to antisense inhibition of the targeted lncRNAs and not to off-target effects. In case of gymnotic delivery we suggest to use the following:

   (a) Negative control.
      • Untreated cells.
      • Cells treated with scrambled LNA GapmeR (to be used at the same concentration of the targeting LNA GapmeR).

(b) Positive control

- Cells treated with a positive (possibly fluorescent) control LNA GapmeR known to efficiently silence a target gene within cells. It allows confirmation that the gymnotic LNA GapmeR delivery process in each experiment is still successful at the time point that you are considering (consider to use the positive control LNA GapmeR at the same concentration of the targeting LNA GapmeR).

## Acknowledgments

This work was financially supported by grants to Antonino Neri [from Associazione Italiana Ricerca sul Cancro (AIRC) (IG16722, IG24365, and the "Special Program Molecular Clinical Oncology-5 per mille" #9980, 2010/15)]; to Pierfrancesco Tassone (from AIRC, IG21588); to Nicola Amodio [from Italian Ministry of Health (GR-2016-02361523) and from AIRC (IG24449)].

## References

1. Mercer TR, Dinger ME, Mattick JS (2009) Long non-coding RNAs: insights into functions. Nat Rev Genet 10(3):155–159. https://doi.org/10.1038/nrg2521

2. Amodio N, Raimondi L, Juli G et al (2018) MALAT1: a druggable long non-coding RNA for targeted anti-cancer approaches. J Hematol Oncol 11(1):63. https://doi.org/10.1186/s13045-018-0606-4

3. Kopp F, Mendell JT (2018) Functional classification and experimental dissection of long noncoding RNAs. Cell 172(3):393–407. https://doi.org/10.1016/j.cell.2018.01.011

4. Slack FJ, Chinnaiyan AM (2019) The role of non-coding RNAs in oncology. Cell 179 (5):1033–1055. https://doi.org/10.1016/j.cell.2019.10.017

5. Arun G, Diermeier SD, Spector DL (2018) Therapeutic targeting of long non-coding RNAs in cancer. Trends Mol Med 24 (3):257–277. https://doi.org/10.1016/j.molmed.2018.01.001

6. Geary RS (2009) Antisense oligonucleotide pharmacokinetics and metabolism. Expert Opin Drug Metab Toxicol 5(4):381–391. https://doi.org/10.1517/17425250902877680

7. Geary RS, Norris D, Yu R et al (2015) Pharmacokinetics, biodistribution and cell uptake of antisense oligonucleotides. Adv Drug Deliv Rev 87:46–51. https://doi.org/10.1016/j.addr.2015.01.008

8. Shen X, Corey DR (2018) Chemistry, mechanism and clinical status of antisense oligonucleotides and duplex RNAs. Nucleic Acids Res 46(4):1584–1600. https://doi.org/10.1093/nar/gkx1239

9. Lundin KE, Hojland T, Hansen BR et al (2013) Biological activity and biotechnological aspects of locked nucleic acids. Adv Genet 82:47–107. https://doi.org/10.1016/B978-0-12-407676-1.00002-0

10. Hagedorn PH, Persson R, Funder ED et al (2018) Locked nucleic acid: modality, diversity, and drug discovery. Drug Discov Today 23 (1):101–114. https://doi.org/10.1016/j.drudis.2017.09.018

11. Amodio N, D'Aquila P, Passarino G et al (2017) Epigenetic modifications in multiple myeloma: recent advances on the role of DNA and histone methylation. Expert Opin Ther Targets 21(1):91–101. https://doi.org/10.1080/14728222.2016.1266339

12. Janssen HL, Kauppinen S, Hodges MR (2013) HCV infection and miravirsen. N Engl J Med 369(9):878. https://doi.org/10.1056/NEJMc1307787

13. Kurreck J, Wyszko E, Gillen C et al (2002) Design of antisense oligonucleotides stabilized by locked nucleic acids. Nucleic Acids Res 30 (9):1911–1918. https://doi.org/10.1093/nar/30.9.1911

14. Wahlestedt C, Salmi P, Good L et al (2000) Potent and nontoxic antisense oligonucleotides containing locked nucleic acids. Proc Natl Acad Sci U S A 97(10):5633–5638. https://doi.org/10.1073/pnas.97.10.5633

15. Stein CA, Hansen JB, Lai J et al (2010) Efficient gene silencing by delivery of locked nucleic acid antisense oligonucleotides, unassisted by transfection reagents. Nucleic Acids Res 38(1):e3. https://doi.org/10.1093/nar/gkp841

16. Amodio N, Stamato MA, Juli G et al (2018) Drugging the lncRNA MALAT1 via LNA gapmeR ASO inhibits gene expression of proteasome subunits and triggers anti-multiple myeloma activity. Leukemia 32 (9):1948–1957. https://doi.org/10.1038/s41375-018-0067-3

17. Morelli E, Biamonte L, Federico C et al (2018) Therapeutic vulnerability of multiple myeloma to MIR17PTi, a first-in-class inhibitor of pri-miR-17-92. Blood 132(10):1050–1063. https://doi.org/10.1182/blood-2018-03-836601

18. Ronchetti D, Todoerti K, Vinci C et al (2020) Expression pattern and biological significance of the lncRNA ST3GAL6-AS1 in multiple myeloma. Cancers (Basel) 12(4):782. https://doi.org/10.3390/cancers12040782

19. Taiana E, Favasuli V, Ronchetti D et al (2020) Long non-coding RNA NEAT1 targeting impairs the DNA repair machinery and triggers anti-tumor activity in multiple myeloma. Leukemia 34(1):234–244. https://doi.org/10.1038/s41375-019-0542-5

20. Zhang Y, Qu Z, Kim S et al (2011) Down-modulation of cancer targets using locked nucleic acid (LNA)-based antisense oligonucleotides without transfection. Gene Ther 18 (4):326–333. https://doi.org/10.1038/gt.2010.133

21. Roux BT, Lindsay MA, Heward JA (2017) Knockdown of nuclear-located enhancer RNAs and long ncRNAs using locked nucleic acid GapmeRs. Methods Mol Biol 1468:11–18. https://doi.org/10.1007/978-1-4939-4035-6_2

# Chapter 11

# Methods Used to Make Lipid Nanoparticles to Deliver LNA Gapmers Against lncRNAs into Acute Myeloid Leukemia (AML) Blasts

## Chun-Tien Kuo, Robert J. Lee, and Ramiro Garzon

### Abstract

Developing strategies to target lncRNAs are needed. In this chapter, we describe in detail a method to deliver antisense oligonucleotides into acute myeloid leukemia cells using lipid nanoparticles tagged with the transferrin receptor. While this chapter is focused on the delivery method, we also discuss important considerations about the design of antisense oligonucleotides (ASOs). The strategy described here has been used successfully to deliver ASOs into leukemic blasts and stem cells.

**Key words** LncRNAs, Therapeutics, Lipid nanoparticles

## 1 Introduction

Cancer is a complex disease where genetic alterations in protein coding genes play a critical role in the initiation and progression of cancer [1]. Over the past 20 years, it become evident that in addition to mutations in protein coding genes, aberrant expression of noncoding RNAs plays also a critical role in carcinogenesis [2]. Following initial studies describing the widespread deregulation of noncoding RNAs in cancer, functional studies proved that non-coding RNAs are also involved in carcinogenesis [2–5]. While there are more than 100 different species of noncoding RNAs, microRNAs (miRs) and long noncoding RNAs (lncRNAs) are the two most frequent noncoding RNA species involved in disease, including cancer [2–5]. Given the lncRNAs are deregulated in many cancers and there is strong in vitro and in vivo evidence that targeting aberrant lncRNAs have profound antitumor effects, it is

---

The original version of this chapter was revised. The correction to this chapter is available at https://doi.org/10.1007/978-1-0716-1581-2_24

Alfons Navarro (ed.), *Long Non-Coding RNAs in Cancer*, Methods in Molecular Biology, vol. 2348, https://doi.org/10.1007/978-1-0716-1581-2_11, © Springer Science+Business Media, LLC, part of Springer Nature 2021, Corrected Publication 2021

reasonable to explore and develop approaches to target lncRNAs in cancer [4, 5]. In this chapter, we will discuss one specific approach to target lncRNAs in cancer by using locked nucleic acid (LNA) gapmers antisense oligonucleotides delivered by lipid nanoparticles.

In our institution, one of the strategies we have chosen to target lncRNAs is using LNA gapmers, which are chimeric molecules, where a central DNA portion is flanked on both sides by LNAs against the desired target lncRNA sequence [6]. Such chimeric LNA-oligonucleotides allow the improved affinity and higher nuclease resistance of LNA to be combined with the ability of gapmers to recruit RNase H and cleave the target [6]. Overall, the efficacy of LNA is further increased by using gapmers. There are several considerations that one need to pay attention in the design of the LNA gapmers such as the potential for off targets effects [7, 8]. Thus, off targets analysis should be performed in silico and in vitro in mice and human to avoid hybridization-dependent toxic/off-target effects [9]. In addition, in general antisense oligonucleotides (ASOs) have been shown to stimulate the immune system both via the phosphorothioate backbone and through binding to nucleic acid sensing toll-like receptors [10]. CpG motifs trigger an innate immune response via binding to Toll like receptor 9 (TLR9) and this can be abrogated by replacing the C in the ASO sequence with 5′ methyl-cytosine in the CpG motif. Thus, one can argue that proper design of the LNA gapmers is critical to avoid off target toxicity effects. Chronic treatment with ASOs may result in accumulation of the ASO compound in the liver and kidney and may lead to kidney and/or liver toxicity [7, 8]. Recently, targeted delivery approaches have been used to improve the therapeutic index of ASO drugs with promising results [11]. For example, conjugation of ASOs with triantennary N-acetyl galactosamine (GalNAc) moieties for hepatocyte-targeted delivery resulted in a 6–10 fold potency increase for 2′-methoxyethyl (MOE)-modified gapmer ASOs and up to 60-fold potency increase for constrained ethyl (cEt)-modified gapmer ASOs [11]. Specific details about the oligos design are out of the scope for this chapter. Here, we will focus on the description of the methods used to make lipid nanoparticles to deliver LNA gapmers against lncRNAs into acute myeloid leukemia (AML) blasts.

To address the insufficient intracellular delivery of naked ASOs, our group has developed a formulation capable of promoting targeted delivery and enhanced pharmacologic activity of ASOs in AML patient cells. We developed transferrin-conjugated pH-sensitive lipopolyplex nanoparticles (Tf-NP). In brief, the LNA gapmer was mixed at a 1:10 weight ratio with lipid nanoparticles (LNPs) consisted of 1,2-dioleoyl-3-trimethylammonium-propane (DOTAP) and 1,2-dioleoyl-sn-glycero-3-phosphocholine (DOPC) at a molar ratio of 1:1. The lipid-oligo formulation was then mixed with a human transferrin solution. The TfR is selectively overexpressed in leukemia cells [12, 13]. The Tf-LNPs protects

ASOs from nucleases and renal clearance and promotes uptake by leukemia cells through Tf receptor-mediated endocytosis. We reported that Tf-NP of this composition effectively delivered functional miR-29b [14], antimiR-126 [15], and the lncRNA *HOXB-AS3B* [16], resulting in target downregulation and antileukemic activity in vivo. Thus, we will describe in detail the protocol we developed and optimized to deliver efficiently LNA gapmers against lncRNAs into AML cells.

## 2    Materials (*See* Note 1)

### 2.1    For the Synthesis of Transferrin-PEG2000-DSPE

1. Maleimide-PEG$_{2000}$-DSPE (1,2-distearoyl-*sn*-glycero-3-phosphoethanolamine-*N*-[maleimide(polyethylene glycol)-2000], ammonium salt) (Avanti Polar Lipids).

2. Holotransferrin, human (Sigma-Aldrich).

3. Traut's reagent (2-iminothiolane) (ThermoFisher Scientific).

4. PD-10 desalting columns (Cytiva Life Sciences).

5. Bio-Rad® Protein Assay (Bio-Rad Protein Assay Dye Reagent Concentrate) (Bio-Rad).

6. 1× PBS.

7. 0.22 μm PVDF syringe filter.

### 2.2    For Preparing Cationic Liposomes

1. DOPC (1,2-dioleoyl-*sn*-glycero-3-phosphocholine) (Avanti Polar Lipids).

2. DOTAP (1,2-dioleoyl-3-trimethylammonium-propane, chloride salt) (Avanti Polar Lipids).

3. Ethanol, molecular biology grade.

4. 20 mM HEPES buffer in ddH$_2$O, pH 7.4.

5. 0.22 μm PES syringe filter.

### 2.3    For Preparing Transferrin-Conjugated LNA Lipid Nanoparticles (Tf-LNPs)

1. Transferrin-PEG$_{2000}$-DSPE as described in Subheading 2.1.

2. Cationic liposomes as described in Subheading 2.2.

3. Locked nucleic acid (LNA) oligonucleotides in sterile DEPC water.

4. 20 mM HEPES buffer in ddH$_2$O, pH 7.4.

### 2.4    Nanoparticle Characterization

*2.4.1    Gel Retardation by Agarose Gel Electrophoresis*

1. Agarose.

2. Ethidium bromide.

3. 1× Tris–Borate–EDTA (TBE) buffer.

<table><tr><td>2.4.2  Dynamic Light
Scattering (DLS) and
Electrophoretic Light
Scattering (ELS)</td><td>Cuvettes of choice according to the instrument manual. An example of a DLS/ELS instrument is a Nicomp® Nano DLS/ZLS Z3000 System from Entegris.</td></tr></table>

# 3  Methods

All procedures are performed under room temperature, unless indicated otherwise.

### 3.1  Preparation of Transferrin-PEG₂₀₀₀-DSPE

*3.1.1  Sulfhydryl Transferrin (Tf-SH) Formation*

1. Dissolve Traut's reagent in PBS (pH 8.0) at 1 mg/mL.
2. Dissolve holotransferrin (Tf) in PBS (pH 8.0) at 5 mg/mL.
3. Mixed 5 mg Tf solution (1 mL of 5 mg/mL) with 0.086 mg (86 µL of 1 mg/mL) Traut's reagent at the molar ratio of 1:10 in a 1.7 mL microcentrifuge tube.
4. Mix the solution on an orbital shaker at room temperature for 2 h to yield Tf-SH.

*3.1.2  Sulfhydryl Transferrin Purification*

1. Wash a PD-10 desalting column with PBS (pH 6.5) at least 3 column volumes.
2. Load Tf/Traut's mixture solution into the PD-10 column, 1 mL per elution process. Discard the flowthrough.
3. Prepare 15 tubes of 1.7 mL microcentrifuge tubes.
4. Add 500 µL PBS (pH 6.5) to the column. Collect the eluent in a microcentrifuge tube and label #1. Repeat this step for 15 times (500 µL PBS per cycle) until 15 tubes of Tf-SH eluent (#1–#15) are collected.
5. Dilute Bio-Rad protein assay dye reagent concentrate 1:4 (v/v) with deionized water. Prepare 15 tubes of 0.6 mL microcentrifuge tube and add 300 µL of diluted dye reagent per tube. Label #1–#15.
6. Mix 10 µL Tf-SH eluent from each collection tube to each corresponding diluted dye. Mix well on vortex.
7. Combine all Tf-SH eluents into a 5 mL centrifuge tube which corresponding dye reagent turn blue, determined by the naked eye.

*3.1.3  Transferrin-PEG₂₀₀₀-DSPE (Tf-PEG₂₀₀₀-DSPE) Conjugation*

1. Dissolve 1.83 mg Maleimide-PEG₂₀₀₀-DSPE in 183 µL PBS buffer (pH 6.5) at 10 mg/mL.
2. Mix Tf-SH with Maleimide-PEG₂₀₀₀-DSPE at the molar ratio of 1:10. 5 mg of Tf-SH is mixed with 1.83 mg Maleimide-PEG₂₀₀₀-DSPE.

3. Mix the reaction solution on an orbital shaker overnight at room temperature to yield Tf-PEG$_{2000}$-DSPE micelle.

4. Filter Tf-PEG$_{2000}$-DSPE with a sterile 0.22µm PVDF syringe filter.

5. Measure the holotransferrin concentration by $A_{280}$ using pure holotransferrin solutions as standards.

6. Store sterile Tf-PEG$_{2000}$-DSPE at 4 °C.

**3.2 Preparation of Cationic Liposomes**

1. Dissolve both lipids (DOPC and DOTAP) in ethanol (molecular biology grade) at the concentration of 50 mg/mL, respectively.

2. Mix two lipid ethanol solutions at the DOPC–DOTAP molar ratio of 50:50. Mix 423.6µL DOPC, 376.4µL DOTAP, and 200µL ethanol in a 1.7 mL microcentrifuge tube up to 1.0 mL solution. The lipid mixture concentration is 40 mg/mL. Mix well by vortex.

3. Prepare a 15 mL conical tube and add 9 mL 20 mM HEPES buffer (pH 7.4) into the conical tube.

4. Draw 1 mL lipid mixture into a 1 mL insulin syringe with 29G × ½″ gauge needle.

5. Put needle tip under the HEPES buffer surface and inject the lipid solution as fast as possible into buffer to form empty cationic liposomes.

6. Mix the solution well by high-speed vortex and sonicate the cationic liposome solution in a water bath sonicator for 10 min. The particle size of the cationic liposomes by dynamic light scattering should be <130 nm at this point.

7. Filter the cationic liposome solution with a 0.22µm PES syringe filter. The final lipid concentration in the liposome solution is 4.0 mg/mL.

8. Store the cationic liposome solution at 4 °C.

**3.3 Transferrin-Conjugated LNA Lipid Nanoparticle Formation**

1. Dissolve LNA selected oligonucleotides in sterile DEPC water at the concentration of 5 mg/mL as stock solutions, respectively.

2. Prepare a 1.7 mL microcentrifuge tube. Add 20µL LNA stock solution (100µg LNA oligonucleotides) into the tube and add 55µL 20 mM HEPES buffer to the LNA solution. Mix well by pipetting gently.

3. Prepare another 1.7 mL microcentrifuge tube and add 250µL cationic liposome solution (mentioned in Subheading 3.2, 1 mg lipids) into the tube. Mix the diluted LNA solution to the cationic liposome at the lipid lipids–LNA oligonucleotide weight ratio of 10/1.

4. Mix the solution well by vortex and sonicate in a bath sonicator for 4 min. Incubate at room temperature for 10 min.

5. Add Tf-PEG$_{2000}$-DSPE into the mixture at the lipid–transferrin weight ratio of 70:8. 114.3 µg transferrin (in Tf-PEG$_{2000}$-DSPE form, mentioned in Subheading 3.1) is added to the LNA–liposome mixture.

6. Mix the final mixture by vortex and incubate at 37 °C for 1 h.

7. Store the transferrin–LNA lipid nanoparticles at 4 °C up to 24 h (*see* **Note 2**).

**3.4 Transferrin-Conjugated LNA Lipid Nanoparticle Characterization**

1. Prepare an agarose gel in TBE buffer at 1.5% (w/w).

2. Load LNA oligonucleotide stocks and transferrin-conjugated LNA lipid nanoparticles in each well.

3. Run the gel in TBE buffer at 100 V (fixed voltage) for 20 min.

4. Stain the gel with EtBr and assay the LNA bands by EtBr fluorescence (*see* **Note 5**).

*3.4.1 LNA Oligonucleotide Encapsulation Assessment by Gel Retardation (*See **Notes 3** *and* **4**)

*3.4.2 Particle Size and Zeta Potential Measurements by DLS and ELS*

Please refer the measuring procedures to the instrument manuals.

A typical particle size (z-average diameter) range of cationic liposomes (prepared in Subheading 3.2) should be 60–80 nm. A typical particle size (z-average diameter) range of Tf-LNPs (prepared in Subheading 3.3) should be 150–250 nm.

The typical mean zeta potential of cationic liposomes should fall within +30 to +40 mV. The typical mean zeta potential of Tf-LNPs should fall within −10 to +20 mV.

**3.5 Application Considerations**

The described protocol could be used for in vitro or in vivo experiments. For in vitro experiments, for example when we intent to silence a lncRNA in primary AML blasts or an AML cell line in culture, the complex of LNP–LNA ASOs are just put into the culture media without using any other procedures. The complexes enter the cells rapidly and we usually asses the target transcript levels at 24 and 48 h using custom quantitative RT-PCR. The amount use for in vitro studies usually ranges from 100 to 300 nM. For in vivo studies, for example patient derived xenograft AML models, we usually give the complexes either intraperitoneally or intravenously through the tail vein using doses and schedules that are variables depending on the target and pharmacokinetics studies.

## 4  Notes

1. The procedures can be adapted to a format using pump-based mixing, especially at scale-up. For example, microfluidics-based mixing can be implemented using a system from Precision Nanosystems for precisely controlled mixing.

2. We recommend preparing the lipid nanoparticles and use it within 24 h as this method has not been optimized for long-term stability and storage.

3. If encapsulation is incomplete (assayed by gel retardation or OliGreen® ssDNA Reagent), increase the lipid/LNA ratio to enhance LNA/cationic lipid complexation by increasing the cationic lipid content. Additional PEGylated agents can be added to the solution if aggregates form.

4. LNA oligonucleotides incorporation can be determined by EtBr/SYBR Green I–staining agarose gel electrophoresis and by gel-permeation chromatography (GPC). The LNA gapmers API and lipid and Tf excipients should be also be analyzed by high-performance liquid chromatography (HPLC) with UV and sodium lauryl sulfate Polyacrylamide Gel Electrophoresis (SDS-PAGE) respectively.

5. Ethidium bromide (EtBr) may have a low binding affinity to LNAs, thus giving low fluorescence signal intensity. In this case, try Quant-iT™ OliGreen® ssDNA Reagent for LNA quantification. To release encapsulated LNAs, lysis buffers such as 3% Triton X-100 or 1% SDS can be used while doing agarose gel electrophoresis.

## References

1. Hanahan RA, Weinberg RA (2011) Hallmarks of cancer: the next generation. Cell 144:646–674

2. Garzon R, Marcucci G, Croce R (2010) Targeting microRNAs in cancer: rationale, strategies and challenges. Nat Rev Drug Dis 9:775–789

3. Derrien T, Johnson R, Bussotti G et al (2012) The GENCODE v7 catalog of human long noncoding RNAs: analysis of their gene structure, evolution, and expression. Genome Res 22:1775–1789

4. Ulitsky I, Bartel DP (2013) lincRNAs: genomics, evolution, and mechanisms. Cell 154:26–46

5. Bartonicek N, Maag JLV, Dinger ME (2016) Long noncoding RNAs in cancer: mechanisms of action and technological advancements. Mol Cancer 15:43

6. Kurreck J, Wyszko E, Gillen C, Erdmann VA (2002) Design of antisense oligonucleotides stabilized by locked nucleic acids. Nucleic Acids Res 30:1911–1918

7. Levin AA (1999) A review of the issues in the pharmacokinetics and toxicology of phosphorothioate antisense oligonucleotides. Biochim Biophys Acta 1489:69–84

8. Bennett CF, Swayze EE (2010) RNA targeting therapeutics: molecular mechanisms of antisense oligonucleotides as a therapeutic platform. Annu Rev Pharmacol Toxicol 50:259–293

9. Kamola PJ, Kitson JDA, Turner G et al (2015) *In silico* and *in vitro* evaluation of exonic and intronic off-target effects form a critical element of therapeutic ASO gamper optimization. Nucl Acid Res 43:8638–8650

10. Tanaka T, Legat A, Adam E et al (2008) DiC14-amidine cationic liposomes stimulate myeloid dendritic cells through toll-like receptor 4. Eur J Immunol 38:1351–1357

11. Prakash TP, Graham MJ, Yu J et al (2014) Targeted delivery of antisense oligonucleotides to hepatocytes using triantennary N- acetyl galactosamine improves potency 10-fold in mice. Nucleic Acids Res 42:8796–8807

12. Wu B, Shi N, Sun L, Liu L (2016) Clinical value of high expression level of CD71 in acute myeloid leukemia. Neoplasma 6:809–815

13. Liu Q, Wang M, Hu Y et al (2014) Significance of CD71 expression by flow cytometry in AML. Leuk Lymphoma 55:892–898

14. Huang X, Schwind S, Yu B et al (2013) Targeted delivery of microRNA-29b by transferring-conjugated anionic lipopolyplex nanoparticles: a novel therapeutic strategy in acute myeloid leukemia. Clin Cancer Res 19:2355–2367

15. Dorrance A, Neviani P, Ferenchak G et al (2015) Targeting leukemia stem cells in vivo with AntagomiR-126 nanoparticles in acute myeloid leukemia. Leukemia 29:2143–2153

16. Papaioannou D, Petri A, Dovey OM et al (2019) The long non-coding RNA HOXB-AS3 regulates ribosomal biogenesis in NPM1-mutated AML. Nat Commun 10:5351

# Chapter 12

## CRISPR/Cas9 to Silence Long Non-Coding RNAs

**Ingrid Arctander Rosenlund, George A. Calin, Mihnea P. Dragomir, and Erik Knutsen**

### Abstract

Knockout (KO) of long non-coding RNAs (lncRNAs) enables functional characterization of this still poorly described group of transcripts. One of the most efficient and simplest methods to achieve complete KO of a lncRNA is by employing CRISPR/Cas gene editing. As most lncRNAs are not well annotated, their individual functional regions are often not defined, and the majority of the transcripts are not affected by single nucleotide mutations. Therefore, CRISPR/Cas KO is more challenging for lncRNAs as compared to KO of protein coding genes. Strategies for lncRNAs KO include complete removal of the entire gene, removal of the promoter and transcriptional start site, abolishing exon–exon junctions, or removing the transcriptional termination site. Here, we describe the methodology to perform CRISPR/Cas9 KO of lncRNAs in vitro using electroporation as the method of transfection of presynthesized single guide RNAs (sgRNAs) and Cas9 enzyme.

**Key words** Long non-coding RNA, CRISPR/Cas9, Knockout, Gene editing, Electroporation

---

## 1  Introduction

Clustered regularly interspaced short palindromic repeats (CRISPR) and CRISPR associated proteins (Cas) is a genome editing technique, established in 2012, that uses RNA molecules to guide nucleases to specific target sites in the DNA [1–3]. The system is a highly specific method for DNA cleavage and allows researchers to create specific modifications to a specific genomic area of interest. The method is based on the adaptive bacterial immune system, where CRISPR and the endonuclease family Cas, make up a defense mechanism against viruses and endogenous plasmids [4–6]. The CRISPR arrays are unique genomic regions in the bacteria where viral DNA and plasmid DNA sequences from previous invasions have been incorporated, and the locus is transcribed into crispr RNAs (crRNAs) [7]. The crRNA is characterized

Mihnea P. Dragomir and Erik Knutsen share senior authorship.

Alfons Navarro (ed.), *Long Non-Coding RNAs in Cancer*, Methods in Molecular Biology, vol. 2348,
https://doi.org/10.1007/978-1-0716-1581-2_12, © Springer Science+Business Media, LLC, part of Springer Nature 2021

by a 20 nucleotide (nt) complementary sequence to the invading viral or plasmid DNA. In experimental research, this region is designed to be complementary to the intended cut site in the target gene. After processing, the mature crRNA binds, via a complementary spacer, to a trans-activating crRNA (tracrRNA), which is either transcribed from the same locus, or from a region in close proximity upstream of the locus [2]. The tracrRNA has the recognition sequence necessary to form a complex with the Cas endonuclease [3]. There are three major types of CRISPR-Cas systems, each characterized by signature genes: Cas3 in type I systems, Cas9 in type II, and Cas10 in type III [8, 9]. The Cas genes are organized in operons under the control of a single promotor, and they are characterized by their use of dual-RNAs for site-specific DNA cleavage [3, 6]. There are 93 known Cas protein families, and multiple and highly diverse Cas proteins have been identified [8]. Cas9 is one of the most commonly used Cas enzymes, and is a dual RNA-guided endonuclease that creates site-specific double-stranded breaks in the target DNA. Cas9 activity requires both a seed sequence in the crRNA as well as a protospacer adjacent motif (PAM) containing a guanine dinucleotide, $5'$-NGG-$3'$, where N is any nucleotide. Cas12 is another commonly used Cas enzyme. In contrast to Cas9, Cas12 targets PAM sequences rich in thymine ($5'$-TTN-$3'$) [10]. Another emerging Cas enzyme in research is Cas13. In contrast to Cas9 and Cas12, Cas13 targets RNA sequences and requires a guide RNA of approximately 64 nt in length [11]. Recently, a hypercompact CRISPR/Cas system was discovered by Pausch et al. in huge bacteriophages [12]. The newly discovered CRISPR associated enzyme CasΦ is about half the size of Cas9 and Cas12, and targets a wider range of genetic sequences. This is a promising finding that could lead to more efficient delivery of the CRISPR/Cas components into cells, and to a broader application of the CRISPR/Cas method for gene editing [12]. The CRISPR/Cas technique for genome editing has shown great potential for applications in biomedical research and biotechnology, and in innovative therapies for diseases [13–16], and multiple clinical trials are currently being conducted [17].

Long non-coding RNAs (lncRNAs) are a class of RNA molecules with no protein coding potential which exceed 200 nt in length [18]. LncRNAs have multiple described functions: guides for proteins or other RNA molecules to specific DNA or RNA regions/sequences; enhancers or inhibitors of transcription; scaffolding RNAs that assemble ribonucleoprotein complexes at specific cellular sites; decoys that inhibit protein or other RNA molecules' function by sequestering or by blocking protein binding sites; or modifiers that can allosterically change proteins or other RNA molecules [19, 20]. Even though great effort has been put into investigating the function of this large class of genes, most lncRNAs are still poorly characterized. We consider that one of the best methods for studying the functionality of lncRNAs is to perform in vitro and in vivo knockout (KO). A simple method to achieve complete KO of a lncRNA is by CRISPR/Cas gene editing. In comparison to CRISPR/Cas KO of other gene types, like protein coding genes, CRISPR/Cas KO of lncRNAs is harder to achieve because of one important challenge: most lncRNA genes are not well characterized and the functional regions of the transcripts are not known. For this reason, it is often necessary to KO the complete lncRNA gene in order to study the functionality of a given lncRNA. In most cases, this will lead to the additional challenge of avoiding alterations of nearby genes, as most classes of lncRNAs are located in close proximity or even overlapping with a protein coding or another non-coding gene.

In this methods section, we will give a detailed description on how to perform CRISPR/Cas9 KO of a lncRNA in the laboratory using presynthesized sgRNAs and Cas9 with electroporation as the transfection method (Note that the term gRNA is used to describe all CRISPR guide RNA formats, while sgRNA is used to describe a guide RNA that is made up of the combination of the crRNA and the tracrRNA elements into a single RNA molecule). In addition, we will give a guide on how to plan and design a KO experiment for different lncRNAs. Cell culturing, flow sorting, DNA isolation, and PCR will only be described in general, as the methods will depend on the cell culture of interest and the availability of kits, reagents, and platforms at the institution where the experiment will be conducted.

## 2    Materials

### 2.1    Electroporation Agent

1. Cell Line Nucleofector™ Kit V (Lonza).

### 2.2    sgRNA

1. CRISPRevolution sgRNA EZ Kit (1.5 nmol) (Modified) (Synthego): sgRNA should be diluted to 100 µM in Low TE buffer upon arrival, aliquoted in separate RNase-free tubes (2.0µl per tube), and stored at −20 °C.

### 2.3    Cas9

1. Cas9 2NLS Nuclease—300 pmol (Synthego).

### 2.4    Electroporation Apparatus

1. Any electroporation apparatus compatible with the Nucleofector™ Kit V is suitable for the CRISPR/Cas9 silencing of lncRNAs. For each cell line, a different electroporation program is recommended.

### 2.5    Cell Culturing Reagent

1. Normal cell culturing reagents and materials are used for the CRISPR/Cas9 silencing of lncRNAs. For the expansion of cells after electroporation, a conditioned growth media is

necessary. Prepare conditioned growth media by sterile filtering growth media used to culture the cell using a 0.2μm filter. The culture media should have been cultivated with the cells for at least 48 h and should not be more than 1 month old at the time of use.

**2.6  Flow Sorting to Establish Single Cell Colonies**

1. Flow tubes with filtering cap.
2. 96-well plates.
3. Propidium iodide.

**2.7  PCR Screening**

1. DNA isolation kit.
2. PCR kit.
3. Specific PCR primers.

## 3  Methods

For generation of a lncRNA KO cell line, a dual sgRNA strategy will be utilized. Here, the two sgRNAs will generate two unique double-stranded DNA breaks within the genomic region of the lncRNA. The sgRNAs will target upstream and downstream of the desired target sequence, allowing a relegation of the two broken ends with the loss of the genomic sequence in between.

**3.1  Establish a Knockout Strategy**

1. Foremost, it is important to get an overview of the genomic organization of the target lncRNA and its residing genes. Annotations of lncRNAs are still poor, and often the annotations will include a large number of potential transcriptional isoforms with different start and termination sites within the gene region. Essential information that will affect the KO strategy includes the following:

   (a) Buildup of gene: gene and transcripts length, number of annotated transcript isoforms, number of exon–intron junctions, and location and number of transcriptional start and termination sites.

   (b) Genomic location of lncRNA and location of overlapping or neighboring genes.

   (c) Validity of promoter region for the lncRNA.

2. Examine the genomic buildup of the lncRNA, by using the UCSC Genome browser (genome.ucsc.edu) or Ensembl (ensembl.org). Both databases include large collections of annotated lncRNAs. If the target lncRNA is a novel transcript, information regarding the gene buildup will not be included in the above-mentioned databases. Regardless of whether the lncRNA is a previously annotated lncRNA or a novel transcript,

the precise organization of the transcript should be further validated.

3. Validate the transcript by using in silico RNA-Seq data analysis. As many lncRNAs are tissue specifically expressed, use RNA-Seq data from tissue with the same origin as the cell line in which lncRNA KO will be performed. Use the RNA-Seq data to examine from which genomic regions RNA transcription is initiated and terminated and the location of exons and introns. If the precise organization of the transcript cannot be validated by RNA-Seq data, conduct 3′ and 5′ RACE and Sanger sequencing of the entire lncRNA transcript to identify the exact DNA region that is being covered by the transcribed lncRNA.

4. After validation of the transcript, choose the most suitable lncRNA KO strategy: (a) remove the entire gene, (b) remove the promoter and transcriptional start site, (c) remove the transcriptional termination site, or (d) abolish exon–intron junctions (Fig. 1). Some of the strategies may only cause a destabilization of the lncRNA (exon and termination) and will therefore not generate a complete KO cell line, but instead a stable knockdown (KD) cell line (*see* **Note 1**).

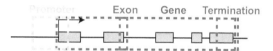

**Fig. 1** Strategies for long non-coding RNAs (lncRNAs) knockout (KO). (**a**) Gene: complete removal of the entire genomic region where the lncRNA transcript resides is the most efficient and secure method for lncRNA KO. However, this often implies removal of a larger genomic area, which might have additional unintended off-target effects. Of major importance, the region must not contain additional genes, as these genes will also be affected. (**b**) Promoter: removal of the promoter and transcriptional start site will prevent transcription of the lncRNA. The method will not completely remove the gene, but only affect initiation of transcription. The promoter region should be examined, as not to be used by neighboring genes. (**c**) Termination: removing the termination site will cause a destabilization of the lncRNA. If the lncRNA is a polyadenylated transcript, removal of the termination site will prevent polyadenylation. Some lncRNAs have alternative stabilizing structures located at their 3′ ends, and these will also be affected by the KO. (**d**) Exon: removal of an exon–intron junction might destabilize the lncRNA transcript, leading to a degradation of the transcript. The method will not completely remove the transcript and will only cause a knockdown (KD) of the lncRNA. The method can also result in a new stable transcript with an inclusion of the intron. This method, as for termination, will only cause a KD of the transcript, and will not generate a complete KO

### 3.2 Identification of Target Region for CRISPR/Cas9

1. After identifying a desired genomic region for KO, use the genomic location of the desired region as an input parameter for target analysis. Analyze the two target regions (upstream and downstream region), separately. Starting with the upstream region, investigate a region of ±500 nt covering the ideal target site in order to get sufficient numbers of targets. For target analysis, use the web tool CHOPCHOP (chopchop. cbu.uib.no). Input parameters are genomic region and species. The format for the genomic region is: chrX:Y–Z, where X = chromosome, Y = lower genomic region for KO, and Z = upper genomic region for KO. The format is case sensitive, so only use lower-case letters. Additional inputs include: for "Using" use "CRISPR/Cas9" and for "For" use "knock-out".

2. Submit these input parameters, and the web tool will generate a ranked list of targets with the most optimal target regions listed at the top. Here, target areas are selected based on their rank and their genomic location. The Cas9 enzyme has a very high specificity, so 3 nt difference should not be considered as off-targets.

3. After identification of a target region for the upstream region, do the same procedure for the downstream region.

4. Export the two identified target sequences, and remove the PAM sequences (the three last nucleotides corresponding to NGG) before using the sequences to order the sgRNAs (named synthetic sgRNA) from the Syntego homepage (synthego.com).

### 3.3 Design of PCR Primers for Validation of Clones

1. Design specific PCR primers for amplification of a region corresponding to 200–500 nt up- and downstream of the two cut sites. Design a forward primer 200–500 nt upstream of the upstream cut site, and a reverse primer 200–500 nt downstream of the downstream cut site. This will give a 400–1000 nt large PCR product if the genomic region of interest has been removed (Fig. 2).

2. In addition, if the KO region is >1 kb, include internal primers (primers located in the region to be removed) giving a PCR product of approximately the same size as your KO PCR product (Fig. 2). In order to separate the two products, it is recommended that the two products have a difference in size of about 100–200 nt.

### 3.4 Cultivation of Cells and Collection of Conditioned Media

1. Cultivate the cells in normal growth media. With every media change and splitting, the old media that has been cultivated with the cells (not including trypsin or PBS) is transferred to a 50 ml falcon tube, centrifuged at $2000 \times g$ for 5 min, and the supernatant is placed at 4 °C. The used media, termed

Region for PCR primer set 1:
Region for PCR primer set 2:
Region for KO:

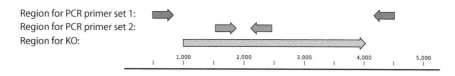

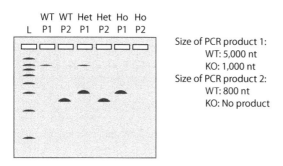

Size of PCR product 1:
     WT: 5,000 nt
     KO: 1,000 nt
Size of PCR product 2:
     WT: 800 nt
     KO: No product

**Fig. 2** For genotype screening of generated knockout (KO) clones, PCR screening is performed on DNA isolated from CRISPR/Cas9 clones. As PCR is more efficient for PCR products <3000 nt in length, KO strategies of larger DNA fragments will require two PCR primer sets. When using two primer sets, homozygous (Ho) wild type (WT), heterozygous (Het) KO, or Ho KO are identified based on the combination of the two PCR products; Ho KO only PCR product by primer set 1, Het KO PCR product from both primer sets, Ho WT only PCR product by primer set 2

conditioned media, will be used during single cell seeding. The later step requires a total of 106 ml conditioned media.

2. On the day of the transfection (Subheading 3.5), the cells should be at 50–80% confluent. The transfection protocol only requires the use of 100,000 cells, so cells can be cultivated in a small (T25) cell culture flask, but pre-cultivation in larger flasks are encouraged for collection of sufficient conditioned media.

**3.5 Transfection of sgRNAs and Cas9**

1. To a 12-well plate, add 450µl complete growth media to two wells and place the plate in the cell incubator.

2. Prepare the Nucleofector mix by combining 43µl of Nucleofector solution with 9.5µl Nucleofector supplement.

3. In a 1.5 ml tube, add 1.8µl of each of the two sgRNAs, 2.0µl Cas9, and 19.4µl Nucleofector mix to a total volume of 25µl. Incubate the solution at room temperature for a minimum of 10 min, but not for more than 1 h.

4. Split the cells and transfer the split cells in growth media to a falcon tube. Take 1 ml aliquot of the cell suspension and transfer to a 1.5 tube. From this tube do a cell counting. The numbers of cells should be in the range of 100,000–500,000 cells per ml. If the cell number is not within this range, dilute the cell suspension and recount the cells. Exact cell number is highly important for the success of the transfection, so care should be taken to prevent errors in cell number.

5. Transfer 100,000 cells to a new 1.5 ml tube and spin down the cells at 100 g for 10 min. The supernatant is carefully removed so not to disrupt the cell pellet. It is important that all liquid is removed. To ensure complete removal of cell media, first use a 1 ml pipette to remove 90% of the media, before changing to a 100μl pipette and do the same. Finally, use a 10μl pipette to remove the remaining liquid. When removing the liquid, be sure not to tilt or do rapid movements of the tube. If the cell pellet is disrupted, do a 5 min spin at 100 g before continuing removing the liquid.

6. Carefully resuspend the cells in 25μl Nucleofector mix, and transfer the cells to the 1.5 ml tube containing the sgRNA-Cas9 mix (mix from **step 3**). Mix by careful pipetting. Continue immediately with the electroporation, as cells should not be kept in the Nucleofector solution for more than 15 min before cells are resuspended in growth media (**step 9**).

7. Transfer the cell mix to an electroporation tube using the included plastic pipettes in the Nucleofector kit. Be careful not to introduce bubbles when placing the solution in the electroporation tube as this will disrupt the electroporation. Bubbles can be removed by gently knocking the electroporation tube onto the bench or by pipetting up the liquid before pipetting it out again into the tube.

8. Place the electroporation tube in the electroporation apparatus and electroporate using a defined electroporation program (Table 1). For instructions on how to program the electroporation apparatus, please refer to the instruction manual of the apparatus.

9. After the electroporation, 50μl of growth media is added to the cell suspension in the electroporation tube, before the cells are seeded out equally into the two wells on the 12-well plate containing 450μl of warm growth media from **step 1**. (50μl

**Table 1**
**Examples of electroporation programs recommended for CRISPR/Cas9 KO in different cell lines with specific characteristics (according to our personal experience). Further suggestions for electroporation program can be acquired form knowledge.lonza.com**

| Cell line characteristic | Example | Electroporation program |
|---|---|---|
| Large epithelial cells | MCF7, T-47D, HN30, HN31 | P-020 |
| Small epithelial cells | KM12SM, COLO320, HCT116 | D-032 |
| Normal suspension cells | MEC1, BM52 | X-005 |
| Small suspension cells | JURKAT | X-001 |

of the cell mix is added to each well). Be sure to transfer all of the cell mixture (*see* **Note 2**).

10. Change growth media after 24 h.

11. 72 h after electroporation, harvest cells from one of the two wells and perform DNA isolation. Follow the same procedure as for genotype screening (Subheading 3.7, **step 6**, expected result is identical as for a heterozygous KO clone).

12. The remaining cells are left to recover for an additional 1–5 days, until they have reached a 10–30% confluence. Do not keep the cells longer before performing single cell seeding.

*3.6 Seeding of Single-Cell Colonies*

1. On the day of the single-cell seeding, it is recommended to include wild-type cells (same cell line as the KO cells) in addition to the CRISPR/Cas9 KO cells, in order to use the wild-type cells for gating for flow sorting. Wild-type cells do not need to be sorted into 96-well plates.

2. Prepare six 96-well plates for the flow sorting. In each well, pipette 200 μl of single cell cultivation media. To make single cell cultivation media, take 106 ml of 0.2 μm sterile filtered conditioned media and mix with 26 ml FBS. If the cells are grown with specific supplements (like insulin), add an equal amount of supplement as to normal growth media to the single cell cultivation media. Place the 96-well plates in the cell incubator.

3. Split the cells from the remaining 12-well and spin down the cells at 100 g for 10 min. Carefully remove the supernatant. Now, excess media can be present, as this will not affect the following procedures. Resuspend the cells in 500 μl warm PBS (This is a higher dilution than for normal flow, giving a lower cell number for the sorting into 96-well plates as additional time is required for changing position between the wells).

4. Pipette the cells through a filter cap on a flow tube to separate clusters of cells into single cells. Here, pipetting should be done in a steady but gentle manner. Too gentle and the cell suspension will not go through the filter, and too hard will cause disruption of cells. Immediately proceed with flow sorting.

5. Add propidium iodide staining just before flow sorting for the separation of dead and live cells.

6. Sort single cells into each well on the six 96-well plates. Use the lowest flow rate applicable for flow sorting, in order to allow for sufficient time for the machine to move between the wells on the 96-well plate without losing too many cells.

7. Place the 96-well plates into the cell culture cabinet and leave the cells for 1 week. Do not examine cells or do excessive moving of the plates during this period (*see* **Note 3**).

*3.7 Expansion of Single-Cell Colonies and Genotype Screening*

1. Expansion of the single cells can take between 1 and 4 weeks before they are ready to be transferred to larger wells. No media change should be conducted during this period. If no experience with single cell seeding of the cell line used is available, perform the first screening of colonies 1 week after single cell sorting (*see* **Note 4**).

2. Take one of the six plates and examine the wells with a normal cell culture microscope. Mark wells where cell colonies can be visualized. The ideal magnification is so that the entire 96-well is visualized without the need to move the plate. The colonies should have reached a cell number of >200 cells, or >40% confluence. For cell lines which has a very low recommended splitting ration (like 1:2 and 1:3), it would be recommended to wait for the cells to become more confluent than the above recommended confluence. However, the cells should not be kept in the 96-well plates for more than 4 weeks before they are split. If no colonies have reached the desired cell number or confluence, place the plate back into the incubator. Continue with a 2–5 days interval to examine the identified colonies on the same plate as first examined, until the desired cell number or confluence has been reached (*see* **Note 5**).

3. At the time when the first colonies have reached a number of >200 cells or a confluence of >40%, split the colonies that have reached these numbers or confluence and transfer them to a 24-well containing 450 μl growth media to allow further expansion of the colonies. To split the colonies, remove the growth media and wash with warm PBS. Add 50 μl of trypsin. Leave the trypsin on until the cells have loosened. This might take up to 45 min as the cells often are strongly attached to the plastic. Be sure to use fresh Trypsin, as to reduce the time the trypsin needs to be on the cells. If the cells have not detached after 45 min, use a 200 μl pipette and pipette up and down the trypsin with a fast release of the trypsin directly above the cell colony in order to loosen the cells by a strong flow of liquid. Repeat this 4–5 times and transfer the trypsin to a 24-well. Examine the 96-well in the microscope and evaluate if the cells are still present in the 96-well or of they have been transferred to the 24-well. If the cells are still present, add new trypsin and wait 15 min before repeating this step.

4. Continue screening the rest of the 96-well plates and transfer colonies that have reached high enough cell numbers or confluence to 24-well plates. Be careful not to mix colonies or to get cross contamination of colonies. From this time point,

96-wells with identified single cell colonies should be screened every 2–5 days in order to identify colonies with desirable confluence.

5. After cells have reached a high confluence (>80%) in the 24-well plates, split the cells and transfer ¾ of the cell suspension to a 12-well containing 900μl growth media and ¼ of the cell suspension is collected for DNA isolation.

6. Isolate DNA from the clone, and perform PCR with the pre-designed PCR primers. Identification of homozygous WT, heterozygous KO, or homozygous KO is done according to Fig. 2 (*see* **Notes 6** and **7**).

7. Continue cultivating and expanding the preferred colonies (*see* **Note 8**).

# 4 Notes

1. The methods for KO should be prioritized in the following order: (a) full gene, (b) promoter, (c) termination, and (d) exon junctions. For KO of entire genes, the gene length will be important as genes larger than 20 KB should be avoided as the efficiency of KO decreases with increased length. In addition, for full length gene KO, the entire lncRNA gene needs to be located in a region that does not overlap with other genes. For the three other strategies, all need to be evaluated based on neighboring genes and how deletions of the specific regions might affect the neighboring genes expression. Identification of strong promoter regions can be examined using the UCSC Genome Browser.

2. Successful electroporation is usually accompanied with partial to high cell death. If no cell debris can be observed immediately after electroporation, electroporation was not successful. Further cell death will be visualized at media change after 24 h.

3. If a low amount of 96-well plates were filled with cells during flow sorting, the following reasons could explain this: insufficient trypsin digestion of cell suspension to generate single cell suspension, high loss of cells during preparation, or wrong flow rate during sorting.

4. If no single cell colonies are generated, the cell line might not be viable when seeded as single cells into a 96-well plate. Before performing KO, a test seeding should be performed on WT cells. Perform single cell sorting of WT cells into 96-wells and estimate number of viable single cells after 3 weeks. Clones should be viable and proliferating in >10% of the wells for the cell line to be appropriate for KO.

5. During the expansion of the colonies, there is a high risk of bacterial contamination. Be careful when handling the plates and plates should be taken out of the incubator only when necessary.

6. No heterozygous or homozygous clones: electroporation was not successful or unknown mutations are present in the sgRNA region of the lncRNA. Hence, we recommend screening of the lncRNA region in all cell lines in which KO is desired before the start of the experiment.

7. If there is a presence of a large population of heterozygous clones (>50%), the genomic region could be highly important for survival of the cells and not allowing for a complete removal of the genomic area. Alternatively, the genomic region could be amplified in the cell line, thereby decreasing the likelihood for removal of all genomic copies of the gene.

8. Additional methods to verify the establishment of complete KO include Northern blotting, RT-qPCR, and FISH.

## References

1. Doudna JA, Charpentier E (2014) Genome editing. The new frontier of genome engineering with CRISPR-Cas9. Science 346 (6213):1258096. https://doi.org/10.1126/science.1258096

2. Deltcheva E, Chylinski K, Sharma CM, Gonzales K, Chao Y, Pirzada ZA, Eckert MR, Vogel J, Charpentier E (2011) CRISPR RNA maturation by trans-encoded small RNA and host factor RNase III. Nature 471 (7340):602–607. https://doi.org/10.1038/nature09886

3. Jinek M, Chylinski K, Fonfara I, Hauer M, Doudna JA, Charpentier E (2012) A programmable dual-RNA-guided DNA endonuclease in adaptive bacterial immunity. Science 337 (6096):816–821. https://doi.org/10.1126/science.1225829

4. Barrangou R, Fremaux C, Deveau H, Richards M, Boyaval P, Moineau S, Romero DA, Horvath P (2007) CRISPR provides acquired resistance against viruses in prokaryotes. Science 315(5819):1709–1712. https://doi.org/10.1126/science.1138140

5. Brouns SJ, Jore MM, Lundgren M, Westra ER, Slijkhuis RJ, Snijders AP, Dickman MJ, Makarova KS, Koonin EV, van der Oost J (2008) Small CRISPR RNAs guide antiviral defense in prokaryotes. Science 321(5891):960–964. https://doi.org/10.1126/science.1159689

6. Wiedenheft B, Sternberg SH, Doudna JA (2012) RNA-guided genetic silencing systems in bacteria and archaea. Nature 482 (7385):331–338. https://doi.org/10.1038/nature10886

7. Haft DH, Selengut J, Mongodin EF, Nelson KE (2005) A guild of 45 CRISPR-associated (Cas) protein families and multiple CRISPR/Cas subtypes exist in prokaryotic genomes. PLoS Comput Biol 1(6):e60. https://doi.org/10.1371/journal.pcbi.0010060

8. Makarova KS, Wolf YI, Alkhnbashi OS, Costa F, Shah SA, Saunders SJ, Barrangou R, Brouns SJ, Charpentier E, Haft DH, Horvath P, Moineau S, Mojica FJ, Terns RM, Terns MP, White MF, Yakunin AF, Garrett RA, van der Oost J, Backofen R, Koonin EV (2015) An updated evolutionary classification of CRISPR-Cas systems. Nat Rev Microbiol 13 (11):722–736. https://doi.org/10.1038/nrmicro3569

9. Makarova KS, Koonin EV (2015) Annotation and classification of CRISPR-Cas systems. Methods Mol Biol 1311:47–75. https://doi.org/10.1007/978-1-4939-2687-9_4

10. Gasiunas G, Barrangou R, Horvath P, Siksnys V (2012) Cas9-crRNA ribonucleoprotein complex mediates specific DNA cleavage for adaptive immunity in bacteria. Proc Natl Acad Sci U S A 109(39):E2579–E2586. https://doi.org/10.1073/pnas.1208507109

11. Yan F, Wang W, Zhang J (2019) CRISPR-Cas12 and Cas13: the lesser known siblings of CRISPR-Cas9. Cell Biol Toxicol 35

(6):489–492.    https://doi.org/10.1007/s10565-019-09489-1

12. Pausch P, Al-Shayeb B, Bisom-Rapp E, Tsuchida CA, Li Z, Cress BF, Knott GJ, Jacobsen SE, Banfield JF, Doudna JA (2020) CRISPR-CasPhi from huge phages is a hypercompact genome editor. Science 369(6501):333–337. https://doi.org/10.1126/science.abb1400

13. Hille F, Richter H, Wong SP, Bratovic M, Ressel S, Charpentier E (2018) The biology of CRISPR-Cas: backward and forward. Cell 172(6):1239–1259.    https://doi.org/10.1016/j.cell.2017.11.032

14. Knott GJ, Doudna JA (2018) CRISPR-Cas guides the future of genetic engineering. Science 361(6405):866–869. https://doi.org/10.1126/science.aat5011

15. Xiao-Jie L, Hui-Ying X, Zun-Ping K, Jin-Lian C, Li-Juan J (2015) CRISPR-Cas9: a new and promising player in gene therapy. J Med Genet 52(5):289–296. https://doi.org/10.1136/jmedgenet-2014-102968

16. Cyranoski D (2016) CRISPR gene-editing tested in a person for the first time. Nature 539(7630):479.    https://doi.org/10.1038/nature.2016.20988

17. Hirakawa MP, Krishnakumar R, Timlin JA, Carney JP, Butler KS (2020) Gene editing and CRISPR in the clinic: current and future perspectives. Biosci Rep 40(4):BSR20200127. https://doi.org/10.1042/BSR20200127

18. Dragomir MP, Kopetz S, Ajani JA, Calin GA (2020) Non-coding RNAs in GI cancers: from cancer hallmarks to clinical utility. Gut 69(4):748–763.    https://doi.org/10.1136/gutjnl-2019-318279

19. Mercer TR, Dinger ME, Mattick JS (2009) Long non-coding RNAs: insights into functions. Nat Rev Genet 10(3):155–159. https://doi.org/10.1038/nrg2521

20. Wang KC, Chang HY (2011) Molecular mechanisms of long noncoding RNAs. Mol Cell 43(6):904–914. https://doi.org/10.1016/j.molcel.2011.08.018

# Chapter 13

## CRISPR Interference (CRISPRi) and CRISPR Activation (CRISPRa) to Explore the Oncogenic lncRNA Network

**Eugenio Morelli, Annamaria Gulla', Nicola Amodio, Elisa Taiana, Antonino Neri, Mariateresa Fulciniti, and Nikhil C. Munshi**

### Abstract

The human genome contains thousands of long noncoding RNAs (lncRNAs), even outnumbering protein-coding genes. These molecules can play a pivotal role in the development and progression of human disease, including cancer, and are susceptible to therapeutic intervention. Evidence of biologic function, however, is still missing for the vast majority of them. Both loss-of-function (LOF) and gain-of-function (GOF) studies are therefore necessary to advance our understanding of lncRNA networks and programs driving tumorigenesis. Here, we describe a protocol to perform lncRNA's LOF or GOF studies in multiple myeloma (MM) cells, using CRISPR interference (CRISPRi) or CRISPR activation (CRISPRa) technologies, respectively. These approaches have many advantages, including applicability to large-scale genetic screens in mammalian cells and possible reversibility of modulating effects; moreover, CRISPRa offers the unique opportunity to enhance lncRNA expression at the site of transcription, with relevant biologic implications.

**Key words** Long noncoding RNA, lncRNA, CRISPR interference, CRISPRi, CRISPR activation, CRISPRa, Cancer, Multiple myeloma

## 1 Introduction

Long noncoding RNAs (lncRNAs) are transcripts with lengths exceeding 200 nucleotides that structurally resemble mRNAs but lack the ability to translate into proteins [1]. The abundance of lncRNA genes (>25,000) outnumber protein-coding genes (~20,000), with a pattern of expression often restricted to specific cell types or conditions [2].

Increasing amount of evidence suggest a pivotal role for lncRNA networks in the development and progression of human diseases, especially cancer, lending support to the importance of their cellular functions [3]. The lncRNA landscape is indeed profoundly affected during malignant transformation, where these molecules have been described as potential drivers, suggesting their use as either biomarkers or therapeutic targets [4–7]. For

Alfons Navarro (ed.), *Long Non-Coding RNAs in Cancer*, Methods in Molecular Biology, vol. 2348,
https://doi.org/10.1007/978-1-0716-1581-2_13, © Springer Science+Business Media, LLC, part of Springer Nature 2021

example, we have recently analyzed the lncRNA landscape in multiple myeloma (MM) patients which resulted significantly different from the lncRNA profile of plasma cells from healthy individuals; and reported their role as independent risk predictors for clinical outcome [8].

With the number of well-characterized cancer-associated lncRNAs growing, the study of lncRNAs in cancer is now generating new hypotheses about the biology of cancer cells. However, their mechanism of action and biological functions are still largely unknown, supporting the need to establish novel methods to study lncRNA networks and programs.

Loss-of (LOF) and gain-of-function (GOF) studies to explore lncRNA expression involve either manipulations at the level of lncRNA gene loci (e.g., gene modification or local recruitment of transcriptional regulators) or manipulations directly involving the RNA transcript (e.g., RNA knockdown or transfection of RNA molecules) [9], as summarized in Table 1. However, biological properties unique to lncRNAs make their genetic manipulation challenging. For instance, several studies have shown that lncRNAs can regulate expression of target genes both *in cis*, in proximity to their site of transcription, and *in trans*, at locations genetically unlinked and spatially distant from their site of production [10–12]. Moreover, lncRNA loci can map to known enhancers or overlap with coding genes [11], making it often difficult to genetically disrupt the lncRNA without affecting local coding genes with possible misinterpretations of data. Therefore, genetic manipulation of lncRNAs need to be supported by knowledge of transcript properties (e.g., its primary sequence, potential isoforms, presence or lack of polyadenylation) and corresponding DNA loci (e.g., accurate mapping of the transcription start site (TSS), genomic relationship to protein coding genes and known enhancers). In most cases, to decipher the function(s) of the lncRNA locus and its transcriptional product, it will be required the use of orthogonal experiments (e.g., epigenetic silencing of lncRNA gene loci and degradation of lncRNA transcripts).

The discovery and continuous development of CRISPR-Cas technologies has rapidly changed the routine for manipulating and studying the coding and noncoding genome [9, 13]. Several Cas proteins can be used to directly target the lncRNA gene loci (i.e., CRISPR/Cas9) [14] or the lncRNA transcripts (i.e., CRISPR/Cas13) [15, 16] with different possible applications including loss-of-function and subcellular localization studies. Moreover, the use of nuclease-dead Cas9 (dCas9) has also emerged as powerful tool to either repress (CRISPRi) [17–21] or activate (CRISPRa) [20–24] the expression of lncRNAs in mammalian cells. As summarized in Table 1, advantages of using dCas9 proteins for LOF or GOF experiments include the need of only one single guide RNA (sgRNA) targeting the TSS of interest (while, for instance, KO

**Table 1**
**Broadly used LOF and GOF approaches to explore lncRNA activity**

| | | Technique | Outcome | *Pros* | *Cons* | References |
|---|---|---|---|---|---|---|
| LncRNA "gene" manipulation | LOF | CRISPRn | KO | · Complete KO possible<br>· Targeting of both *cis* acting and *trans* acting lncRNAs<br>· Large-scale screening application<br>· Relatively few off-target effects | · May require paired sgRNAs<br>· Cannot discriminate *cis* and *trans* acting lncRNAs<br>· Stochastic outcome in individual cells (mono or biallelic KO)<br>· Cannot discriminate lncRNA isoforms | [13, 14, 26] |
| | | CRISPRi | KD | · One sgRNA required;<br>· Reversible KD using inducible dCas9 fusion proteins<br>· Targeting of both *cis* acting and *trans* acting lncRNAs<br>· Large-scale screening application<br>· Relatively few off-target effects | · Cannot discriminate *cis* and *trans* acting lncRNAs<br>· Cannot discriminate lncRNA isoforms (except if derived from alternative TSS)<br>· Requires precise information about TSS and gene neighborhood | [9, 13, 17–21, 24, 26] |
| | GOF | Lentiviral ORF | Ectopic expression | · Can discriminate lncRNA isoforms | · Does not reproduce activity in *cis*<br>· Cannot be used for very long lncRNAs (generally >5000 nt) | [26] |
| | | CRISPRa | Enhanced endogenous expression | · One single gRNA required<br>· Increases | · Cannot discriminate *cis* and *trans* acting | [13, 20–23, 25, 26] |

(continued)

**Table 1**
**(continued)**

| | | Technique | Outcome | *Pros* | *Cons* | References |
|---|---|---|---|---|---|---|
| | | | | lncRNA expression at proper site of transcription<br>· Works on lncRNAs independently of transcript length<br>· Large-scale screening application<br>· Relatively few off-target effects | lncRNAs<br>· Cannot discriminate lncRNA isoforms (except if derived from alternative TSS) | |
| LncRNA "transcript" manipulation | LOF | RNAi (siRNAs or shRNAs) | RISC-mediated KD | · Can discriminate lncRNA isoforms<br>· Large-scale screening<br>· application using lentiviral shRNAs | · Low or no activity on nuclear lncRNAs (including all cis acting lncRNAs)<br>· Many off-targets<br>· Expansive (siRNAs) | [7, 26] |
| | | ASOs | RNase H-mediated KD | · Targeting of both *cis* acting and *trans* acting lncRNAs<br>· Use in transfection-free conditions (gymnosis), avoiding transfection-related toxicity<br>· Gymnosis can be used in primary samples form patients | · Cannot discriminate lncRNA isoforms<br>· Many off-targets<br>· Not available for large-scale screenings<br>· Expansive | [6] |
| | | Cas13 (-A, -B or -D) | KD | · Targeting of both *cis* acting and *trans* acting lncRNAs | · gRNA design web portals not yet available | [15, 16] |

(continued)

**Table 1**
**(continued)**

| | Technique | Outcome | Pros | Cons | References |
|---|---|---|---|---|---|
| GOF | Transfection of lncRNA transcript | Ectopic expression | · Very specific<br>· Large-scale screening application<br>· Can discriminate lncRNA isoforms<br>· Can discriminate activity in nucleus and cytosol<br>· Can discriminate lncRNA isoforms | · Does not reproduce activity in *cis*<br>· Requires in vitro transcription | [9] |

*LOF* loss-of-function, *GOF* gain-of-function, *CRISPRn* CRISPR nuclease (canonical CRISPR-Cas9), *CRISPRi* CRISPR interference, *CRISPRa* CRISPR activation, *RNAi* RNA interference, *ASOs* antisense oligonucleotides, specifically referring to gapmeRs in this table, *KO* knockout, *KD* knockdown

using CRISPR/Cas9 may require paired sgRNAs); applicability in genetic screens in mammalian cells; and reversibility of modulating effect using inducible Cas9 vectors. Moreover, compared to other GOF approaches, CRISPRa offers the unique opportunity to enhance lncRNA expression at its own site of transcription, allowing to investigate activity *in cis* [25].

CRISPRi is based on the use of dCas9 protein fused to the Kruppel-associated box (KRAB) transcriptional repressor domain (dCas9-KRAB) [17, 20, 21] (Fig. 1a). The CRISPRi system represses transcription in part through dCas9's ability to block RNA polymerase elongation and in part through the KRAB domain that recruits KRAB-Associated Protein 1 (KAP1), Heterochromatin Protein 1-Alpha (HP1α) and other proteins to edit the epigenome by deposition of H3k9me3 [18]. This approach minimally requires expression of the dCas9-KRAB fusion protein and a customizable targeting sgRNA directed at the TSS of lncRNAs of interest. The expression of both coding and noncoding genes can be efficiently repressed [17, 19]; and applications span from the investigation of specific lncRNA candidates to large scale loss-of-function screenings [26]. With a precise and relatively narrow window of activity between −50 and +300 bp relative to the TSS of the target gene, CRISPRi can repress lncRNA expression while minimizing disruption to the activity of cis regulatory regions or neighboring genes.

On the other hand, CRISPRa is based on the use of dCas9 protein fused to transcriptional activator domains and customizable sgRNAs designed to bind upstream of TSS of genes of interest (−300 to +50 bp) [9, 13]. This approach can be applied to enhance transcription of both coding and noncoding genes, in either targeted experiments or screening approaches [9, 13]. Three main CRISPRa approaches have been optimized so far, each based on the use of single gRNAs and dCas9 fusion proteins recruiting more than one activator domain: (1) the VPR (VP64-p65-Rta) system [24] (Fig. 1b), (2) the SunTag system [22], and (3) the SAM (Synergistic Activation Mediator) system [23]. These CRISPRa approaches have been extensively reviewed by others. In this chapter, we will only focus on the use of the VPR system for the activation of lncRNAs expression. In the VPR system, the dCas9 is fused to three transcriptional activator domains: VP64 (an engineered tetramer of the herpes simplex VP16 transcriptional activator domain), p65 (subunit of NF-kB) and Epstein−Barr virus R transactivator Rta [24]. Compared to other CRISPRa systems, VPR minimally requires one vector for the dCas9 fusion protein and one vector to express customizable sgRNAs.

The following protocol details the use of CRISPRi or CRISPRa to modulate the expression of candidate lncRNAs in human MM cell lines; along with troubleshooting tips, explanations, and recommendations for the successful execution and analysis of experiments.

## 2    Materials

Prepare all solutions with ultrapure water and molecular biology grade reagents.

### 2.1  dCAS9 and gRNA Vectors

1. dCas9 plasmid for CRISPRi pHR-SFFV-dCas9-BFP-KRAB (Plasmid #46911, Addgene).

2. dCas9 plasmid for CRISPRa pXPR_120 (Plasmid #96917, Addgene).

3. Human gRNA plasmid pU6-sgRNA EF1Alpha-puro-T2A-BFP (Plasmid #60955, Addgene).

4. pLenti-CMV-GFP-Puro (658-5) (Plasmid #17448, Addgene) to be used as positive control for transfection and transduction experiments.

5. Restriction enzymes *BstXI* and *BlpI* (New England Biolabs).

6. NEBuffer™ 2.1 (New England Biolabs).

7. QIAquick gel extraction kit (Qiagen).

## A    CRISPRi

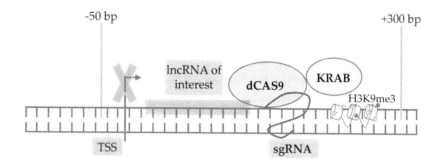

## B

## CRISPRa

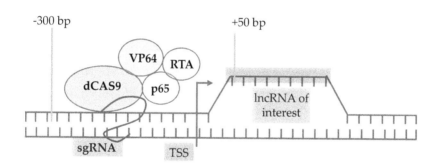

**Fig. 1** CRISPRi and CRISPRa to modulate lncRNA expression. (**a**) CRISPRi: sgRNA recruits dCas9-KRAB fusion protein at the genomic locus of lncRNA of interest, in a region ranging from −50 to +300 bp relative to TSS. dCas9-KRAB fusion protein antagonizes lncRNA transcription in part through dCas9's ability to block RNA polymerase elongation and in part through the KRAB domain that mediates deposition of H3K9me3 (**b**) CRISPRa: sgRNA recruits dCas9-VPR fusion protein at the genomic locus of lncRNA of interest, in a region ranging from −300 to +50 bp relative to TSS. dCas9-VPR fusion protein enhances lncRNA transcription via combined activity of VP64, p65 and RTA

8. UltraPure 10× TAE buffer (Invitrogen).

9. UltraPure agarose (Invitrogen).

10. GelRed® Nucleic Acid Gel Stain (Biotium).

11. PCR primers for sgRNA cloning.

12. Oligo Annealing buffer: 10 mM Tris–HCl, 50 mM NaCl.

13. Quick Ligation™ Kit (New England Biolabs).

14. One Shot™ Stbl3™ Chemically Competent *E. coli* (Invitrogen).

15. LB medium (Sigma-Aldrich).

16. LB agar medium (Sigma-Aldrich).

17. Ampicillin, sterile filtered, 100 mg mL$^{-1}$ (Sigma-Aldrich).

18. QIAGEN Plasmid Mini Kit (Qiagen).

19. ddH$_2$O, sterile.

**2.2   Virus Generation**

1. Lenti-X™ 293T Cell Line (Takara).

2. DMEM (Dulbecco's Modified Eagle Medium), FBS-free, antibiotic-free.

3. Lipofectamine 2000 Transfection Reagent (Thermo Fisher Scientific).

4. pMD2.G (Plasmid #12259, Addgene).

5. psPAX2 (Plasmid #12260, Addgene).

6. DNA vector of interest (dCas9 or gRNA).

7. Complete Medium (DMEM).

8. Lenti-X™ Concentrator (Takara).

9. Phosphate buffered saline (PBS).

10. Trypsin-EDTA (0.05%), phenol red (Gibco).

**2.3   Testing CRISPRi/a in Multiple Myeloma (MM) Cells**

1. MM cell line (e.g., AMO1, available at DSMZ).

2. Complete growth medium (RPMI-1640, 10% FBS, 1% Pen-Strep) supplemented with L-glutamine 300 mg/L (*see* **Note 1**).

3. Polybrene (SantaCruz Biotechnology).

4. Phosphate buffered saline (PBS).

5. Puromycin dihydrochloride (Sigma Aldrich).

6. Blasticidin (Thermo fisher Scientific).

7. Fluorescence microscope.

8. Cell sorter.

9. Quantitative RT-PCR reagents.

**2.4   Equipment**

1. RNase-free microfuge tubes (1.5 mL).

2. Thermocycler with programmable temperature control.

3. PCR plates, 96 wells.

4. Real-time PCR System.

5. 0.2 mL PCR tubes.

6. Gel electrophoresis system.

7. T75 cm$^2$ cell culture flasks.

8. Incubator for bacteria plates or warm room.

9. Microplate shaking incubator for bacteria suspension culture.

10. NanoDrop 8000 UV-visible spectrophotometer (Thermo Scientific).

11. Multiwell tissue culture plates.

12. Digital gel imaging system.

13. BD-LSR II (BD Biosciences) or alternate flow cytometer.

# 3  Methods

## 3.1  Stable Expression of dCAS9 Fusion Proteins in MM Cell Lines

The following protocol can be used to generate lentiviral particles using either CRISPRi or CRISPRa dCAS9 vectors, as well as gRNA vectors. Each time, it is strongly recommended the use of pLenti-CMV-GFP-Puro as positive control (*see* **Note 2**).

### 3.1.1  Production of Lentiviral Particles

1. *Day 1*: seed $5 \times 10^6$ Lenti-X™ 293T cells per T75 flask in 12 mL culture media.

2. *Day 2*: change medium on the Lenti-X™ 293T cells (11 mL DMEM) 1 h prior to transfection.

3. Prepare the transfection mix as follows:
   (a) Solution "A": 500μL of FBS-free DMEM (*see* **Note 3**) and 40μL Lipofectamine 2000.
   (b) Solution "B": 500μL of FBS-free DMEM (*see* **Note 3**), 4μg of DNA vector, 4μg psPAX.2 and 2μg pMD2.G.

4. Mix solution A and B by vortexing and incubate 5′ at RT.

5. Add transfection mix to Lenti-X™ 293T cells.

6. *Day 3*: remove the medium from the T75 flask and add 10 mL fresh media (*see* **Note 4**).

7. Check the transfection efficiency (optional): on *Day 3* you can evaluate the transfection efficiency by fluorescence microscopy. If you estimate the transfection efficiency to be below 70%, consider starting over.

8. *Day 4*: collect the supernatant from the T75 flask; if you are planning on doing a second harvest on day 5, add 10 mL fresh medium and incubate for another 24 h.

9. Filter the pooled supernatant through a 0.45μm filter.

10. Concentrate lentiviral particles using Lenti-X™ Concentrator, according to manufacturer's protocol available at the following link: https://www.takarabio.com/assets/documents/User%20Manual/PT4421-2.pdf.

### 3.1.2  Transduction of MM Cells

The following protocol can be used to generate either CRISPRi or CRISPRa dCAS9-expressing MM cell lines (AMO1 for this protocol). Each time, it is strongly recommended the use of pLenti-CMV-GFP-Puro as positive control (*see* **Note 2**). It is recommended to transduce at a low multiplicity of infection (MOI) of

0.1–0.3. The low MOI helps control the number of inserted copies of the dCas9 fusion proteins-encoding cassette per cell, reducing the overall heterogeneity of the population in terms of dCas9 expression levels. Therefore, before to generate dCas9-expressing cells, assess the titer of lentiviral particles (*see* **Note 5**).

1. *Day 1*: seed $1 \times 10^6$ cells per well in a 6-well plate or in another suitable culture format, in a final volume of 2 mL. Seed cells in three wells in total: cells in the first well will be used as negative control (transduced without any vector), cells in the second well will be used as positive control (transduced with pLenti-CMV-GFP-Puro), cells in the third well will be infected with dCas9 lentiviral particles (either for CRISPRi or CRISPRa).

2. *Day 1* (same day): transduce using a viral particle load ensuring low MOI. Transduction of MM cells requires Spinoculation: spin in a balanced tabletop centrifuge for 1 h at 1000 rpm at 32 °C. Collect cells, wash twice with 1× sterile PBS, and resuspend in 4 mL of complete culture media.

3. *Day 5*: protocol will differ if generating stable cell line for CRISPRi or CRISPRa.
   (a) Option 1 (generation of CRISPRi cell line using pHR-SFFV-dCas9-BFP-KRAB vector), select BFP+ cells using cell sorter. The first well serves as control (BFP negative population).

   (b) Option 2 (generation of CRISPRa cell line using pXPR_120), replace culture media with media containing blasticidin (*see* **Note 6**); the first well serves as a control for blasticidin selection.

4. From *Day 5* to *Day 20*: proceed by culturing cells in a larger appropriate culture volume. For Option 1, you may perform another round of cell sorting to ensure a >99% BFP+ population; for option 2, maintain cells under blasticidin selection and passage as required.

5. *Day 21*: freeze down several aliquots of the population and proceed to test the functionality of dCas9 fusion proteins (as detailed in Subheading 3.3).

6. (Optional) To establish and characterize individual dCas9-expressing clones, seed cells individually to start generating expanded cell clones.

### 3.2 gRNA Design and Cloning

#### 3.2.1 Design

gRNAs for either CRISPRi or CRISPRa can be designed using the Broad Institute's Genetic Perturbation Platform (GPP) web portal (https://portals.broadinstitute.org/gpp/public/analysis-tools/sgrna-design-crisprai). For well-investigated lncRNAs (e.g., MALAT1 or XIST), it is sufficient to input gene ID. For novel lncRNAs, or to target alternative TSSs, it is required to input a syntax indicating chromosome, strand and TSS position (*see* **Note 7**). As general rule, CRISPRi works better if gRNAs bind between −50 and +300 bp relative to the TSS of the target lncRNA; while CRISPRa works better if gRNAs bind between −300 and +50 bp relative to the TSS of the target lncRNA. Oligonucleotides (oligo) for gRNAs to be cloned into the pU6-sgRNA EF1Alpha-puro-T2A-BFP vector should be designed as follows.

1. Top oligo
   (a) 5′ end, add "TTG."
   (b) Protospacer sequence (this is the output provided by Broad Institute's Genetic GPP web portal).
   (c) 3′ end, add "GTTTAAGAGC."

2. Bottom oligo
   (a) 5′ end, add "TTAGCTCTTAAAC."
   (b) "Reverse complement" of protospacer sequence (*see* **Note 8**).
   (c) 3′ end, add "CAACAAG."

*3.2.2 Cloning*

1. Perform the oligo annealing. For oligo annealing prepare the following mix: 5μL of 100μM Top oligo, 5μL of 100μM Top oligo, and 40μL of Annealing buffer.

2. Place it in the thermocycler with the following program: 30 min at 37 °C, 10 min at 97 °C, and let oligos gradually anneal while cooling to RT (take the plate out and set it on your bench).

3. Make a 1:20 dilution of annealed oligos in ddH2O. Annealed oligos can be stored at −20 °C and are stable through at least 2–3 freeze thaws.

4. Perform the vector digestion. Prepare following mix to digest backbone vector (pU6-sgRNA EF1Alpha-puro-T2A-BFP): 1μL of *BstXI* and 1μL *BlpI*, 1μg of DNA vector, 5μL of 10× NEBuffer (2.1) and 42μL of ddH$_2$O. Incubate for 15′ at 37 °C.

5. Separate the restriction enzyme–digested samples by electrophoresis in a 1% (wt/vol) agarose gel using standard protocols. Verify the fragment size using a suitable DNA ladder; the correct band is at ~9 kb. Extract the ~9000-bp-long vector DNA using the gel purification kit.

6. Perform the Ligation. Prepare the following mix (total volume = 20μL): 100 ng of digested vector backbone (pU6-sgRNA EF1Alpha-puro-T2A-BFP), 2μL of 1:20 diluted annealed oligos, 10μL of Quick Ligase Reaction Buffer (2×), 1μL Quick Ligase and ddH$_2$O up to 20μL. Gently mix the reaction by pipetting up and down and microfuge briefly. Incubate at room temperature (25 °C) for 5 min.

7. Chill on ice and transform 1–5µL of the reaction into 50µL competent cells using standard protocols. Alternatively, Store at −20 °C. Do not heat-inactivate—heat inactivation dramatically reduces transformation efficiency.

8. Pick one colony per gRNA construct and miniprep.

9. Sanger sequence (*see* **Note 9**).

10. Lentiviral particles can be generated as described above (Subheading 3.1.1).

### 3.3 Modulation of lncRNA Expression in MM Cells

Assessing the functionality and efficiency of dCas9 fusion proteins in the cells can be done by delivering a sgRNA to the cells. We recommend doing this by transducing the cells with gRNAs targeting a very highly expressed gene for CRISPRi, such as the metabolic enzyme Enolase 1 (ENO1); or with gRNAs targeting a very poorly expressed gene for CRISPRa, such as the POU Class 5 Homeobox 1 (*POU5F1*) gene. In Fig. 2, we provide examples for both CRISPRi and CRISPRa efficiency in different MM cell lines. Protocol below can be applied to both CRISPRi and CRISPRa MM cell lines.

1. *Day 1*: seed 2–5 × $10^5$ cells per well in a 6-well dish or in another suitable culture format. Seed cells in three wells in total: cells in the first well will be used as negative control (transduced without any vector), cells in the second well will be used as positive control (transduced with pLenti-CMV-GFP-Puro), cells in the third well will be infected with sgRNAs.

2. *Day 1* (same day): transduce MM cells using Spinoculation protocol as detailed above. We usually use MOI ~ 2 for transduction with gRNAs.

3. *Day 3*: apply puromycin to all wells (*see* **Note 6**); the first well will serve as a control for puromycin selection.

4. *Day 5*: harvest cells for downstream application (q-RT-PCR).

## 4  Notes

1. MM cells are dependent on glutamine for their growth and survival. Make sure to purchase RPMI-1640 medium already supplemented with glutamine; otherwise provide to supplementation by yourself.

2. Using the pLenti-CMV-GFP-Puro as positive control will definitively result in a save of time for your experiments. Each time, 24 h after transfection of Lenti-X™ 293T cells or 24–48 h after transduction of MM cells, check GFP at fluorescence microscope to assess transfection or transduction efficiency. This will allow to easily identify errors occurred during transfection or transduction.

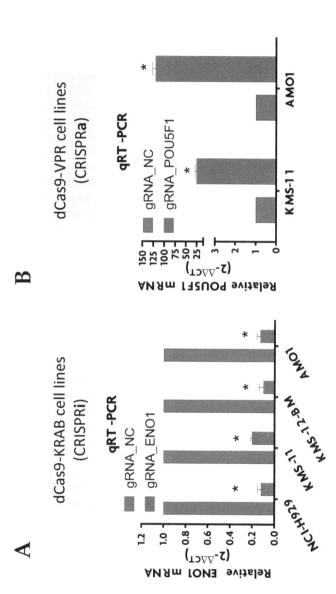

**Fig. 2** Functionality of CRISPRi and CRISPRa dCas9 fusion proteins in MM cell lines. (**a**) Knockdown of ENO1 expression obtained in four MM cell lines (NCI-H929, KMS-11, KMS-12-BM and AMO1) engineered to express a dCas9-KRAB fusion protein. ENO1 mRNA expression was investigated by qRT-PCR 5 days after infection with gRNA vectors, according to protocol. The results shown are relative mRNA expression levels after normalization with GAPDH and $\Delta\Delta$Ct calculations. gRNA sequence for ENO1 (gRNA_ENO1): CCGGCGAGATCTCCGTGCTC. gRNA sequence used as nontargeting negative control (gRNA_NC): GATGTGGTCATTCGTCATGA. (**b**) Enhancement of POU5F1 expression obtained in two MM cell lines (KMS-11 and AMO1) engineered to express a dCas9-VPR fusion protein. POU5F1 mRNA expression was investigated by qRT-PCR 5 days after infection with gRNA vectors, according to protocol. The results shown are relative mRNA expression levels after normalization with GAPDH and $\Delta\Delta C_t$ calculations. gRNAs were obtained from Dharmacon. * $p < 0.05$

3. Presence of serum in the transfection mix will strongly reduce transfection efficiency.

4. This step is important to reduce the "carryover" of plasmid along with lentiviral particles. However, it can become optional if planning to concentrate the virus.

5. The titering of lentiviral particles can be performed either by flow-cytometry (if the lentiviral vector has a fluorescent marker) or by antibiotic selection (if the lentiviral vector has an antibiotic-resistance marker). Use the following protocol from Cellecta: https://manuals.cellecta.com/crispr-pooled-lentiviral-sgrna-libraries/.

6. Calculate killing curve before starting the experiment. MM cells are sensitive to blasticidin concentrations ranging 5–10μg/mL and puromycin concentrations ranging from 0.25 to 1.5μg/mL.

7. For the syntax, input the following lncRNA's information in the gene input box of Broad Institute's Genetic Perturbation Platform (GPP) web portal (URL has been provided above, Subheading 3.2.1):

   (a) chromosome NCBI's RefSeq identifiers (e.g., NC_000001.11 for chromosome 1).

   (b) Strand (+ or −).

   (c) TSS.

   As example, we here provide the syntax to design gRNAs targeting the transcript MALAT1.1. This transcript, according to LNCipedia version 5.2 (https://lnci-pedia.org/db/search?search_id=malat1), is located on chr11:65496267-65509085, positive strand.

   (a) Chr11 becomes "NC_000011.10".

   (b) Positive strand becomes "+".

   (c) TTS is 6549626.

   The correct syntax is "NC_000011.10:+:65496267".
   Note that, if the transcript was produced at the negative strand, the TSS would have been 65509085.

8. To obtain reverse complement, use online tools such as https://www.bioinformatics.org/sms/rev_comp.html.

9. Use human U6 promoter forward primer LKO.1 5′ (Weinberg Lab): GACTATCATATGCTTACCGT.

## Acknowledgments

This work was supported by National Institutes of Health Grants No. P01 CA155258 and P50 CA100707, and VA Healthcare System Grant No. 5I01BX001584. This work was also supported by Italian Ministry of Health (GR-2016-02361523). Annamaria Gulla' is a Fellow of The Leukemia & Lymphoma Society and a Scholar of the American Society of Hematology (ASH).

**Grant Funding**

E.M. is supported by the Brian D. Novis Junior Grant from the International Myeloma Foundation (IMF) and by the Dana Farber/Harvard Cancer Center SPORE in Multiple Myeloma Career Enhancement Award (SPORE-P50CA100707).

We thank the "8th Annual Miracles for Myeloma 5K Virtual Run/Walk" organizers and attendees for the fundraising in support to this research project.

## References

1. Ulitsky I, Bartel DP (2013) lincRNAs: genomics, evolution, and mechanisms. Cell 154 (1):26–46. https://doi.org/10.1016/j.cell.2013.06.020

2. Hon CC, Ramilowski JA, Harshbarger J, Bertin N, Rackham OJ, Gough J, Denisenko E, Schmeier S, Poulsen TM, Severin J, Lizio M, Kawaji H, Kasukawa T, Itoh M, Burroughs AM, Noma S, Djebali S, Alam T, Medvedeva YA, Testa AC, Lipovich L, Yip CW, Abugessaisa I, Mendez M, Hasegawa A, Tang D, Lassmann T, Heutink P, Babina M, Wells CA, Kojima S, Nakamura Y, Suzuki H, Daub CO, de Hoon MJ, Arner E, Hayashizaki Y, Carninci P, Forrest AR (2017) An atlas of human long non-coding RNAs with accurate 5′ ends. Nature 543(7644):199–204. https://doi.org/10.1038/nature21374

3. Wapinski O, Chang HY (2011) Long noncoding RNAs and human disease. Trends Cell Biol 21(6):354–361. https://doi.org/10.1016/j.tcb.2011.04.001

4. Schmitt AM, Chang HY (2016) Long noncoding RNAs in cancer pathways. Cancer Cell 29 (4):452–463. https://doi.org/10.1016/j.ccell.2016.03.010

5. Morelli E, Gulla A, Rocca R, Federico C, Raimondi L, Malvestiti S, Agosti V, Rossi M, Costa G, Giavaresi G, Azab KA, Cagnetta A, Cea M, Tagliaferri P, Neri A, Munshi NC, Viglietto G, Tassone P, Amodio N (2020) The non-coding RNA landscape of plasma cell Dyscrasias. Cancers (Basel) 12(2):320. https://doi.org/10.3390/cancers12020320

6. Amodio N, Stamato MA, Juli G, Morelli E, Fulciniti M, Manzoni M, Taiana E, Agnelli L, Cantafio MEG, Romeo E, Raimondi L, Caracciolo D, Zuccala V, Rossi M, Neri A, Munshi NC, Tagliaferri P, Tassone P (2018) Drugging the lncRNA MALAT1 via LNA gapmeR ASO inhibits gene expression of proteasome subunits and triggers anti-multiple myeloma activity. Leukemia 32 (9):1948–1957. https://doi.org/10.1038/s41375-018-0067-3

7. Tseng YY, Moriarity BS, Gong W, Akiyama R, Tiwari A, Kawakami H, Ronning P, Reuland B, Guenther K, Beadnell TC, Essig J, Otto GM, O'Sullivan MG, Largaespada DA, Schwertfeger KL, Marahrens Y, Kawakami Y, Bagchi A (2014) PVT1 dependence in cancer with MYC copy-number increase. Nature 512 (7512):82–86. https://doi.org/10.1038/nature13311

8. Samur MK, Minvielle S, Gulla A, Fulciniti M, Cleynen A, Aktas Samur A, Szalat R, Shammas M, Magrangeas F, Tai YT, Auclair D, Keats J, Richardson P, Attal M, Moreau P, Anderson KC, Parmigiani G, Avet-Loiseau H, Munshi NC (2018) Long intergenic non-coding RNAs have an independent impact on survival in multiple myeloma. Leukemia 32(12):2626–2635. https://doi.org/10.1038/s41375-018-0116-y

9. Liu SJ, Lim DA (2018) Modulating the expression of long non-coding RNAs for functional studies. EMBO Rep 19(12):e46955. https://doi.org/10.15252/embr.201846955

10. Engreitz JM, Ollikainen N, Guttman M (2016) Long non-coding RNAs: spatial amplifiers that control nuclear structure and gene expression. Nat Rev Mol Cell Biol 17 (12):756–770. https://doi.org/10.1038/nrm.2016.126

11. Engreitz JM, Haines JE, Perez EM, Munson G, Chen J, Kane M, McDonel PE, Guttman M, Lander ES (2016) Local regulation of gene expression by lncRNA promoters, transcription and splicing. Nature 539 (7629):452–455. https://doi.org/10.1038/nature20149

12. Hacisuleyman E, Goff LA, Trapnell C, Williams A, Henao-Mejia J, Sun L, McClanahan P, Hendrickson DG, Sauvageau M, Kelley DR, Morse M, Engreitz J, Lander ES, Guttman M, Lodish HF, Flavell R, Raj A, Rinn JL (2014) Topological organization of multichromosomal regions by the long intergenic noncoding RNA firre. Nat Struct Mol Biol 21(2):198–206. https://doi.org/10.1038/nsmb.2764

13. Engreitz J, Abudayyeh O, Gootenberg J, Zhang F (2019) CRISPR tools for systematic studies of RNA regulation. Cold Spring Harb Perspect Biol 11(8):a035386. https://doi.org/10.1101/cshperspect.a035386

14. Zhu S, Li W, Liu J, Chen CH, Liao Q, Xu P, Xu H, Xiao T, Cao Z, Peng J, Yuan P, Brown M, Liu XS, Wei W (2016) Genome-scale deletion screening of human long non-coding RNAs using a paired-guide RNA CRISPR-Cas9 library. Nat Biotechnol 34 (12):1279–1286. https://doi.org/10.1038/nbt.3715

15. Abudayyeh OO, Gootenberg JS, Essletzbichler P, Han S, Joung J, Belanto JJ, Verdine V, Cox DBT, Kellner MJ, Regev A, Lander ES, Voytas DF, Ting AY, Zhang F (2017) RNA targeting with CRISPR-Cas13. Nature 550(7675):280–284. https://doi.org/10.1038/nature24049

16. Konermann S, Lotfy P, Brideau NJ, Oki J, Shokhirev MN, Hsu PD (2018) Transcriptome engineering with RNA-targeting type VI-D CRISPR effectors. Cell 173(3):665–676. e614. https://doi.org/10.1016/j.cell.2018.02.033

17. Larson MH, Gilbert LA, Wang X, Lim WA, Weissman JS, Qi LS (2013) CRISPR interference (CRISPRi) for sequence-specific control of gene expression. Nat Protoc 8 (11):2180–2196. https://doi.org/10.1038/nprot.2013.132

18. Thakore PI, D'Ippolito AM, Song L, Safi A, Shivakumar NK, Kabadi AM, Reddy TE, Crawford GE, Gersbach CA (2015) Highly specific epigenome editing by CRISPR-Cas9 repressors for silencing of distal regulatory elements. Nat Methods 12(12):1143–1149. https://doi.org/10.1038/nmeth.3630

19. Liu SJ, Horlbeck MA, Cho SW, Birk HS, Malatesta M, He D, Attenello FJ, Villalta JE, Cho MY, Chen Y, Mandegar MA, Olvera MP, Gilbert LA, Conklin BR, Chang HY, Weissman JS, Lim DA (2017) CRISPRi-based genome-scale identification of functional long noncoding RNA loci in human cells. Science 355 (6320):aah7111. https://doi.org/10.1126/science.aah7111

20. Gilbert LA, Larson MH, Morsut L, Liu Z, Brar GA, Torres SE, Stern-Ginossar N, Brandman O, Whitehead EH, Doudna JA, Lim WA, Weissman JS, Qi LS (2013) CRISPR-mediated modular RNA-guided regulation of transcription in eukaryotes. Cell 154 (2):442–451. https://doi.org/10.1016/j.cell.2013.06.044

21. Gilbert LA, Horlbeck MA, Adamson B, Villalta JE, Chen Y, Whitehead EH, Guimaraes C, Panning B, Ploegh HL, Bassik MC, Qi LS, Kampmann M, Weissman JS (2014) Genome-scale CRISPR-mediated control of gene repression and activation. Cell 159(3):647–661. https://doi.org/10.1016/j.cell.2014.09.029

22. Tanenbaum ME, Gilbert LA, Qi LS, Weissman JS, Vale RD (2014) A protein-tagging system for signal amplification in gene expression and fluorescence imaging. Cell 159(3):635–646. https://doi.org/10.1016/j.cell.2014.09.039

23. Konermann S, Brigham MD, Trevino AE, Joung J, Abudayyeh OO, Barcena C, Hsu PD, Habib N, Gootenberg JS, Nishimasu H, Nureki O, Zhang F (2015) Genome-scale transcriptional activation by an engineered CRISPR-Cas9 complex. Nature 517 (7536):583–588. https://doi.org/10.1038/nature14136

24. Chavez A, Scheiman J, Vora S, Pruitt BW, Tuttle M, PRI E, Lin S, Kiani S, Guzman CD, Wiegand DJ, Ter-Ovanesyan D, Braff JL, Davidsohn N, Housden BE, Perrimon N, Weiss R, Aach J, Collins JJ, Church GM (2015) Highly efficient Cas9-mediated transcriptional programming. Nat Methods 12 (4):326–328. https://doi.org/10.1038/nmeth.3312

25. Joung J, Engreitz JM, Konermann S, Abudayyeh OO, Verdine VK, Aguet F, Gootenberg JS, Sanjana NE, Wright JB, Fulco CP, Tseng YY, Yoon CH, Boehm JS, Lander ES, Zhang F (2017) Genome-scale activation screen identifies a lncRNA locus regulating a gene neighbourhood. Nature 548(7667):343–346. https://doi.org/10.1038/nature23451

26. Kampmann M (2018) CRISPRi and CRISPRa screens in mammalian cells for precision biology and medicine. ACS Chem Biol 13 (2):406–416. https://doi.org/10.1021/acschembio.7b00657

# Chapter 14

## In Vivo Silencing/Overexpression of lncRNAs by CRISPR/Cas System

**Marianna Vitiello, Laura Poliseno, and Pier Paolo Pandolfi**

### Abstract

Long noncoding RNAs (lncRNAs) are implicated in several biological processes and it has been observed that their expression is altered in several diseases. The generation of animal models where selective silencing or overexpression of lncRNAs can be attained is crucial for their biological characterization, since it offers the opportunity to analyze their function at the tissue specific or organismal level. CRISPR/Cas technology is a newly developed tool that allows to easily manipulate the mouse genome, in turn allowing to discover lncRNAs functions in an in vivo context. Here, we provide an overview of how CRISPR/Cas technology can be used to generate transgenic mouse models in which lncRNAs can be studied.

**Key words** lncRNA, CRISPR/Cas system, Genetically engineered mouse model

## 1 Introduction

### 1.1 LncRNAs

LncRNAs are RNA molecules longer than 200 nucleotides. They are not translated, but can bind to DNA, RNA, and proteins. Thanks to high-throughput sequencing techniques, thousands of lncRNAs have been identified and their involvement in cellular and biological processes gets clearer every day.

LncRNAs can be divided in three main groups: intronic lncRNAs, long intergenic noncoding RNAs (lincRNAs), host genes of other lncRNAs or microRNAs (*see* Chapter 1).

Intronic lncRNAs are localized within introns of coding or noncoding genes and an important aspect that needs to be considered, while modeling their function in the mouse, is if the intronic lncRNA is independently transcribed or not from the host gene. An example of lncRNA belonging to this group is Panct1 [1].

LincRNAs are defined as autonomously transcribed noncoding RNAs that do not overlap with annotated coding genes. For lincRNAs, a polyA signal plus a strong transcriptional terminator sequence can be introduced to interrupt transcription.

Alfons Navarro (ed.), *Long Non-Coding RNAs in Cancer*, Methods in Molecular Biology, vol. 2348,
https://doi.org/10.1007/978-1-0716-1581-2_14, © Springer Science+Business Media, LLC, part of Springer Nature 2021

LncRNAs can also be host genes of other lncRNAs or micro-RNAs. An example is Carmn, the host gene for miR143/145 [2, 3].

The number of lncRNAs has not been established yet. However, several studies and databases (*see* Chapter 1), such as LNCi-pedia (https://lncipedia.org/), estimate a number that ranges from more than 10.000 [4] to almost 50.000 [5] human lncRNA genes [6]. In addition, only few of them are described and functionally annotated. During the last decade, several pipelines have in fact been developed to facilitate the identification of lncRNAs from high-throughput sequencing data (e.g., PLAR [7]).

LncRNAs transcripts are localized both in the nucleus and in the cytoplasm, although the majority of them exert their function in the nucleus, close to their transcription start site. Furthermore, they usually act through their secondary structures, rather than their primary sequence. This aspect is very important, since secondary structure is usually more conserved among species [8]. Indeed, several lncRNAs are conserved between different vertebrates: thousands of human lncRNAs have an orthologous in other mammals [7]. Conversely, some lncRNAs are not shared by all species, suggesting a high turnover and genetic drift of this kind of genes along speciation.

So far, lncRNAs have been implicated, among other processes, in chromosome remodeling, chromatin modifier recruitment, transcriptional regulation, transport of intracellular material, and microRNA sponging, leading to derepression of microRNA-target expression. A well-known example of an epigenetic modifier is Xist lncRNA, which acts in *cis* by silencing the genes located on the same X chromosome from which it is transcribed [9]. Conversely, an example of lncRNA working as competing endogenous RNA (ceRNA) [10] is CDR1as, a circular RNA that contains 73 binding sites for miR-7 [11].

The more lncRNA functions are discovered, the longer is the list of alterations in their expression that are linked with disease, including cancer (a noticeable example is HOTAIR, a lncRNA overexpressed in breast cancer [12]). Therefore, there is a clear need of further investigations in order to fully decipher the functions of this large class of noncoding RNAs. To this end, in vivo studies are of crucial importance.

**1.2  CRISPR/Cas System**

CRISPR (Clustered Regularly Interspaced Short Palindromic Repeats)/Cas (CRISPR-associated) system has been employed for mouse genome editing for the first time less than 10 years ago, but its use in this field is growing steadily, both in terms of number of papers and in terms of types of approaches used [13–15].

CRISPR/Cas system is a process originally used by prokaryotic organisms to cut foreign nucleic acids and protect themselves against viruses. Later on, it has been adapted by scientists to the manipulation of the eukaryotic genome. CRISPR/Cas system is a dual system composed by a Cas enzyme and a guide RNA (gRNA). In turn, gRNAs are composed by a Cas-specific scaffold RNA (tracrRNA), which drives enzyme recognition and nuclease activation, and a 20 nt long CRISPR RNA (crRNA), which drives target identification and confers target specificity to the system. crRNA is customizable and can be exploited to target a DNA or RNA sequence of interest. When this system was adapted to scientific research, tracrRNA and crRNA molecules were fused in one, generating a single guide RNA (sgRNA). Cas9 derived from *Streptococcus pyogenes* (SpyCas9) is one of the most used enzyme of the CRISPR/Cas system, given its efficiency and precision. Cas9 enzyme needs a Protospacer-Adjacent Motif (PAM), a short DNA sequence juxtaposed to the region targeted by the sgRNA, to work. PAM is Cas9-specific (for example PAM sequence of SpyCas9 is 5′-NGG-3′) and acts as an allosteric regulator of Cas9, driving DNA binding and cleavage by Cas9 enzyme [16]. Cas9 enzyme cuts 4–5 nt around the PAM sequence, introducing a double strand break (DSB). By default, cells repair the DSB by nonhomologous end joining (NHEJ), so that insertions or deletions (indels) are introduced. However, cells can be "forced" to use homology-directed repair (HDR), if a donor filament (containing two homology arms flanking the DSB region and the specific sequence that should be modified or introduced) is provided.

During the years, the in vivo application of CRISPR/Cas system has been greatly improved. Initially, it consisted of a first step of gRNA design and in vitro validation, followed by a second step performed in vivo. Nowadays several online tools exist for gRNA design and several gRNAs are already published. Moreover, companies provide ready-to-use synthetic gRNAs. In addition, many studies describe approaches for in vivo injection of the CRISPR/Cas ribonucleoprotein (RNP) complex composed by Cas enzyme protein and the synthetic gRNA. In this way, genome editing occurs in a very short time (almost 1 h) [17]. This is very important to minimize mosaicism and, later on, to enhance germline transmission of the DNA edit [18, 19]. Indeed, if Cas is administered as DNA or RNA, it needs to be transcribed, exported into the cytoplasm where it is translated and then imported again as protein into the nucleus. This process takes a long time, with two main negative consequences. First, the delay decreases editing efficacy and, second, the time required is longer than that required for zygotic or cell division, in turn favoring mosaicism, and hence affecting germline transmission [18, 19]. Conversely, when the Cas enzyme is injected/transfected as protein, the enzyme is ready to cut DNA, as strongly supported by the rapid and effective NHEJ and NHEJ-mediated knockout of the target [18, 19]. To improve HR-mediated knockin efficacy, it has been shown that chemically synthetized crRNA and tracrRNA molecules, rather than the "all in one" sgRNA, should be used together with the "ready to cut" Cas protein [18].

An additional advantage of in vivo CRISPR/Cas application is the low rate of off-target effects. CRISPR/Cas system is highly specific for the on-target locus, with little or no signs of off-targets [18]. Furthermore, Cas9 enzymes have been engineered to further reduce off-targets (high fidelity Cas9) [19, 20]. It should also be noted that, due to mouse breeding, even a rare off-target can be segregated from the on-target editing [19]. In addition, a method for in vivo off-target identification has been recently reported [21]. We can thus conclude that the number of CRISPR/Cas-induced off-target events in the mouse can be kept to a minimum [18, 22, 23].

**1.3  Mouse Models**

In vivo studies allow to take into account the environment, interactions with other organs and non–cell autonomous stimuli that are important for gene expression and function. For these reasons, they are usually more meaningful compared to in vitro studies. Animal models also offer the possibility to compare the expression among organs and to follow gene expression in time.

Different animal models exist. They differ in terms of biological complexity and their choice depends on type of study, budget, timing and ethical considerations. The most common animal models are *Caenorhabditis elegans*, *Drosophila melanogaster*, *Dario rerio*, *Xenopus laevis*, *Rattus norvegicus*, *Mus musculus*, and nonhuman primates.

LncRNAs have been found in all the above-listed animal models. Their primary sequence is not highly conserved. However, cross-species comparisons have highlighted the presence of conserved regions. Furthermore, secondary structure is sometimes conserved [8]. These aspects point toward conserved function and support the use of animal models for lncRNA studies. It should also be considered that, if the animal model lacks the orthologue lncRNA, it is possible to restore it by knockin.

In vivo studies can be schematically divided into two main groups: xenograft and allograft approaches, which principally consist in the transplantation of cells previously treated in vitro, and genetically engineered animals, where the disease or the phenotype are directly developed by the organism. This second approach allows to study the initiation and the progression of the disease and also to analyze and study the natural microenvironment and the interactions with other organs.

Mice are usually preferred as animal model given their short life cycle and their genetic similarity to humans. Three different approaches are mainly used to generate genetically engineered mice (Fig. 1): (1) zygotic microinjection, (2) mESCs in vitro manipulation and blastocyst transplantation, and (3) embryos electroporation.

| | |
|---|---|
| *1.3.1 Zygotic Microinjection* | Zygotic microinjection (Fig. 1i) is one of the most used techniques for transgenic mouse generation. This approach consists in the injection of a nucleic acid into the pronucleus of fertilized oocytes, which are then implanted in pseudopregnant females (foster mothers). Offspring are then genotyped for the presence of the transgenic DNA or DNA mutation and its expression is generally tested. Then, founders with the desired DNA editing are bred with wildtype mice to generate a stable transgenic mouse line. Initially, this technique did not allow to generate transgenic mice by homologous recombination and the insertion of the transgene was random, with several consequent drawbacks. Today, it is possible to associate zygotic microinjection with CRISPR/Cas system [24]. This allows to overcome the problems related to random insertion of the transgene, as well as those related to uncontrolled number of integrated copies of the transgene. Moreover, it allows knockout studies and those based on precise gene editing. |
| *1.3.2 mESC In Vitro Manipulation and Blastocyst Transplantation* | mESCs in vitro manipulation and blastocyst transplantation approach (Fig. 1ii) consists in in vitro modification of mESCs and then, once cell clones carrying the desired modification are selected, few cells are injected into a mouse blastocyst, which in turn is transferred into pseudopregnant females. Contrary to the zygotic approach, this approach results in a chimeric mouse. Chimeric mice are then bred with wildtype mice to obtain a stable transgenic mouse line. This approach is much longer than the zygotic approach, but it allows to build on already highly complex genome modifications [25]. |
| *1.3.3 Embryos Electroporation* | Embryos electroporation (Fig. 1iii) is a sophisticated technique that allows to inject nucleic acids into various embryonic tissues in a spatiotemporally restricted manner [26]. This approach has been recently associated with CRISPR/Cas technology to develop a method termed GONAD (genome editing via oviductal nucleic acids delivery) [27, 28]. GONAD consists in the injection of CRISPR components (Cas9 mRNA or protein and gRNA) into the oviducts of pregnant females post conception, coupled with electroporation of the components into zygotes in situ. GONAD allows to further reduce the time needed to generate transgenic founder lines, as it takes ~6 weeks [27]. |

## 2 In Vivo Studies of lncRNAs by CRISPR/Cas System

CRISPR/Cas system is a powerful tool to generate transgenic mice for lncRNA studies. Particularly, CRISPR/Cas system can be used for in vivo lncRNA loss-of-function studies, knockin of lncRNAs, and lncRNA transcriptional regulation by CRISPRi and CRISPRa.

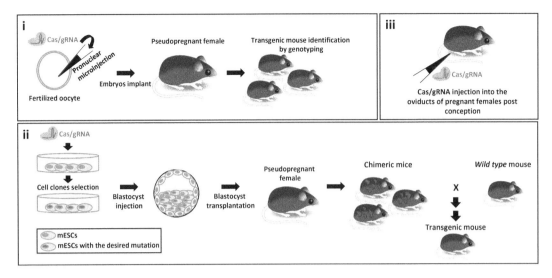

**Fig. 1** Approaches for transgenic mouse generation. (**i**) Zygotic microinjection. (**ii**) mESCs in vitro manipulation and blastocyst transpantation. (**iii**) Embryos electroporation. See text for details

*2.1 In Vivo Loss-of-Function Studies of lncRNAs Using CRISPR/Cas-Mediated Genome Editing*

Silencing of lncRNA is considered a challenge given that they act as transcripts. RNA interference (RNAi), using siRNAs/shRNAs or antisense oligos such as morpholinos, is sometimes used for in vivo lncRNA loss-of-function studies. RNA interference leads to RNA degradation. Instead, morpholinos usually prevent the translation or correct splicing of mature RNAs. An example of shRNA used for in vivo lncRNA inhibition is the one used to inhibit Arid2-IR in the mouse [29]. Conversely, the downregulation of Malat1 in mice has been achieved using an antisense oligonucleotide [30]. A drawback of RNAi is that it is effective for RNA molecules localized into the cytoplasm, but it is usually much less effective for RNA molecules localized into the nucleus, where several lncRNAs act [31]. Furthermore, siRNAs/shRNAs and antisense oligonucleotides only downregulate and do not completely eliminate the expression of lncRNA targets [30].

To completely eliminate the expression of the gene of interest, it is better to act on the DNA sequence and CRISPR/Cas system offers many straightforward ways to do it.

Since lncRNAs are not translated and act as RNAs, it is generally ineffective to introduce indels in the gene sequence by the canonical CRISPR/Cas9 system, as usually carried out for coding genes. However, it is necessary to analyze the lncRNA of interest and to know as much as possible about its regulatory regions and its sequence (e.g., promoter, enhancer, transcription start site, and potential overlap of its gene sequence with other genes). This analysis is essential to decide which CRISPR/Cas strategies should be used. Although it has been recently reported that sometimes CRISPR has serious limitations for lncRNA editing [32], it is still

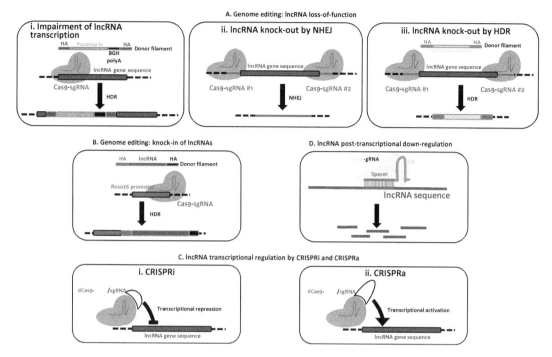

**Fig. 2** Manipulation of lncRNAs expression by CRISPR/Cas technology. (**a**) lncRNA loss-of-function by genome editing. (**i**) Impairment of lncRNA transcription. Cas9/sgRNA system introduces a DSB in the lncRNA gene sequence, which is repaired by HDR in presence of a donor filament. The donor filament contains two target gene homology arms flanking the DSB region (HA, dark green) and the sequence that should be introduced. In this case, an antibiotic selection marker (puromycin, dark yellow) is introduced together with a BGH polyA signal that causes the termination of gene transcription (black). (**ii–iii**) Complete elimination of lncRNA gene sequence (knockout). Using a pair of sgRNAs that recognize regions located at the extremities of the lncRNA gene sequence, it is possible to completely eliminate the lncRNA gene sequence itself. The DSB is repaired (**ii**) by NHEJ in the absence of a donor filament or (**iii**) by HDR in presence of a donor filament. (**b**) lncRNA knockin. lncRNA gene sequence can be introduced by knockin in the genome using an sgRNA that targets an endogenous promoter (such as Rosa26 promoter, blue), plus a donor filament containing the 5′ and 3′ homology arms flanking the DSB region and the sequence of the lncRNA that we want to introduce (HA, blue and black). (**c**) lncRNAs transcriptional regulation by CRISPRi and CRISPRa. Dead mutant Cas9 (dCas9, purple) is fused with (**i**) transcriptional inhibitors (such as KRAB, yellow) or (**ii**) activators (such as VP64, yellow) to manipulate target lncRNA transcription. (**d**) lncRNA post-transcriptional downregulation. A lncRNA transcript can be downregulated using Cas13 enzyme. In this case, the gRNA is composed by a spacer sequence (red), which is about 20 nt in length and recognizes target sequence, and a direct repeat scaffold sequence (DR, light blue)

possible to exploit several strategies based on the use of CRISPR technology.

As summarized in (Fig. 2a), the CRISPR/Cas system can be used to achieve (1) impairment of lncRNA transcription and (2) elimination of lncRNA sequence from the genome.

*2.1.1 Impairment of lncRNA Transcription*

An example of impairment of lncRNA transcription is the one recently described by us [33]. *PTENP1* is a processed and not translated pseudogene that acts as ceRNA for *PTEN*-targeting microRNAs. To impair its transcription, we inserted a GFP expression cassette in the opposite orientation compared to *PTENP1* gene, using the SpyCas9 enzyme and an sgRNA specific for *PTENP1* gene, localized between *PTENP1* promoter and its transcribed region [33]. The insertion of this cassette by homology directed repair (HDR) has been possible thanks to the presence of *PTENP1* homologous arms cloned upstream and downstream the GFP gene [33]. The construct containing plasmid has been transfected in DU145 cells stably expressing the inducible Cas9 enzyme and the sgRNA. Once the enzyme was induced by doxycycline treatment, positive clones were selected by genotyping and qRT-PCR [33].

Another strategy based on the use of CRISPR/Cas technology for lncRNA silencing is the one described in [34] for *MALAT1* silencing. The termination of gene expression has been achieved by introducing an upstream bovine growth hormone (BGH) polyA signal within the transcriptional unit of *MALAT1*, thanks to HDR into both alleles (Fig. 2ai). To this end, a donor fragment has been designed, containing a 5′ homology arm, the puromycin resistance gene (or another gene selection marker, such as NeoR, GFP, etc.), the BGH polyA and a 3′ homology arm [34]. The gRNA used targets a region immediately downstream the *MALAT1* promoter. Silencing of lncRNA by biallelic integration of the polyA signal was confirmed by genotyping analysis and by qRT-PCR [34].

*2.1.2  Elimination of lncRNA Sequence from the Genome (Knockout)*

The complete deletion (knockout) of the lncRNA gene is not always feasible, since very often this kind of genes show partial overlap with coding genes or other noncoding genes, also in their regulatory regions. For this reason, an in silico analysis of gene sequence is a crucial starting point. The elimination of a lncRNA gene of interest can be obtained using a pair of sgRNAs targeting the 5′ and 3′ flanking sequences. It is possible to use two approaches: to push cells toward NHEJ in the absence of a donor filament (Fig. 2aii); or to push cells toward HDR, using a donor filament that contains 5′ and 3′ homology arms (Fig. 2aiii). In the first strategy, cells repair the break by insertion of indels and up to 10 kbp of DNA can be eliminated [35, 36]. The second strategy allows to insert a puromycin resistance gene (or another gene selection marker, such as NeoR, GFP etc.) that facilitates the selection of cells where the cassette is inserted.

An example of the first strategy is the knockout of *Gm15441* lncRNA in the mouse [24]. This lncRNA is a liver-enriched transcript, downregulated during the development of metabolic diseases and induced during feeding/fasting transition [24]. *Gm15441* gene overlaps with the protein-coding gene *Txnip*. For this reason, it is not possible to completely eliminate the lncRNA gene sequence and only the transcription start site plus exon 1 (a region of about 400 bp) were eliminated. This genome portion is unique to *Gm15441* and its elimination was indeed enough to abrogate the lncRNA expression [24]. Specifically, Hansmeier and colleagues used two sgRNAs located at the 5' and at the 3' of the selected region. They first analyzed several sgRNAs and selected those 2 showing maximum activity in vitro, using cell lines with a high proliferative capacity and transfection efficiency: C57BL/6 mice-derived mouse motor neuron-like hybrid cells (NSC-34). Then, they employed zygotic microinjection of CRISPR/Cas9 components (Cas9 mRNA/protein, crRNA, tracrRNA) into C57BL/6NRj zygotes. Finally, two-cell stage embryos were implanted into pseudopregnant foster mothers and the genotyping of founder litters was performed, revealing multiple successful random alterations in *Gm15441* locus.

Another example of the use of CRISPR/Cas9 system for NHEJ-mediated knockout of a lncRNA is the deletion of *NANOGP8* [37]. *NANOG* has 10 pseudogenes and the selective knockdown of *NANOGP8* using RNAi is almost impossible, given that the sequence of *NANOG* and *NANOGP8* are highly homologous. To evaluate the specific function of *NANOG* and *NANOGP8*, each of them was deleted in DU145 cells using CRISPR/Cas9 technology. Particularly, the deletion of *NANOG* was performed using two sgRNAs targeting exon 2, which is a region only present in this gene, resulting in a premature stop codon [37]. Conversely, the deletion of *NANOGP8* was performed using two sgRNAs targeting regions outside *NANOGP8* gene sequence. *NANOGP8*-knockout cells were identified by genotyping [37].

As far as the second strategy is concerned (the lncRNA of interest is replaced with a reporter gene sequence), if the promoter region is preserved, then the expression of the lncRNA under study can be followed spatiotemporally. Moreover, since sometimes the lncRNA is essential for embryo survival (e.g., Meg3 [38] and Tsix [39] lncRNAs), the Cre-lox system can be utilized to induce gene deletion at a specific time point or in a specific tissue.

An additional approach consists in mutagenizing functionally relevant elements within a lncRNA. As an example, in the case of lncRNAs that act as ceRNA for microRNAs, it is possible to edit specific microRNA binding elements (MRE) within the lncRNA. If multiple MREs are present, it is possible to replace the entire sequence introducing mutations in multiple MREs at once, by using the appropriate donor filament.

### 2.2 In Vivo Knockin of lncRNAs by CRISPR/Cas System

The knockin of entire lncRNAs is more complicated than knockout in terms of experimental design and efficacy [18] and its use for in vivo studies is rare. We resort to lncRNA knockin in the case the animal model does not express the lncRNA of interest. Therefore, the expression of such lncRNA is necessarily ectopic (for example, a human lncRNA is expressed in a mouse model that normally does not express that human lncRNA). Clearly, the introduction of the lncRNA gene in a different genome locus from the original one prevents its use to study possible cis-acting mechanisms (surrounding loci are different).

An example of lncRNA add-back approach used for in vivo studies is the one described for Fendrr, a lncRNA essential for proper heart and body wall development in the mouse. This lncRNA was reintroduced through a bacterial artificial chromosomes (BAC), to rescue Fendrr-null mice phenotype [40].

When CRISPR/Cas system is used to knockin a sequence in the mouse genome, a donor filament is injected together with Cas enzyme and a gRNA. Nowadays, it is possible to use a linearized dsDNA of up to 6 kb that can be integrated [41]. Conversely, if the sequence to be introduced is very long, a BAC is used as donor filament [19]. The donor filament, which contains the lncRNA sequence and the 5′ and 3′ homology arms (surrounding the gRNA target locus), is inserted into the genome by HDR, which repairs the DSB induced by Cas enzyme activity (Fig. 2b).

Analogously to knockout constructs, knockin constructs can be designed for total body or cell type specific expression. In the first case, a ubiquitous promoter should be used, such as Rosa26 gene promoter [42]. In the second case, a tissue specific promoter should be used, such as TYR promoter for melanocytic lineage cells. The knockin of hSIRPA coding gene is an example of knockin performed by the introduction of the gene sequence of interest under the control of Rosa26 promoter [43]. It has been performed using a cassette containing Rosa26 homologous arms and the hSIRPA sequence. The gRNA used targets intron 1 of the mouse Rosa26 locus [42]. An advantage of the use of the endogenous Rosa26 promoter is that the gRNA to be used is potentially the same, irrespectively of the gene that should be introduced, simplifying experimental procedures.

As mentioned above for knockout experiments, also for knockin experiments it is very important to evaluate if the ectopic expression of the lncRNA affects embryonic development and, to overcome this problem, the Cre-lox recombinase system can be used. Particularly, a lox-STOP codon-lox sequence can be introduced upstream the lncRNA sequence. This allows to prevent the expression of the lncRNA, until the CRE enzyme is expressed in a temporal or tissue-specific manner, and hence the lox-STOP codon-lox cassette is excised.

### 2.3 In Vivo Transcriptional Regulation of lncRNAs by CRISPRi and CRISPRa

CRISPR/Cas system has also been adapted for negative and positive regulation of gene transcription. For this purpose, a mutant form of Cas9 (dCas9) enzyme, characterized by point mutations in its catalytic domain, has been fused with transcriptional inhibitors (CRISPRi) or with transcriptional activators (CRISPRa) domains (Fig. 2c) [44]. This system is also applied to the study of lncRNAs in vivo, and this is remarkable because it allows to manipulate the expression of endogenous genes. For in vivo studies, both dCas9 and the gRNA can be stably inserted into the mouse genome by various approaches.

In CRISPRi, Kruppel associated box (KRAB) domain or KRAB-MeCP2 domain are among the most used transcriptional repressor domains fused to dCas9 (Fig. 2ci). These domains induce heterochromatin formation, leading to the inhibition of gene transcription, and have been used as alternative to the Cre-loxP system for loss-of-function studies in mice [45]. Interestingly, this system has been recently used to assess the function of ~17,000 lncRNAs in seven different human cell lines. In this way, ~500 of tested lncRNAs have been found to influence biological processes and most of them were previously unknown [46].

CRISPRa system is particularly important for lncRNA studies since they are very often expressed at low level: it allows to boost the expression of endogenous genes, avoiding problems related to ectopic gene expression. An example of transcriptional activator fused to dCas9 is VP64, which facilitates transcription factors and/or RNA polymerase recruitment (Fig. 2cii). In a recent study by our group, this system has been used in vitro to identify lncRNAs involved in drug-resistance mechanisms [47]. An example of CRISPRa used for in vivo studies is the one described in [48]. Loss-of-function mutation in the protein-coding gene Sim1 causes an obesity phenotype. Using obesity as readout, the authors tested in mice a CRISPR-mediated activation of endogenous Sim1 gene, targeting its promoter or its enhancer. Indeed, Sim1 upregulation was sufficient to rescue the obesity phenotype observed in $Sim1^{+/-}$ heterozygous mice without any off-target effect [48].

In CRISPRi and CRISPRa, the gRNA used has the same features as the one used for Cas9-mediated DNA editing, but it is located close to the transcription start site: at $-500$ to $+300$ bp compared to transcription start site for CRISPRi and at $-400$ to $-50$ bp compared to transcription start site for CRISPRa [49]. Moreover, the dCas9 used for CRISPRi and CRISPRa requires a PAM sequence ($5'$-NGG-$3'$) to work [44, 45, 50, 51].

A drawback of loss or gain of function of lncRNA by CRISPRi and CRISPRa is the current lack of information about the transcriptional regulation of lncRNAs: regulatory regions of several lncRNA genes remain uncharacterized, limiting the use of this technique. Consequently, it is often not easy to position the gRNA target sequence along the promoter or other regulatory regions of the lncRNA of interest. An additional drawback is that the regulatory regions of lncRNAs often overlap with those of other genes or overlap with antisense transcripts (e.g., the regulatory region of *PTENP1* sense transcripts partially overlaps with *PTENP1* antisense transcripts [52]). Therefore, although there is much room for improvement, CRISPRi and CRISPRa use for lncRNA study is still limited and complex.

## 3    Conclusions and Future Perspectives

The number of lncRNAs identified in the last years thanks to high throughput techniques is extremely high. They were believed "junk DNA" at beginning, but by now their involvement in several biological processes and diseases, including cancer development and progression, gets clearer every day. For this reason, their identification and study is crucial both to better understand the molecular mechanisms that govern physiological processes and to better understand disease pathogenesis, in turn uncovering new possible targets for therapy.

For a long time lncRNA study was very limited, since the analysis and modulation of their expression were not easy to accomplish with the available techniques (such as qRT-PCR and RNA interference). This was principally due to the fact that they are highly homologous and/or extensively overlapping with other genes, as well as to the fact that they work as noncoding RNAs. However, in the last years the advent of CRISPR/Cas system has enormously contributed to move this field forward. Indeed, CRISPR/Cas technology allows to perform genome editing (knockout or knockin of lncRNA genes, insertion of specific mutations or deletions in lncRNA gene sequence) (Fig. 2aii, 2aiii, b); to inhibit transcription by the introduction of a cassette in the lncRNA gene sequence (Fig. 2ai) or by the use of CRISPRi (Fig. 2ci); conversely, to enhance transcription by CRISPRa (Fig. 2cii). As described in this review, this is particularly important because these methodologies can also be adapted for in vivo studies, providing a powerful tool to study lncRNA role at an organismal level. By using CRISPR/Cas system, it is also possible to edit RNA sequence, to identify RNA or protein molecules bound to the lncRNA of interest, and even to track the lncRNA transcript for live imaging. Another novel and important application of CRISPR/Cas system is the downregulation of lncRNA expression at posttranscriptional level using the Cas13 enzyme [53] (Fig. 2d). This system allows to knockdown desired noncoding RNA transcripts with high efficiency and specificity, as recently described in [33, 53, 54] [https://doi.org/10.1101/2020.03.23.002238]. As far as in vivo applications are concerned, Cas13 has been already proposed for the manipulation of gene expression in zebrafish [https://doi.org/10.1101/2020.01.13.904763] and in the mouse [55]. It is very likely that in the next years this approach will be widely applied for in vivo studies of lncRNAs, possibly by Cas13 and sgRNA adenovirus delivery [56]. This is because this approach will permit to manipulate gene expression spatiotemporally without affecting genome sequence. Overall, CRISPR/Cas technology represents an essential tool for studying lncRNAs in vivo and will certainly contribute to greatly increase their functionalization, as well as to expedite their therapeutic exploitation in human disease.

## References

1. Chakraborty D, Paszkowski-Rogacz M, Berger N, Ding L, Mircetic J, Fu J, Iesmantavicius V, Choudhary C, Anastassiadis K, Stewart AF, Buchholz F (2017) lncRNA Panct1 Maintains Mouse Embryonic Stem Cell Identity by Regulating TOBF1 Recruitment to Oct-Sox Sequences in Early G1. Cell Rep 21(11):3012–3021. https://doi.org/10.1016/j.celrep.2017.11.045

2. Cheng Y, Liu X, Yang J, Lin Y, Xu DZ, Lu Q, Deitch EA, Huo Y, Delphin ES, Zhang C (2009) MicroRNA-145, a novel smooth muscle cell phenotypic marker and modulator, controls vascular neointimal lesion formation. Circ Res 105(2):158–166. https://doi.org/10.1161/CIRCRESAHA.109.197517

3. Cordes KR, Sheehy NT, White MP, Berry EC, Morton SU, Muth AN, Lee TH, Miano JM, Ivey KN, Srivastava D (2009) miR-145 and miR-143 regulate smooth muscle cell fate and plasticity. Nature 460(7256):705–710. https://doi.org/10.1038/nature08195

4. Hon CC, Ramilowski JA, Harshbarger J, Bertin N, Rackham OJ, Gough J, Denisenko E, Schmeier S, Poulsen TM, Severin J, Lizio M, Kawaji H, Kasukawa T, Itoh M, Burroughs AM, Noma S, Djebali S, Alam T, Medvedeva YA, Testa AC, Lipovich L, Yip CW, Abugessaisa I, Mendez M, Hasegawa A, Tang D, Lassmann T, Heutink P, Babina M, Wells CA, Kojima S, Nakamura Y, Suzuki H, Daub CO, de Hoon MJ, Arner E, Hayashizaki Y, Carninci P, Forrest AR (2017) An atlas of human long non-coding RNAs with accurate 5′ ends. Nature 543(7644):199–204. https://doi.org/10.1038/nature21374

5. Volders PJ, Anckaert J, Verheggen K, Nuytens J, Martens L, Mestdagh P, Vandesompele J (2019) LNCipedia 5: towards a reference set of human long non-coding RNAs. Nucleic Acids Res 47(D1):D135–D139. https://doi.org/10.1093/nar/gky1031

6. Iyer MK, Niknafs YS, Malik R, Singhal U, Sahu A, Hosono Y, Barrette TR, Prensner JR, Evans JR, Zhao S, Poliakov A, Cao X, Dhanasekaran SM, Wu YM, Robinson DR, Beer DG, Feng FY, Iyer HK, Chinnaiyan AM (2015) The landscape of long noncoding RNAs in the human transcriptome. Nat Genet 47(3):199–208. https://doi.org/10.1038/ng.3192

7. Hezroni H, Koppstein D, Schwartz MG, Avrutin A, Bartel DP, Ulitsky I (2015) Principles of long noncoding RNA evolution derived from direct comparison of transcriptomes in 17 species. Cell Rep 11(7):1110–1122. https://doi.org/10.1016/j.celrep.2015.04.023

8. Washietl S, Hofacker IL, Lukasser M, Huttenhofer A, Stadler PF (2005) Mapping of conserved RNA secondary structures predicts thousands of functional noncoding RNAs in the human genome. Nat Biotechnol 23(11):1383–1390. https://doi.org/10.1038/nbt1144

9. Froberg JE, Yang L, Lee JT (2013) Guided by RNAs: X-inactivation as a model for lncRNA function. J Mol Biol 425(19):3698–3706. https://doi.org/10.1016/j.jmb.2013.06.031

10. Salmena L, Poliseno L, Tay Y, Kats L, Pandolfi PP (2011) A ceRNA hypothesis: the Rosetta stone of a hidden RNA language? Cell 146(3):353–358. https://doi.org/10.1016/j.cell.2011.07.014

11. Hansen TB, Jensen TI, Clausen BH, Bramsen JB, Finsen B, Damgaard CK, Kjems J (2013) Natural RNA circles function as efficient microRNA sponges. Nature 495(7441):384–388. https://doi.org/10.1038/nature11993

12. Gupta RA, Shah N, Wang KC, Kim J, Horlings HM, Wong DJ, Tsai MC, Hung T, Argani P, Rinn JL, Wang Y, Brzoska P, Kong B, Li R,

West RB, van de Vijver MJ, Sukumar S, Chang HY (2010) Long non-coding RNA HOTAIR reprograms chromatin state to promote cancer metastasis. Nature 464(7291):1071–1076. https://doi.org/10.1038/nature08975

13. Mashiko D, Fujihara Y, Satouh Y, Miyata H, Isotani A, Ikawa M (2013) Generation of mutant mice by pronuclear injection of circular plasmid expressing Cas9 and single guided RNA. Sci Rep 3:3355. https://doi.org/10.1038/srep03355

14. Wang H, Yang H, Shivalila CS, Dawlaty MM, Cheng AW, Zhang F, Jaenisch R (2013) One-step generation of mice carrying mutations in multiple genes by CRISPR/Cas-mediated genome engineering. Cell 153(4):910–918. https://doi.org/10.1016/j.cell.2013.04.025

15. Ran FA, Hsu PD, Lin CY, Gootenberg JS, Konermann S, Trevino AE, Scott DA, Inoue A, Matoba S, Zhang Y, Zhang F (2013) Double nicking by RNA-guided CRISPR Cas9 for enhanced genome editing specificity. Cell 154(6):1380–1389. https://doi.org/10.1016/j.cell.2013.08.021

16. Sternberg SH, Redding S, Jinek M, Greene EC, Doudna JA (2014) DNA interrogation by the CRISPR RNA-guided endonuclease Cas9. Nature 507(7490):62–67. https://doi.org/10.1038/nature13011

17. Kim S, Kim D, Cho SW, Kim J, Kim JS (2014) Highly efficient RNA-guided genome editing in human cells via delivery of purified Cas9 ribonucleoproteins. Genome Res 24(6):1012–1019. https://doi.org/10.1101/gr.171322.113

18. Aida T, Chiyo K, Usami T, Ishikubo H, Imahashi R, Wada Y, Tanaka KF, Sakuma T, Yamamoto T, Tanaka K (2015) Cloning-free CRISPR/Cas system facilitates functional cassette knock-in in mice. Genome Biol 16:87. https://doi.org/10.1186/s13059-015-0653-x

19. Miano JM, Long X, Lyu Q (2019) CRISPR links to long noncoding RNA function in mice: a practical approach. Vasc Pharmacol 114:1–12. https://doi.org/10.1016/j.vph.2019.02.004

20. Kleinstiver BP, Pattanayak V, Prew MS, Tsai SQ, Nguyen NT, Zheng Z, Joung JK (2016) High-fidelity CRISPR-Cas9 nucleases with no detectable genome-wide off-target effects. Nature 529(7587):490–495. https://doi.org/10.1038/nature16526

21. Akcakaya P, Bobbin ML, Guo JA, Malagon-Lopez J, Clement K, Garcia SP, Fellows MD, Porritt MJ, Firth MA, Carreras A, Baccega T, Seeliger F, Bjursell M, Tsai SQ, Nguyen NT, Nitsch R, Mayr LM, Pinello L, Bohlooly YM, Aryee MJ, Maresca M, Joung JK (2018) In vivo CRISPR editing with no detectable genome-wide off-target mutations. Nature 561(7723):416–419. https://doi.org/10.1038/s41586-018-0500-9

22. Iyer V, Boroviak K, Thomas M, Doe B, Riva L, Ryder E, Adams DJ (2018) No unexpected CRISPR-Cas9 off-target activity revealed by trio sequencing of gene-edited mice. PLoS Genet 14(7):e1007503. https://doi.org/10.1371/journal.pgen.1007503

23. Anderson KR, Haeussler M, Watanabe C, Janakiraman V, Lund J, Modrusan Z, Stinson J, Bei Q, Buechler A, Yu C, Thamminana SR, Tam L, Sowick MA, Alcantar T, O'Neil N, Li J, Ta L, Lima L, Roose-Girma M, Rairdan X, Durinck S, Warming S (2018) CRISPR off-target analysis in genetically engineered rats and mice. Nat Methods 15(7):512–514. https://doi.org/10.1038/s41592-018-0011-5

24. Hansmeier NR, Widdershooven PJM, Khani S, Kornfeld JW (2019) Rapid generation of Long noncoding RNA knockout mice using CRISPR/Cas9 technology. Noncoding RNA 5(1):12. https://doi.org/10.3390/ncrna5010012

25. Bok I, Vera O, Xu X, Jasani N, Nakamura K, Reff J, Nenci A, Gonzalez JG, Karreth FA (2020) A versatile ES cell-based melanoma mouse modeling platform. Cancer Res 80(4):912–921. https://doi.org/10.1158/0008-5472.CAN-19-2924

26. Saito T (2010) Embryonic in vivo electroporation in the mouse. Methods Enzymol 477:37–50. https://doi.org/10.1016/S0076-6879(10)77003-8

27. Gurumurthy CB, Sato M, Nakamura A, Inui M, Kawano N, Islam MA, Ogiwara S, Takabayashi S, Matsuyama M, Nakagawa S, Miura H, Ohtsuka M (2019) Creation of CRISPR-based germline-genome-engineered mice without ex vivo handling of zygotes by i-GONAD. Nat Protoc 14(8):2452–2482. https://doi.org/10.1038/s41596-019-0187-x

28. Ohtsuka M, Sato M, Miura H, Takabayashi S, Matsuyama M, Koyano T, Arifin N, Nakamura S, Wada K, Gurumurthy CB (2018) I-GONAD: a robust method for in situ germline genome engineering using CRISPR nucleases. Genome Biol 19(1):25. https://doi.org/10.1186/s13059-018-1400-x

29. Zhou Q, Huang XR, Yu J, Yu X, Lan HY (2015) Long noncoding RNA Arid2-IR is a novel therapeutic target for renal

inflammation. Mol Ther 23(6):1034–1043. https://doi.org/10.1038/mt.2015.31

30. Wheeler TM, Leger AJ, Pandey SK, MacLeod AR, Nakamori M, Cheng SH, Wentworth BM, Bennett CF, Thornton CA (2012) Targeting nuclear RNA for in vivo correction of myotonic dystrophy. Nature 488(7409):111–115. https://doi.org/10.1038/nature11362

31. Zeng Y, Cullen BR (2002) RNA interference in human cells is restricted to the cytoplasm. RNA 8(7):855–860. https://doi.org/10.1017/s1355838202020071

32. Goyal A, Myacheva K, Gross M, Klingenberg M, Duran Arque B, Diederichs S (2017) Challenges of CRISPR/Cas9 applications for long non-coding RNA genes. Nucleic Acids Res 45(3):e12. https://doi.org/10.1093/nar/gkw883

33. Vitiello M, Evangelista M, Zhang Y, Salmena L, Pandolfi PP, Poliseno L (2020) PTENP1 is a ceRNA for PTEN: it's CRISPR clear. J Hematol Oncol 13(1):73. https://doi.org/10.1186/s13045-020-00894-2

34. Liu Y, Han X, Yuan J, Geng T, Chen S, Hu X, Cui IH, Cui H (2017) Biallelic insertion of a transcriptional terminator via the CRISPR/Cas9 system efficiently silences expression of protein-coding and non-coding RNA genes. J Biol Chem 292(14):5624–5633. https://doi.org/10.1074/jbc.M116.769034

35. Zheng Q, Cai X, Tan MH, Schaffert S, Arnold CP, Gong X, Chen CZ, Huang S (2014) Precise gene deletion and replacement using the CRISPR/Cas9 system in human cells. BioTechniques 57(3):115–124. https://doi.org/10.2144/000114196

36. Han J, Zhang J, Chen L, Shen B, Zhou J, Hu B, Du Y, Tate PH, Huang X, Zhang W (2014) Efficient in vivo deletion of a large imprinted lncRNA by CRISPR/Cas9. RNA Biol 11(7):829–835. https://doi.org/10.4161/rna.29624

37. Kawamura N, Nimura K, Nagano H, Yamaguchi S, Nonomura N, Kaneda Y (2015) CRISPR/Cas9-mediated gene knockout of NANOG and NANOGP8 decreases the malignant potential of prostate cancer cells. Oncotarget 6(26):22361–22374. https://doi.org/10.18632/oncotarget.4293

38. Zhou Y, Cheunsuchon P, Nakayama Y, Lawlor MW, Zhong Y, Rice KA, Zhang L, Zhang X, Gordon FE, Lidov HG, Bronson RT, Klibanski A (2010) Activation of paternally expressed genes and perinatal death caused by deletion of the Gtl2 gene. Development 137 (16):2643–2652. https://doi.org/10.1242/dev.045724

39. Sado T, Wang Z, Sasaki H, Li E (2001) Regulation of imprinted X-chromosome inactivation in mice by Tsix. Development 128 (8):1275–1286

40. Grote P, Wittler L, Hendrix D, Koch F, Wahrisch S, Beisaw A, Macura K, Blass G, Kellis M, Werber M, Herrmann BG (2013) The tissue-specific lncRNA Fendrr is an essential regulator of heart and body wall development in the mouse. Dev Cell 24(2):206–214. https://doi.org/10.1016/j.devcel.2012.12.012

41. Yao X, Zhang M, Wang X, Ying W, Hu X, Dai P, Meng F, Shi L, Sun Y, Yao N, Zhong W, Li Y, Wu K, Li W, Chen ZJ, Yang H (2018) Tild-CRISPR allows for efficient and precise gene Knockin in mouse and human cells. Dev Cell 45(4):526–536. e525. https://doi.org/10.1016/j.devcel.2018.04.021

42. Menoret S, De Cian A, Tesson L, Remy S, Usal C, Boule JB, Boix C, Fontaniere S, Creneguy A, Nguyen TH, Brusselle L, Thinard R, Gauguier D, Concordet JP, Cherifi Y, Fraichard A, Giovannangeli C, Anegon I (2015) Homology-directed repair in rodent zygotes using Cas9 and TALEN engineered proteins. Sci Rep 5:14410. https://doi.org/10.1038/srep14410

43. Jung CJ, Menoret S, Brusselle L, Tesson L, Usal C, Chenouard V, Remy S, Ouisse LH, Poirier N, Vanhove B, de Jong PJ, Anegon I (2016) Comparative analysis of piggyBac, CRISPR/Cas9 and TALEN mediated BAC Transgenesis in the zygote for the generation of humanized SIRPA rats. Sci Rep 6:31455. https://doi.org/10.1038/srep31455

44. Qi LS, Larson MH, Gilbert LA, Doudna JA, Weissman JS, Arkin AP, Lim WA (2013) Repurposing CRISPR as an RNA-guided platform for sequence-specific control of gene expression. Cell 152(5):1173–1183. https://doi.org/10.1016/j.cell.2013.02.022

45. MacLeod RS, Cawley KM, Gubrij I, Nookaew I, Onal M, O'Brien CA (2019) Effective CRISPR interference of an endogenous gene via a single transgene in mice. Sci Rep 9(1):17312. https://doi.org/10.1038/s41598-019-53611-6

46. Liu SJ, Horlbeck MA, Cho SW, Birk HS, Malatesta M, He D, Attenello FJ, Villalta JE, Cho MY, Chen Y, Mandegar MA, Olvera MP, Gilbert LA, Conklin BR, Chang HY, Weissman JS, Lim DA (2017) CRISPRi-based genome-scale identification of functional long noncoding RNA loci in human cells. Science 355 (6320):aah7111. https://doi.org/10.1126/science.aah7111

47. Bester AC, Lee JD, Chavez A, Lee YR, Nachmani D, Vora S, Victor J, Sauvageau M, Monteleone E, Rinn JL, Provero P, Church GM, Clohessy JG, Pandolfi PP (2018) An integrated genome-wide CRISPRa approach to functionalize lncRNAs in drug resistance. Cell 173(3):649–664. e620. https://doi.org/10.1016/j.cell.2018.03.052

48. Matharu N, Rattanasopha S, Tamura S, Maliskova L, Wang Y, Bernard A, Hardin A, Eckalbar WL, Vaisse C, Ahituv N (2019) CRISPR-mediated activation of a promoter or enhancer rescues obesity caused by haploinsufficiency. Science 363(6424):eaau0629. https://doi.org/10.1126/science.aau0629

49. Gilbert LA, Horlbeck MA, Adamson B, Villalta JE, Chen Y, Whitehead EH, Guimaraes C, Panning B, Ploegh HL, Bassik MC, Qi LS, Kampmann M, Weissman JS (2014) Genome-scale CRISPR-mediated control of gene repression and activation. Cell 159(3):647–661. https://doi.org/10.1016/j.cell.2014.09.029

50. Chavez A, Scheiman J, Vora S, Pruitt BW, Tuttle M, PRI E, Lin S, Kiani S, Guzman CD, Wiegand DJ, Ter-Ovanesyan D, Braff JL, Davidsohn N, Housden BE, Perrimon N, Weiss R, Aach J, Collins JJ, Church GM (2015) Highly efficient Cas9-mediated transcriptional programming. Nat Methods 12 (4):326–328. https://doi.org/10.1038/nmeth.3312

51. Yeo NC, Chavez A, Lance-Byrne A, Chan Y, Menn D, Milanova D, Kuo CC, Guo X, Sharma S, Tung A, Cecchi RJ, Tuttle M, Pradhan S, Lim ET, Davidsohn N, Ebrahimkhani MR, Collins JJ, Lewis NE, Kiani S, Church GM (2018) An enhanced CRISPR repressor for targeted mammalian gene regulation. Nat Methods 15(8):611–616. https://doi.org/10.1038/s41592-018-0048-5

52. Johnsson P, Ackley A, Vidarsdottir L, Lui WO, Corcoran M, Grander D, Morris KV (2013) A pseudogene long-noncoding-RNA network regulates PTEN transcription and translation in human cells. Nat Struct Mol Biol 20 (4):440–446. https://doi.org/10.1038/nsmb.2516

53. Konermann S, Lotfy P, Brideau NJ, Oki J, Shokhirev MN, Hsu PD (2018) Transcriptome engineering with RNA-targeting type VI-D CRISPR effectors. Cell 173(3):665–676. e614. https://doi.org/10.1016/j.cell.2018.02.033

54. Abudayyeh OO, Gootenberg JS, Essletzbichler P, Han S, Joung J, Belanto JJ, Verdine V, Cox DBT, Kellner MJ, Regev A, Lander ES, Voytas DF, Ting AY, Zhang F (2017) RNA targeting with CRISPR-Cas13. Nature 550(7675):280–284. https://doi.org/10.1038/nature24049

55. He B, Peng W, Huang J, Zhang H, Zhou Y, Yang X, Liu J, Li Z, Xu C, Xue M, Yang H, Huang P (2020) Modulation of metabolic functions through Cas13d-mediated gene knockdown in liver. Protein Cell 11 (7):518–524. https://doi.org/10.1007/s13238-020-00700-2

56. Nguyen TM, Zhang Y, Pandolfi PP (2020) Virus against virus: a potential treatment for 2019-nCov (SARS-CoV-2) and other RNA viruses. Cell Res 30(3):189–190. https://doi.org/10.1038/s41422-020-0290-0

# Chapter 15

# Experimental Validation of the Noncoding Potential for lncRNAs

## Emily A. Dangelmaier and Ashish Lal

## Abstract

In recent years, long noncoding RNAs (lncRNAs) have been increasingly recognized as critical regulators of a broad spectrum of cellular processes. Recent advancements in proteomic technologies have uncovered that an abundance of noncoding genes, including lncRNAs, have been misannotated and in reality encode proteins. This revelation underscores the need to accurately determine the coding potential of lncRNAs prior to assessment of their functional mechanisms. Here, we detail numerous experimental techniques useful in the determination of lncRNA coding potential. Several of these methods are doubly useful in that they may also be employed in studying the function of a lncRNA, be it via an RNA, protein, or both.

**Key words** lncRNAs, Long noncoding RNAs, Micropeptides, Coding potential, Translation

## 1    Introduction

In recent years, long noncoding RNAs (lncRNAs) have been increasingly characterized in a variety of cellular contexts. These studies have revealed lncRNAs to regulate diverse cellular processes [1, 2], many of which play important roles in human diseases [3], including cancer [4]. However, despite these advances the vast majority of lncRNAs remain uncharacterized and the precise biological mechanisms of action of most lncRNAs are unknown. A potential key in bridging this knowledge gap may lie in recent studies demonstrating that some lncRNAs have been misannotated and, surprisingly, encode small proteins also called micropeptides [5–12]. This misannotation may, in part, be due to the prevailing definition of an open reading frame (ORF), which denotes a eukaryotic ORF as greater than 100 codons long [13]. As a result, genes containing small ORFs (sORFs) and have the potential to encode small proteins, or micropeptides, are often misannotated as noncoding [10, 14]. Therefore, it is critical for future lncRNA studies to consider the tools available to establish the noncoding potential of novel lncRNAs.

Alfons Navarro (ed.), *Long Non-Coding RNAs in Cancer*, Methods in Molecular Biology, vol. 2348,
https://doi.org/10.1007/978-1-0716-1581-2_15, © Springer Science+Business Media, LLC, part of Springer Nature 2021

lncRNAs are a subclass of noncoding RNAs that are defined as transcripts >200 nucleotides long and often contain many of the same structural features of messenger RNAs (mRNAs), such as a poly(A) tail and 5′ cap. In contrast to mRNAs, however, most lncRNAs tend to be expressed at lower levels and are often nuclear localized. Despite this trend, several lncRNAs are localized to the cytoplasm and expressed at levels comparable to that of mRNAs, which can make it difficult to differentiate between the two. There are many additional features of lncRNAs that inform coding potential, which can be assessed both biochemically and computationally. For example, regions of the genome that code for protein tend to be more evolutionarily conserved and evolve under different selective pressures compared to noncoding regions. Additionally, the sequence of protein-coding regions is often similar to that of other proteins, particularly if they contain specific functional domains. Finally, in order to encode protein a transcript must associate with translation machinery at an ORF, although the existence of this association is not sufficient to prove that the transcript is, in fact, translated. If a lncRNA is found to code for protein it does not mean that the protein produced is abundant or stable enough to be present at biologically significant levels, as mRNA levels are often poorly correlated to protein levels [15]. Considering these important considerations, we herein describe a variety of methods to validate the potential of lncRNAs to code for small proteins.

## 2    Experimental Methods to Determine the Translation Status of lncRNAs

*2.1 Polysome Fractionation and Ribosome Profiling*

Reliable assessment of lncRNA coding potential depends on combined application of a variety of experimental approaches. Polysome fractionation and Ribo-seq are examples of complimentary methods commonly used to assess RNA translational status by identifying transcripts that associate with ribosomes (Fig. 1). Polysome fractionation can quantitatively determine the proportion of actively translated copies of a transcript by separating polysome fractions by size using a sucrose density gradient. Methods for polysome fractionation are commonly described for cell culture for technical reasons [16, 17]; however, it has also been successively conducted from solid tissue extracts [18]. In performing polysome fractionation, cells are first treated with cycloheximide (CHX) to freeze translation. Then, cytoplasmic lysates are prepared and loaded on to a 10–50% sucrose gradient and polysome fractions are collected using a fraction collector. Finally, RNA is isolated from the various fractions and can be analyzed using a variety of methods. For global analyses, deep RNA-sequencing or microarray analyses can be conducted. Analysis of the association of specific lncRNAs with ribosomes can be performed using quantitative real-time PCR (qRT-PCR) or northern blotting. lncRNAs found

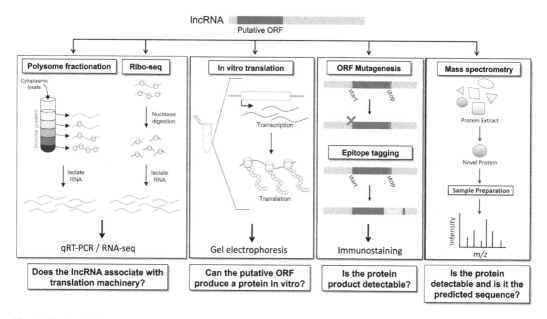

**Fig. 1** Methods for accessing lncRNA coding potential. Schematic representation of experimental methods used to identify and characterize novel proteins encoded by lncRNAs and questions addressed by corresponding methods

in heavy polysome fractions have the potential to be robustly translated [16].

Although polysome fractionation is useful in that it provides information about the fraction of transcripts of an lncRNA that may be actively translated, it does not provide any information about what region of the transcript is translated, which can be identified using ribosome profiling, or Ribo-seq. This information is significant as although a great number of annotated lncRNAs have been found to associate with polysomes [6], global applications of Ribo-seq have revealed that many of these associations do not occur within regions of a transcript that have the potential to be translated; specifically regions between a start and stop codon [19].

Ribo-seq is a genome-wide method used to identify transcripts that associate with actively translating 80S ribosomes by performing deep sequencing of ribosome-protected regions of RNA, or ribosome "footprints" [5]. This method has been successfully applied to a variety of biological systems, including yeast [5], zebrafish [20], plants [21], and mice [6]. These studies have revealed that a significant number of annotated lncRNAs associate with ribosomes, although many of these associations do not occur within sORFs [19]. Similar to polysome fractionation, early protocols for Ribo-seq describe an initial incubation with CHX to halt translation [5]; however, more recent versions report the use of other translation-disrupting drugs such as harringtonine, lactimidomycin, or puromycin [6, 22], which can be used in combination with CHX. After incubation with the drug(s), RNA is extracted, purified, and fragmented [5]. Next, footprinting is performed by digesting RNA with a nuclease, generally RNase I, which is the preferred nuclease due to its low sequence bias. RNA can then be size-selected and finally sequenced using a preprepared library to identify ribosome-protected footprints on RNA. More recently, methods that expand upon the capabilities of Ribo-seq have been described. These include TRAP-seq [23] which allows for cell-specific in vivo analysis of translation and Proximity-specific Ribo-seq [24] which can reveal subcellular localized translation [25].

Publicly available Ribo-seq data can be found on a variety of databases, which include RPFdb [26], RiboStreamR [27], and PR OTEOFORMER [28]. These databases can be useful for characterizing some lncRNAs; however, because many lncRNAs have remarkably cell-type and tissue-specific expression, use of these databases to access the coding potential of a specific lncRNA may be limited. For example, using single-cell analysis in the developing human neocortex, it was found that lncRNAs tended to have ~10-fold lower expression in a pool of cells compared to single cells [29]. Therefore, certain lncRNAs may be found to not associate with ribosomes in Ribo-seq experiments simply because the experiments were not performed in a cell type with robust expression of the lncRNA being investigated.

Although lack of association of an lncRNA with ribosomes confirms the noncoding status of a transcript, the presence of an association does not necessarily mean that a lncRNA is translated or that it encodes a functional protein. This is an important point. For example, bona fide lncRNAs such as *HULC* and the *H19* mouse transcript have been found to associate with polysomes despite being established noncoding transcripts [30, 31]. Therefore, to establish a lncRNA found to associate with polysomes as protein-coding, this association should be shown to occur within an ORF and the definitive evidence of the existence of the predicted protein in nature is required, which can, in turn be established by techniques such as mass spectrometry or using an antibody against the novel protein as described below after the CRISPR/Cas9 section.

*2.2   CRISPR/*
*Cas9-Based*
*Approaches*

Recent advancements in gene editing technology have yielded countless new techniques with a myriad of applications. In combination with polysome fractionation and Ribo-seq, additional approaches utilizing the CRISPR/Cas9-based technology can be used to determine if a lncRNA encodes a protein. This technology is particularly significant as it allows for editing of an lncRNA at its endogenous locus, which yields more biologically relevant results. Though CRISPR/Cas9-based techniques are most commonly used to characterize candidate lncRNAs on a case-by-case basis, this technology can also be developed for more global analyses of the translatome.

To start, CRISPR/Cas9 can be used to knockout a candidate lncRNA followed by detection of the protein in the lncRNA wild-type and knockout (KO) cells using an antibody generated from a predicted peptide of that protein. If the lncRNA is protein-coding, a protein of approximately the predicted size should be detected in wild-type cells, but not in KO cells, which can be determined by immunoblotting. Another method calls for mutating the start codon of the sORF within the lncRNA locus using a guide RNA targeting the start codon, then again using the predicted antibody to detect the protein in wild-type versus mutant cells (Fig. 1). Mutagenesis of the start codon or insertion of a premature stop codon is often the preferred approach as it is more precise and can be used for downstream loss-of-function studies. If the function or phenotype associated with a lncRNA is known, it is important to determine whether the function of this lncRNA is dependent on the RNA, the protein, or both. If cells expressing the transcript containing a mutant start codon display a similar phenotype to that of the KO, this suggests that the function of the lncRNA is most likely carried out by its encoded protein.

Although these approaches represent useful applications of CRISPR/Cas9 technology, they depend on the use of immunohistochemistry which has limited sensitivity compared to other methods such as mass spectrometry. Despite this, immunohistochemistry and immunostaining can be used to determine the subcellular localization of the protein in both tissues and cell lines, which often is critical to further elucidate the function of the protein in question. Additionally, performing immunoprecipitation for the protein of interest followed by mass spectrometry (IP-MS) allows for the identification of its interacting partners, which can also help determine its function and mechanism of action. Both techniques also depend on the use of an antibody generated from a predicted peptide of the expected protein product, which are notoriously nonspecific and difficult to use. To compensate for this, CRISPR/Cas9-generated KO cells can serve as an effective control for any nonspecific binding of the antibody.

To avoid the usage of such an antibody, CRISPR/Cas9 technology can also be used to knock in an epitope tag at the endogenous locus [7], detectable by microscopy or immunoblotting (Fig. 1). It is important to keep in mind that proteins produced from misannotated transcripts are usually small and the presence of an epitope tag, particularly a large tag, can confound functional studies or alter the stability and/or localization of the protein. Also, while CRISPR/Cas9 is praised for its high efficiency in knockout experiments, it generally has much lower efficiency for knockin experiments. Knockin using CRISPR/Cas9 harnesses the cell's DNA repair system, traditionally relying on homology directed repair (HDR) to introduce the knockin, which is less error prone but inefficient compared to nonhomologous end joining (NHEJ).

A recent study, however, describes a method to hijack NHEJ for knockin using CRISPR/Cas9 with markedly increased efficiency compared to HDR-mediated methods with minimal error [32]. Future investigations of lncRNAs may utilize this technology, in combination with other previously described applications of CRISPR/Cas9, to assess the coding potential and function of lncRNAs.

The applications of CRISPR/Cas9 for experimental validation of the non-coding potential of lncRNAs described thus far represent candidate gene-based approaches. Moving beyond these methods, CRISPR/Cas9 has also been applied for global analysis of noncanonical ORFs, which can validate findings from other global analyses such as Ribo-seq, polysome fractionation, or mass spectrometry. For example, Chen et al. performed a functional CRISPR/Cas9-based screen using a single guide RNA designed to knockout thousands of noncanonical ORFs that were previously identified by ribosome profiling [33]. This study demonstrates the immense and largely untapped power of CRISPR/Cas9-based methodologies for the validation of lncRNA non-coding potential.

## 2.3 Additional Methods to Access lncRNA Coding Potential

There are several other available methods used to validate lncRNA coding status that do not require the use of CRISPR/Cas9. Many of these approaches achieve results similar to those using CRISPR/Cas9 but rather utilize an overexpression system. This system can either use a plasmid transiently transfected or stably expressed using a lentiviral-based system. A plasmid expressing the lncRNA containing an epitope tag in its ORF with or without a mutant start codon can be used, rendering the protein detectable by microscopy or immunoblotting. In many cases a knockout, though preferable, is difficult to achieve and therefore a knockdown using RNA interference (RNAi) can be used to deplete either the endogenous or the tagged construct. An antibody against either the epitope tag or the protein can then be used to examine whether the detected protein is depleted upon knockdown of the lncRNA. Although these overexpression-based systems can be useful, overexpression of lncRNAs with low endogenous expression could result in the production of a protein product that is not typically expressed at biologically significant levels. Additionally, use of these systems for functional studies may result in aberrant localization or confound functional studies as they do not accurately reflect basal conditions.

Another method used to assess lncRNA coding potential is coupled in vitro transcription and translation [7]. This technique allows for radiolabeling of the peptide of interest with $^{35}$S-methionine during protein synthesize, which can then be detected by SDS-PAGE [7, 34] (Fig. 1). While in vitro translation can be useful, a protein that is translated in vitro may not necessarily be translated in vivo, and vice versa. As a result, findings obtained using this method should be validated using other methods described in this chapter.

## 2.4 Proteomics-Based Techniques to Study Translation

Mass spectrometry (MS)-based proteomics are currently the leading methodologies for protein detection used to validate the noncoding status of lncRNAs. Generally, MS functions by ionizing compounds via bombardment with an electron beam in order to create charged fragments, which are then separated by their mass-to-charge (m/z) ratio in a magnetic field. The relative abundance of each fragment measured by detectors and can later be associated with libraries of MS spectra of known compounds or macromolecules. Specifically, for application for targeted proteomics, proteins are extracted and digested using a protease to produce peptide fragments. Peptide fragments are then separated and purified using liquid chromatography, ionized using electrospray ionization, and finally the m/z ratio of the different peptides is determined by MS and reported on a spectrum [35] (Fig. 1). Analysis is often refined by integration of data obtained by MS with RNA-seq data and various bioinformatic tools.

Due to its high sensitivity, MS has frequently been used to detect peptides from proteins encoded by lncRNAs [36–38], which often have low expression levels. Most notably, peptides originating from 69 largely misannotated lncRNAs were detected in K562 and GM12878 human cell lines after cross referencing tandem MS (MS/MS) data with RNA-seq data from ENCODE [36]. While this study was limited to sORFs at a minimum of 23 amino acids in length, another study designed a more comprehensive database integrating RefSeq, MS/MS, and tandem MS coupled with liquid chromatography (LC-MS/MS). Cross-reference of this data revealed 86 novel proteins originating from genes annotated as lncRNAs in K562 cells [37].

Although MS represents a powerful tool for identifying misannotated lncRNAs, there are a few drawbacks in the application of this technique for lncRNAs specifically that must be considered. First, analysis of MS data using a reference database of peptide sequences poses many issues when specifically looking for novel proteins. To combat this, bioinformatic tools that can predict peptide sequences from MS spectra, such as SMSNet [39], can be used. Also, when mapping MS spectra globally, the use of search parameters with different levels of stringency can yield wildly different findings for the same spectra [40]. Although MS is highly sensitive compared to other methods that may be used, extraordinarily low expression, as is characteristic of many lncRNAs, can cause some proteins to remain undetectable by MS. This problem may be resolved by overexpressing a specific lncRNA of interest. However, detection of peptides originating from an overexpressed lncRNA does not prove that it is translated within a cell. Low expression and small protein size can also cause peptides produced from lncRNAs to be lost in the sample preparation process. In addition to these potential issues for lncRNA studies, there are also more general technical problems that can arise when using MS. For example, peptide fragments produced following digestion with a protease may be undetectable if they are either too small or too large. Taken together, these obstacles greatly encourage the use of MS-based approaches in combination with other approaches described in this chapter for reliable experimental validation of the lncRNA protein-coding potential.

## 3 Summary

lncRNAs are a rapidly expanding and exciting field; however, due to the potential misannotation of many lncRNAs, it is important to validate the noncoding potential of novel lncRNAs. Hereto unknown mechanisms of lncRNA function may be more thoroughly understood if a function can be attributed to either the lncRNA itself or its encoded protein. The tools described in this chapter, when used in concert, offer a comprehensive assessment of lncRNA coding potential. Although application of these techniques serves to validate the translation of a lncRNA, it is important to note that the same tools can be further used to investigate the function and mechanism of the lncRNA and/or the protein. While no technique is without its drawbacks, future advancements in proteomic technology will undoubtedly improve our ability to make such determinations regarding lncRNAs and more clearly resolve the line between coding and noncoding.

## Acknowledgments

This research to A.L and E.D was supported by the Intramural Research Program of the National Cancer Institute (NCI), Center for Cancer Research (CCR), National Institutes of Health (NIH).

## References

1. Kopp F, Mendell JT (2018) Functional classification and experimental dissection of long noncoding RNAs. Cell 172(3):393–407. https://doi.org/10.1016/j.cell.2018.01.011

2. Yao RW, Wang Y, Chen LL (2019) Cellular functions of long noncoding RNAs. Nat Cell Biol 21(5):542–551. https://doi.org/10.1038/s41556-019-0311-8

3. Wapinski O, Chang HY (2011) Long noncoding RNAs and human disease. Trends Cell Biol 21(6):354–361. https://doi.org/10.1016/j.tcb.2011.04.001

4. Schmitt AM, Chang HY (2016) Long noncoding RNAs in cancer pathways. Cancer Cell 29(4):452–463. https://doi.org/10.1016/j.ccell.2016.03.010

5. Ingolia NT, Ghaemmaghami S, Newman JR, Weissman JS (2009) Genome-wide analysis in vivo of translation with nucleotide resolution using ribosome profiling. Science 324

(5924):218–223. https://doi.org/10.1126/science.1168978

6. Ingolia NT, Lareau LF, Weissman JS (2011) Ribosome profiling of mouse embryonic stem cells reveals the complexity and dynamics of mammalian proteomes. Cell 147(4):789–802. https://doi.org/10.1016/j.cell.2011.10.002

7. Anderson DM, Anderson KM, Chang CL, Makarewich CA, Nelson BR, McAnally JR, Kasaragod P, Shelton JM, Liou J, Bassel-Duby R, Olson EN (2015) A micropeptide encoded by a putative long noncoding RNA regulates muscle performance. Cell 160 (4):595–606. https://doi.org/10.1016/j.cell.2015.01.009

8. Cai B, Li Z, Ma M, Wang Z, Han P, Abdalla BA, Nie Q, Zhang X (2017) LncRNA-Six1 encodes a micropeptide to activate Six1 in cis and is involved in cell proliferation and muscle growth. Front Physiol 8:230. https://doi.org/10.3389/fphys.2017.00230

9. Huang JZ, Chen M, Chen D, Gao XC, Zhu S, Huang H, Hu M, Zhu H, Yan GR (2017) A peptide encoded by a putative lncRNA HOXB-AS3 suppresses colon cancer growth. Mol Cell 68(1):171–184. e176. https://doi.org/10.1016/j.molcel.2017.09.015

10. Andrews SJ, Rothnagel JA (2014) Emerging evidence for functional peptides encoded by short open reading frames. Nat Rev Genet 15 (3):193–204. https://doi.org/10.1038/nrg3520

11. Rossi M, Bucci G, Rizzotto D, Bordo D, Marzi MJ, Puppo M, Flinois A, Spadaro D, Citi S, Emionite L, Cilli M, Nicassio F, Inga A, Briata P, Gherzi R (2019) LncRNA EPR controls epithelial proliferation by coordinating Cdkn1a transcription and mRNA decay response to TGF-beta. Nat Commun 10 (1):1969. https://doi.org/10.1038/s41467-019-09754-1

12. Makarewich CA, Olson EN (2017) Mining for Micropeptides. Trends Cell Biol 27 (9):685–696. https://doi.org/10.1016/j.tcb.2017.04.006

13. Harrow J, Frankish A, Gonzalez JM, Tapanari E, Diekhans M, Kokocinski F, Aken BL, Barrell D, Zadissa A, Searle S, Barnes I, Bignell A, Boychenko V, Hunt T, Kay M, Mukherjee G, Rajan J, Despacio-Reyes G, Saunders G, Steward C, Harte R, Lin M, Howald C, Tanzer A, Derrien T, Chrast J, Walters N, Balasubramanian S, Pei B, Tress M, Rodriguez JM, Ezkurdia I, van Baren J, Brent M, Haussler D, Kellis M, Valencia A, Reymond A, Gerstein M, Guigo R, Hubbard TJ (2012) GENCODE: the reference human genome annotation for the ENCODE project. Genome Res 22 (9):1760–1774. https://doi.org/10.1101/gr.135350.111

14. Hartford CCR, Lal A (2020) When long noncoding becomes protein coding. Mol Cell Biol 40(6):e00528-19. https://doi.org/10.1128/MCB.00528-19

15. Schwanhausser B, Busse D, Li N, Dittmar G, Schuchhardt J, Wolf J, Chen W, Selbach M (2011) Global quantification of mammalian gene expression control. Nature 473 (7347):337–342. https://doi.org/10.1038/nature10098

16. Panda AC, Martindale JL, Gorospe M (2017) Polysome fractionation to analyze mRNA distribution profiles. Bio Protoc 7(3). https://doi.org/10.21769/BioProtoc.2126

17. Gandin V, Sikstrom K, Alain T, Morita M, McLaughlan S, Larsson O, Topisirovic I (2014) Polysome fractionation and analysis of mammalian translatomes on a genome-wide scale. J Vis Exp 87:51455. https://doi.org/10.3791/51455

18. del Prete MJ, Vernal R, Dolznig H, Mullner EW, Garcia-Sanz JA (2007) Isolation of polysome-bound mRNA from solid tissues amenable for RT-PCR and profiling experiments. RNA 13(3):414–421. https://doi.org/10.1261/rna.79407

19. Guttman M, Russell P, Ingolia NT, Weissman JS, Lander ES (2013) Ribosome profiling provides evidence that large noncoding RNAs do not encode proteins. Cell 154(1):240–251. https://doi.org/10.1016/j.cell.2013.06.009

20. Bazzini AA, Johnstone TG, Christiano R, Mackowiak SD, Obermayer B, Fleming ES, Vejnar CE, Lee MT, Rajewsky N, Walther TC, Giraldez AJ (2014) Identification of small ORFs in vertebrates using ribosome footprinting and evolutionary conservation. EMBO J 33 (9):981–993. https://doi.org/10.1002/embj.201488411

21. Juntawong P, Girke T, Bazin J, Bailey-Serres J (2014) Translational dynamics revealed by genome-wide profiling of ribosome footprints in Arabidopsis. Proc Natl Acad Sci U S A 111 (1):E203–E212. https://doi.org/10.1073/pnas.1317811111

22. Gao X, Wan J, Liu B, Ma M, Shen B, Qian SB (2015) Quantitative profiling of initiating ribosomes in vivo. Nat Methods 12(2):147–153. https://doi.org/10.1038/nmeth.3208

23. Heiman M, Kulicke R, Fenster RJ, Greengard P, Heintz N (2014) Cell type-specific mRNA purification by translating ribosome affinity purification (TRAP). Nat Protoc

9(6):1282–1291. https://doi.org/10.1038/nprot.2014.085

24. Jan CH, Williams CC, Weissman JS (2014) Principles of ER cotranslational translocation revealed by proximity-specific ribosome profiling. Science 346(6210):1257521. https://doi.org/10.1126/science.1257521

25. Dermit M, Dodel M, Mardakheh FK (2017) Methods for monitoring and measurement of protein translation in time and space. Mol BioSyst 13(12):2477–2488. https://doi.org/10.1039/c7mb00476a

26. Wang H, Yang L, Wang Y, Chen L, Li H, Xie Z (2019) RPFdb v2.0: an updated database for genome-wide information of translated mRNA generated from ribosome profiling. Nucleic Acids Res 47(D1):D230–D234. https://doi.org/10.1093/nar/gky978

27. Perkins P, Mazzoni-Putman S, Stepanova A, Alonso J, Heber S (2019) RiboStreamR: a web application for quality control, analysis, and visualization of Ribo-seq data. BMC Genomics 20(Suppl 5):422. https://doi.org/10.1186/s12864-019-5700-7

28. Crappe J, Ndah E, Koch A, Steyaert S, Gawron D, De Keulenaer S, De Meester E, De Meyer T, Van Criekinge W, Van Damme P, Menschaert G (2015) PROTEOFORMER: deep proteome coverage through ribosome profiling and MS integration. Nucleic Acids Res 43(5):e29. https://doi.org/10.1093/nar/gku1283

29. Liu SJ, Nowakowski TJ, Pollen AA, Lui JH, Horlbeck MA, Attenello FJ, He D, Weissman JS, Kriegstein AR, Diaz AA, Lim DA (2016) Single-cell analysis of long non-coding RNAs in the developing human neocortex. Genome Biol 17:67. https://doi.org/10.1186/s13059-016-0932-1

30. Panzitt K, Tschernatsch MM, Guelly C, Moustafa T, Stradner M, Strohmaier HM, Buck CR, Denk H, Schroeder R, Trauner M, Zatloukal K (2007) Characterization of HULC, a novel gene with striking up-regulation in hepatocellular carcinoma, as noncoding RNA. Gastroenterology 132(1):330–342. https://doi.org/10.1053/j.gastro.2006.08.026

31. Li YM, Franklin G, Cui HM, Svensson K, He XB, Adam G, Ohlsson R, Pfeifer S (1998) The H19 transcript is associated with polysomes and may regulate IGF2 expression in trans. J Biol Chem 273(43):28247–28252. https://doi.org/10.1074/jbc.273.43.28247

32. Artegiani B, Hendriks D, Beumer J, Kok R, Zheng X, Joore I, Chuva de Sousa Lopes S, van Zon J, Tans S, Clevers H (2020) Fast and efficient generation of knock-in human organoids using homology-independent CRISPR-Cas9 precision genome editing. Nat Cell Biol 22(3):321–331. https://doi.org/10.1038/s41556-020-0472-5

33. Chen J, Brunner AD, Cogan JZ, Nunez JK, Fields AP, Adamson B, Itzhak DN, Li JY, Mann M, Leonetti MD, Weissman JS (2020) Pervasive functional translation of noncanonical human open reading frames. Science 367(6482):1140–1146. https://doi.org/10.1126/science.aay0262

34. Esposito AM, Kinzy TG (2014) In vivo [35S]-methionine incorporation. Methods Enzymol 536:55–64. https://doi.org/10.1016/B978-0-12-420070-8.00005-2

35. Doerr A (2013) Mass spectrometry-based targeted proteomics. Nat Methods 10(1):23. https://doi.org/10.1038/nmeth.2286

36. Banfai B, Jia H, Khatun J, Wood E, Risk B, Gundling WE Jr, Kundaje A, Gunawardena HP, Yu Y, Xie L, Krajewski K, Strahl BD, Chen X, Bickel P, Giddings MC, Brown JB, Lipovich L (2012) Long noncoding RNAs are rarely translated in two human cell lines. Genome Res 22(9):1646–1657. https://doi.org/10.1101/gr.134767.111

37. Slavoff SA, Mitchell AJ, Schwaid AG, Cabili MN, Ma J, Levin JZ, Karger AD, Budnik BA, Rinn JL, Saghatelian A (2013) Peptidomic discovery of short open reading frame-encoded peptides in human cells. Nat Chem Biol 9(1):59–64. https://doi.org/10.1038/nchembio.1120

38. Wilhelm M, Schlegl J, Hahne H, Gholami AM, Lieberenz M, Savitski MM, Ziegler E, Butzmann L, Gessulat S, Marx H, Mathieson T, Lemeer S, Schnatbaum K, Reimer U, Wenschuh H, Mollenhauer M, Slotta-Huspenina J, Boese JH, Bantscheff M, Gerstmair A, Faerber F, Kuster B (2014) Mass-spectrometry-based draft of the human proteome. Nature 509(7502):582–587. https://doi.org/10.1038/nature13319

39. Karunratanakul K, Tang HY, Speicher DW, Chuangsuwanich E, Sriswasdi S (2019) Uncovering thousands of new peptides with sequence-mask-search hybrid De novo peptide sequencing framework. Mol Cell Proteomics 18(12):2478–2491. https://doi.org/10.1074/mcp.TIR119.001656

40. Housman G, Ulitsky I (2016) Methods for distinguishing between protein-coding and long noncoding RNAs and the elusive biological purpose of translation of long noncoding RNAs. Biochim Biophys Acta 1859(1):31–40. https://doi.org/10.1016/j.bbagrm.2015.07.017

# Chapter 16

# Identification of lncRNA–Protein Interactions by CLIP and RNA Pull-Down Assays

## Kunming Zhao, Xingwen Wang, and Ying Hu

## Abstract

The emerging data indicates that long noncoding RNAs (lncRNAs) are involved in fundamental biological processes, and their deregulation may lead to oncogenesis and other diseases. LncRNA fulfil its biological functions at least in part by interacting with distinctive proteins. Here, we described two methods to identify the direct or indirect interactions between lncRNA and proteins: cross-linking and immunoprecipitation (CLIP) and RNA pull-down assay. CLIP methods enable yield a list of lncRNAs that directly interact target protein in living cells, whereas immunoprecipitation of biotin-labeled RNA (RNA pull-down) assay represents a method for identification of proteins that directly and indirectly bind with a particular target lncRNA of interest.

**Key words** lncRNA, UV cross-linking, CLIP, Immunoprecipitation, RNA pull-down, Immunoblots

## 1 Introduction

Long noncoding RNAs (lncRNAs) represent a class of transcribed RNA molecules that are longer than 200 nucleotides with low potential to encode proteins [1]. LncRNAs have been long considered transcript noise. Until recently, mounting evidence has indicated that lncRNAs are involved in multiple essential biological processes and the dysregulated lncRNA expression is associated with various diseases, such as cancer, cardiovascular disease, and neurodegenerative diseases [2]. LncRNAs localize either in the cytoplasm or in the nucleus, where they elicit their biological functions by binding with protein, DNA, or RNA. There is an urgent need to understand the underlying mechanisms of lncRNAs action [1]. Techniques have been developed for the purpose of identification of lncRNA–protein [3], –DNA [4], and –RNA [5] interactions. In this chapter, we describe two methods our laboratory used to identify the direct or indirect interactions between lncRNA and protein either in vivo or in vitro (Fig. 1).

Alfons Navarro (ed.), *Long Non-Coding RNAs in Cancer*, Methods in Molecular Biology, vol. 2348,
https://doi.org/10.1007/978-1-0716-1581-2_16, © Springer Science+Business Media, LLC, part of Springer Nature 2021

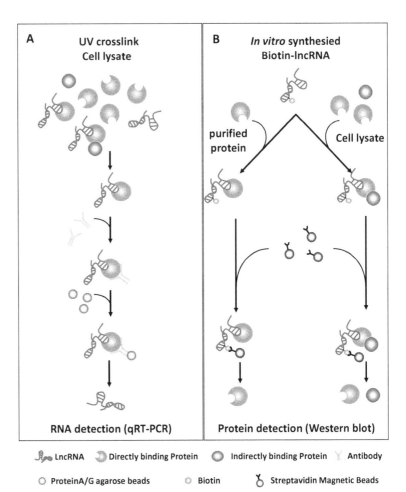

**Fig. 1** Schematic model of the lncRNA–protein interaction assays ((**a**) CLIP and (**b**) RNA pull-down assay). (**a**) after UV cross-linking, the direct lncRNA and protein interaction is analyzed by immunoprecipitation after incubating with specific antibody targeted to the protein of interest. Coprecipitated lncRNAs were detected by qRT-PCR. (**b**) RNA pull-down assay is an in vitro assay used to detect a direct lncRNA–protein interaction by mixing in vitro synthesized biotin-lncRNA and purified protein. It can be also used to reveal novel protein binding partners by mixing in vitro synthesized biotin-lncRNA and cell lysate. The complex is purified by using streptavidin magnetic beads and the protein is detected by Western blot

One method is cross-linking and immunoprecipitation (CLIP) that enable the identification of RNAs, including lncRNA that bind with particular protein of interest [6]. CLIPs involves cross-linking of proteins to target RNAs. UV cross-linking during the CLIP procedure results in the formation of a covalent bond between the RNA and the nearby amino acid moiety and therefore generally used to reveal direct lncRNA–protein interaction in living cell. Following cross-linking, immunoprecipitation of the protein of interest and its associated RNAs with specific antibodies enable further detection of protein-bound RNA fragments [6]. Here, we use quantitative RT-PCR after digesting proteins in the immunoprecipitates (Fig. 1a). High-throughput sequencing of the protein-bound RNA fragments is also reported in the literatures [7].

Another method is an in vitro technique used to detect the interactions between lncRNA of interest and protein binding partners and an invaluable tool for confirming a predicted lncRNA–protein interaction or identifying possible novel interacting partners in cell lysates [8]. This method in detection of lncRNA–protein interaction typically takes advantage of high-affinity tags, such as biotin. For example, biotinylated lncRNA is synthesized in vitro and then complexed with either in vitro synthesized proteins to confirm a direct interaction or protein in cell lysates to reveal both direct and indirect binding partners. After that, the biotin–RNA–protein complex is purified using magnetic beads. The protein binding partners can be detected by Western blot (Fig. 1b). For a high-throughput assay, the resulting proteins from the immunoprecipitates also can be subjected to a mass-spectrum assay [9].

# 2 Materials

Prepare all solutions using RNase-free water, and all materials, such as microcentrifuge tubes and pipette tips are RNase-free. Add protease inhibitor cocktail and/or RNase inhibitor into the indicated solutions before use. Prepare and store all reagents at room temperature, unless otherwise specified.

## 2.1 Cross-Linking and Immuno-precipitation (IP)

### 2.1.1 Lysis Buffers

1. Buffer A:
   5 mM PIPES (PH8.0).
   85 mM KCl.
   0.5% NP40.
   1× protease inhibitor cocktail.
   RNase inhibitor.

2. Buffer B:
   1% SDS.
   10 mM EDTA.
   50 mM Tris–HCl pH (8.1).
   1× protease inhibitor cocktail.
   RNase inhibitor.

3. IP Buffer:
   0.01% SDS.
   1.1% Triton X-100.

1.2 mM EDTA.

16.7 mM Tris (pH 8.1).

167 mM NaCl.

1× protease inhibitor cocktail.

RNase inhibitor.

*2.1.2 Wash Buffers and Elution Buffer*

1. Low-salt wash buffer.
   0.1% SDS.

   1% Triton X-100.

   2 mM EDTA.

   20 mM Tris–HCl (pH 8.1).

   150 mM NaCl.

2. High-salt wash buffer B.
   0.1% SDS.

   1% Triton X-100.

   2 mM EDTA.

   20 mM Tris–HCl (pH 8.1).

   500 mM NaCl.

3. TE buffer (pH 8.0).
   0.01 M Tris–HCl (pH 8.1).

   1 mM EDTA.

4. Elution buffer.
   1% SDS.

   0.1 M $NaHCO_3$.

   RNase inhibitor.

**2.2 RNA Pull-Down**

1. 2× RNA structure buffer.
   20 mM Tris (pH 7.4).

   200 mM KCl.

   20 mM $MgCl_2$.

   RNase inhibitor

2. NETN buffer.
   50 mM Tris–HCl (pH 8.0).

   150 mM NaCl.

   1% NP40.

   1 mM EDTA.

   1× protease inhibitor cocktail.

   RNase inhibitor.

**2.3 Additional Reagents and Equipment**

1. Proteinase Inhibitor Cocktail (MedChemExpress).
2. Protein G Sepharose beads 4 Fast Flow (GE Healthcare).
3. Streptavidin Magnetic Beads (MedChemExpress).
4. RiboLock RNase Inhibitor (Thermo Fisher).
5. Cross Linker (Gene Company Limited).
6. TRIzol (Thermo Fisher).
7. PrimeScript reverse transcription (RT) reagent kit (Takara).
8. SYBR Premix Ex Taq II kit (Takara).

# 3 Methods

**3.1 Cross-Linking and Immunoprecipitation**

*3.1.1 Protein–RNA Cross-Linking*

1. Grow HeLa cells on 10 cm$^2$ tissue culture petri dish to reach 70–80% confluence (*see* **Note 1**).
2. Remove culture medium from the dish and wash cells twice in ice-cold 1× PBS.
3. UV cross-link plate of cells in Cross Linker at 254 nm wavelength with 400 mJ/cm$^2$ of UVB (*see* **Notes 2** and **3**).
4. Remove plate of cells from crosslinker and immediately put on ice.

*3.1.2 Lysates Preparation*

1. Add 500 μL ice-cold Buffer A (supplemented with 1X proteinase inhibitor cocktail and RNase inhibitor (*see* **Notes 4** and **5** to lyse HeLa cells after cross-link).
2. Scrape cells from plate, gently pipette the lysate upside down 5–10 times and then keep the lysates on ice for an additional 10 min.
3. Transfer cell lysates into a 1.5 mL microcentrifuge tubes and centrifuge samples at 5000 × *g* for 5 min at 4 °C. Collect supernatants as cytosolic fraction.
4. Wash cell pellet once with 1 mL Buffer A. Resuspend the pellet in 500 μL Buffer B (supplemented with 1× proteinase inhibitor cocktail and RNase inhibitor, *see* **Notes 4** and **5**). Beak the pellet harshly and keep the lysates on ice for an additional 10 min.
5. Sonicate lysates with 4 short burst of 20 s followed by intervals of 1 min to reestablish a low temperature (*see* **Note 6**). During the sonication, turn the output level 40% and then return it to 0.
6. Remove cell debris by centrifuge at 16,000 × *g* for 10 min at 4 °C. Label the resulting supernatants as nuclear fraction (*see* **Note** 7).

*3.1.3 Beads Preparation*

1. Wash protein G Sepharose beads 4 Fast Flow with 1 mL ice-cold 1× PBS for four times and store it in IP buffer (volume ratio = 1:1), namely, precleaned protein G Sepharose beads.

2. Block precleaned protein G Sepharose beads 1 mL with DMEM cell culture medium (contain 10% FBS) for 1 h at 4 °C on rotation.

3. Centrifuge at 800 × *g* for 5 min at 4 °C.

4. Aspirate the blocking solution and wash the blocked protein G Sepharose beads with 1 mL ice cold 1× PBS for four times and store it in IP buffer (volume ratio = 1:1) (*see* **Note 8**).

*3.1.4 RNA*
*Immunoprecipitation*

1. Dilute the targeted lysates in IP buffer by 1:10. Mix well and aliquot 500 µL as an input control. Froze it at −80 °C to avoid degradation.

2. Preclean cell lysates with 40 µL precleaned protein G Sepharose beads for 1 h at 4 °C on rotation. Centrifuge samples at 1000 × *g* for 2 min at 4 °C.

3. Aliquot same volume of precleaned cell lysates into two 1.5 mL microcentrifuge tubes and incubate with the indicated antibody (0.5–2 µg/IP) and same amount of IgG derived from the same species, respectively (*see* **Note 9**).

4. To allow the antibody bind with the target protein, incubate the mixture on a rotator at 4 °C overnight for at least 20 h.

5. Next day, add 50 µL blocked protein G Sepharose beads into each mixture. Incubate for additional 2 h under the same conditions.

6. Centrifuge at 800 × *g* for 5 min at 4 °C to pellet protein G Sepharose beads bound with immune complex.

*3.1.5 Immune Complex*
*Washes*

Sequentially wash the obtained protein G Sepharose beads with the following.

1. Low-salt washing buffer.

2. High-salt washing buffer.

3. LiCl washing buffer.

4. TE buffer (pH 8.0).

5. TE buffer (pH 8.0).

For each wash, add 1 mL of the indicated washing buffer and rotate the mixture on a rotator for 5 min following centrifuge at 800 × *g* for 5 min at 4 °C. Aspirate or pipette washing buffer carefully without disturbing beads (*see* **Note 10**).

**3.1.6 Complex Elution and Decrosslink**

1. Incubate 250 μL fresh Elution Buffer with protein G Sepharose beads on a shaker for 15 min to elute RNA–protein complexes from agarose beads. Centrifuge samples at $4000 \times g$ for 2 min at 4 °C. Collect supernatants,

2. Repeat the elution step and obtain 500 μL elutes in total.

3. Decrosslink RNA–protein of the eluted samples and previous aliquot input samples that have been stored at −80 °C, with 200 mM NaCl at 65 °C for 2 h.

4. Denature proteins in input sample and 5% elutes with SDS loading buffer and then analysis protein pull-down efficiency by Western blot analysis.

5. Next, isolate RNA from left elucidate (95%) by TRIzol RNA extraction reagent following standard RNA isolation procedures.

**3.1.7 RNA Detection**

1. Reverse transcript RNA to cDNA by PrimeScript reverse transcription (RT) reagent kit in the presence of gDNA Eraser.

2. Determine the presence of the targeted RNA in the immunoprecipitates by quantitative RT-PCR using SYBR Premix Ex Taq II kit with GAPDH or 18S as negative controls. An example of the results of the assay obtained by CLIP is shown in Fig. 2a. The protein pull-down of the same experiments is shown in Fig. 2b.

**3.2 RNA Pull-Down Assay**

**3.2.1 In Vitro Biotin-Labeled RNA Synthesis**

1. Prepare the endonuclease reaction as follow: 1 μL of 10× Buffer, 1 μg DNA plasmids, 1 μL (10 U) of restriction endonuclease, and RNase-free MilliQ $H_2O$ up to 10 μL.

2. Linearize plasmids DNA containing sense or antisense lncRNA sequence and T7 promoter sequence by using restriction

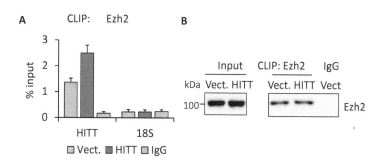

**Fig. 2 (a)** CLIP is a method to investigate the direct interaction between lncRNA and protein in living cells. After UV cross-linking, the lncRNA HITT-Ezh2 complex is purified by using anti-Ezh2 antibody. IgG was used as a antibody control. The presence of lncRNA HITT in the immunoprecipitates was detected using qRT-PCR. 18s was used as a negative control. **(b)** The efficiency of Ezh2 immunoprecipitation was confirmed by Western blot

endonuclease and allow reaction happened at 37 °C for 5–10 min in a water bath.

3. After the reaction, load 5 µL sample into agarose gel and run electrophoresis to test linearization efficiency of the plasmid DNA.

4. Isolate the linearized plasmid by phenol-chloroform method as described previously [10].

5. Prepare the RNA synthesis reaction in a 200 µL Eppendorf tube as follows: 6.5 µL of 10× transcription Buffer, 1 µL of Bio-RNA Labeling Mix, 500 ng of linear plasmid, 0.5 µL (20 U) of RNase inhibitor, 1 µL (20 U) of T7 RNA polymerase, and RNase-free MilliQ $H_2O$ up to 10 µL.

6. Run the reaction in a water bath at 37 °C for 2 h.

7. Add 1 µL DNase I into the reaction mixture and incubate the mixture in a water bath at 37 °C for 15 min to digest the template (DNA plasmid).

8. Stop the reaction by adding 1 µL 0.2 M EDTA (PH 8.0) into the mixture.

9. Alcohol precipitation: add 1.2 µL 4 M LiCl and 30 µL 100% alcohol into the mixture, mix well and incubate the samples at −20 °C for 30 min.

10. Centrifuge samples at $13,000 \times g$ for 15 min at 4 °C (*see* **Note 11**).

11. Aspirate the supernatant. Add 50–100 µL precooled 70% alcohol, mix well and centrifuge samples at $13,000 \times g$ for 15 min at 4 °C.

12. Remove the supernatant and dry RNA samples at room temperature (*see* **Note 12**).

13. Dissolve RNA with 40 µL RNase-free water. Measure RNA concentration by nanodrop and adjust RNA concentration to 100 ng/mL by adding RNase-free water.

14. Denature 500 ng RNA at 65 °C for 10 min, and run agarose gel electrophoresis to test the quality of RNA samples (*see* **Notes 13** and **14**) (Fig. 3).

*3.2.2  RNA and Protein Binding Reaction*

1. Denature biotin-labeled RNA at 70 °C for 10 min.

2. Place the mixture on ice immediately after the reaction and kept it on ice for an additional 2 min.

3. Add the same volume 2× RNA structure buffer and mix well. Allow the reaction occurred at room temperature for 30 min to form structure.

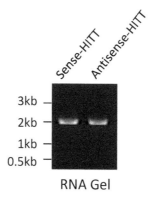

RNA Gel

**Fig. 3** Sense and antisense biotin-labeled *HITT* is synthesized by using T7 RNA polymerase kit. The presence of 2 kb biotin-*HITT* transcripts confirmed using RNA electrophoresis

4. Add 1 pmol Biotin-RNA and proteins (2 mg total cell lysate in NETN buffer or 5–10 pmol purified protein) in a 1.5 mL RNase-free tube in 500 μL NETN.

5. Place the microcentrifuge tubes at 4 °C on a rotator for 2 h, and then ready for future use.

*3.2.3 RNA Pull-Down*

1. Streptavidin magnetic beads was washed once with cold NETN buffer, and then block with 2 mg/mL BSA and 1 mg/mL Yeast tRNA for 1 h at 4 °C.

2. Add 20 μL blocked streptavidin magnetic beads into the prepared RNA–protein mixture, allow the reaction on a rotator at 4 °C for additional 1 h.

3. Place the tubes on the magnetic stand and remove the supernatant with pipette carefully without disturbing beads.

4. Wash the beads with 1 mL NETN buffer four times (*see* **Note 15**).

5. Denature proteins in the immunoprecipitates by adding 30 μL 2× SDS-loading buffer and boil the samples at 100 °C for 5 min.

6. Analyze RNA-binding protein by Western blot (*see* Subheading 3.2.4).

*3.2.4 Protein Detection*

1. Load 10 μL samples (include input antisense and sense three groups) and run SDS-PAGE gel.

2. Transfer the protein from SDS-PAGE gel to the PVDF membrane.

3. Block the membrane with 5% skim milk in TBS-T for 1 h at room temperature.

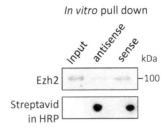

**Fig. 4** In an in vitro RNA pull-down assay, Sense and antisense biotin-labeled *HITT* is mixed with purified Ezh2 protein, add streptavidin magnetic beads, and detect the binding of Ezh2 and *HITT* by WB (top lane). The presence of RNA transcripts was confirmed using streptavidin-HRP by dot-blot assay (bottom lane)

4. Incubate the membrane with the primary antibody specifically target protein or tag protein overnight at 4 °C.

5. Wash the membrane with TBS-T, 5 min, three times.

6. Incubate the membrane with secondary antibody for 1 h at room temperature.

7. Wash the membrane with TBS-T, 15 min, three times.

8. After finishing all steps, detect the signal of immune complex by ECL kit. An example of the results of the assay obtained by RNA pull-down assay is shown in Fig. 4. The RNA pull-down of the same experiments is shown in Fig. 4 (bottom blot).

## 4   Notes

1. The number of cells used for this assay was variable, according to cell types, the expression levels of target protein and lncRNA.

2. Because of the easily degradation character of RNA, make sure all materials are RNase free and precool all solutions before use.

3. The time of cross-link reversing can be varied with experiment condition.

4. RNA is very susceptible to degradation, so special care must be taken not to introduce RNases into the reaction.

5. The type of lysis buffer depends on whether nuclear, cytoplasmic or whole cell lysates are needed.

6. Ultrasound temperature is high, and the protein is easy to denature under such conditions. Thus, it must be operated on ice.

7. Whether the cytosolic, nuclear or total protein are deemed to be used in the assay, it dependents the localization of the target protein or lncRNA.

8. Insufficient blocking of the beads will cause nonspecific proteins to bind to the beads.

9. Antibody should be tested before used in this assay to be sure that it can recognize and pulldown the target protein efficiently.

10. Beads should be suspended well with wash buffer during every washing step to remove unbound protein.

11. After centrifugation, white precipitate can be found at the bottom of the microcentrifuge tubes.

12. After drying at room temperature for 2–3 min, add RNase-free water to 1.5 mL microcentrifuge tubes.

13. In vitro synthesized RNA should be aliquot and stored at −80 °C, to avoid repeated freeze–thaw cycles.

14. After in vitro RNA synthesis, run an RNA agarose gel to test the quality of RNA. The TAE running buffer should be prepared with RNase-free water (we use DEPC treated MilliQ water), and all materials should be pretreated with DEPC.

15. Please remove the supernatant carefully following each wash, avoid disturbing the magnetic beads.

## Acknowledgments

This work was funded by the National Nature Science Foundation of China (No. 31301131, 31741084, and 31871389) and Basic Science Foundation of Science and Technology Innovation Commission in Shenzhen (No. JCYJ20170811154452255).

## References

1. Kopp F, Mendell JT (2018) Functional classification and experimental dissection of long noncoding RNAs. Cell 172(3):393–407. https://doi.org/10.1016/j.cell.2018.01.011

2. Batista PJ, Chang HY (2013) Long noncoding RNAs: cellular address codes in development and disease. Cell 152(6):1298–1307. https://doi.org/10.1016/j.cell.2013.02.012

3. Zhang Y, Feng Y, Hu Z, Hu X, Yuan C-X, Fan Y, Zhang L (2016) Characterization of long noncoding RNA-associated proteins by RNA-immunoprecipitation. Methods Mol Biol 1402:19–26. https://doi.org/10.1007/978-1-4939-3378-5_3

4. Besch R, Giovannangeli C, Schuh T, Kammerbauer C, Degitz K (2004) Characterization and quantification of triple helix formation in chromosomal DNA. J Mol Biol 341 (4):979–989

5. Cai Z, Cao C, Ji L, Ye R, Wang D, Xia C, Wang S, Du Z, Hu N, Yu X, Chen J, Wang L, Yang X, He S, Xue Y (2020) RIC-seq for global in situ profiling of RNA-RNA spatial interactions. Nature 582(7812):432–437. https://doi.org/10.1038/s41586-020-2249-1

6. Darnell JC, Mele A, Hung KYS, Darnell RB (2018) Immunoprecipitation and SDS-PAGE for cross-linking immunoprecipitation (CLIP). Cold Spring Harb Protoc 2018(12). https://doi.org/10.1101/pdb.prot097956

7. Grozdanov PN, Macdonald CC (2014) High-throughput sequencing of RNA isolated by cross-linking and immunoprecipitation (HITS-CLIP) to determine sites of binding of CstF-64 on nascent RNAs. Methods Mol Biol 1125:187–208. https://doi.org/10.1007/978-1-62703-971-0_17

8. Feng Y, Hu X, Zhang Y, Zhang D, Li C, Zhang L (2014) Methods for the study of long non-coding RNA in cancer cell signaling. Methods Mol Biol 1165:115–143. https://doi.org/10.1007/978-1-4939-0856-1_10

9. Shan M, Gregory BD (2020) Using RNA affinity purification followed by mass spectrometry to identify RNA-binding proteins (RBPs). Methods Mol Biol 2166:241–253. https://doi.org/10.1007/978-1-0716-0712-1_14

10. Koshy L, Anju AL, Harikrishnan S, Kutty VR, Jissa VT, Kurikesu I, Jayachandran P, Nair AJ, Gangaprasad A, Nair GM, Sudhakaran PR (2017) Evaluating genomic DNA extraction methods from human whole blood using end-point and real-time PCR assays. Mol Biol Rep 44(1):97–108. https://doi.org/10.1007/s11033-016-4085-9

# Chapter 17

# Empirical Validation of Overlapping Virus lncRNAs and Coding Transcripts by Northern Blot

## Mehmet Kara and Scott A. Tibbetts

## Abstract

Viruses, like their metazoan hosts, have evolved to utilize intricate transcriptional mechanisms to generate a vast array of both coding and noncoding RNA transcripts. The resolution of specific noncoding RNA transcripts produced by viruses, particularly herpesviruses, presents a particularly difficult challenge due to their highly dense dsDNA genomes and their complex, overlapping, and context-dependent network of transcripts. While new long read sequencing platforms have facilitated the resolution of some noncoding transcripts from virus genomes, empirical molecular validation of transcripts from individual regions is essential. Herein, we demonstrate that the use of strand specific northern blots is essential for true validation of specific viral noncoding RNAs, and provide here a detailed molecular method for such an approach.

**Key words** Viral lncRNAs, Herpesviruses, Strand specific northern blot

## 1  Introduction

Over the last 15 years, the rapid advance of new sequencing technologies has greatly expanded our understanding of the vast complexity of host and pathogen transcriptomes and has led to the identification of thousands of new noncoding RNA transcripts [1, 2]. Through this work it has become clear that a large number unannotated regions of metazoan genomes are actively transcribed [3, 4]. However, perhaps most emblematic of such complexity are the highly dense dsDNA genomes of herpesviruses. Despite their small genomic sizes, ranging from 100 to 250 kb, herpesviruses carry up to 235 protein coding genes which are expressed bidirectionally [5]. Moreover, these viruses have demonstrated the capacity to generate hundreds of additional coding and noncoding RNA molecules through antisense, intergenic, and readthrough transcription, as well as alternative splicing and alternate promoter usage [6–9].

Alfons Navarro (ed.), *Long Non-Coding RNAs in Cancer*, Methods in Molecular Biology, vol. 2348,
https://doi.org/10.1007/978-1-0716-1581-2_17, © Springer Science+Business Media, LLC, part of Springer Nature 2021

The vast majority of the noncoding RNAs that have been identified in viruses are derived from herpesvirus family members [10]. Thus, it has been presumed that these viruses harbor numerous other noncoding transcripts that have yet to be discovered. However, the transcriptional intricacy of herpesviruses has provided an enormous obstacle for resolution of individual noncoding RNA isoforms. Recently though, the advent of single molecule long read sequencing has provided a catalyst for global resolution of RNAs from many of these genomes. For example, we have recently used the TRIMD pipeline [11] to integrate parallel data sets from Pacific Biosciences SMRT Iso-Seq long read sequencing, Illumina short read RNA-Seq, and 5′ cap analysis of gene expression (deepCAGE) platforms to globally resolve transcript structures from murine gammaherpesvirus 68 (MHV68) [12]. Not surprisingly, 25 putative long noncoding RNAs (lncRNAs) were among the transcripts identified using this approach.

As with metazoan lncRNAs, ascribing a biological role for such newly discovered viral lncRNAs provides a significant challenge [13–15]. In the field, the study of viral lncRNA function typically begins with examination of expression levels at different time points, in varying conditions, or in specific cell types [16–18]. Assessment of lncRNA expression level is most frequently accomplished using qRT-PCR assays using primers purposely designed for a short region thought to span the transcript of interest. However, this method requires the a priori knowledge of every transcript spanning the region of interest—comprehensive information that is not always available using even the most robust long read platforms for discovery. Thus, it is our experience that detailed molecular validation through northern blot should be undertaken for any individual region under study.

Here we provide a specific example of this approach using parallel qRT-PCR and northern blot analyses of viral noncoding RNA isoforms discovered through integrated long read sequencing of RNA from MHV68-infected cells [12].These putative noncoding transcripts, which range in size from 1.9 to 5.4 kb (Fig. 1a), lie directly antisense to open reading frames (ORFs) 63 and 64, and utilize multiple 5′ transcription initiation sites as well as alternative splicing. qRT-PCR analysis clearly identified robust expression of at least one of these transcripts (Fig. 1b), generating a single amplicon (Fig. 1c). Although northern blot analysis using probes directed to the same exact region validated the presence of the four transcripts predicted to be most abundant (Fig. 1d), this approach also revealed that a major surprise: the single most abundant RNA in this region is an approximately 10 kb transcript not previously identified through modern transcriptomics methods. Such information is essential not only for qRT-PCR-based assessment of

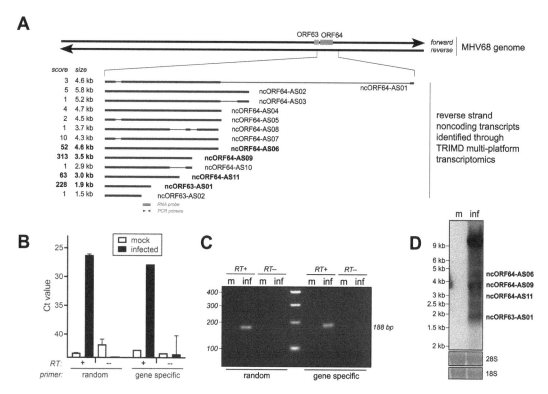

**Fig. 1** Comparison of northern blot and qRT-PCR analyses of noncoding RNA transcripts identified through modern transcriptomics. (**a**) *Noncoding RNA transcripts identified using TRIMD pipeline integration of data from multiple transcriptomics platforms.* A schematic of the MHV68 dsDNA genome is depicted to emphasize the location of ORF63 and ORF64 on the forward strand. TRIMD-identified RNA transcripts which lie antisense to ORF63 and ORF64 indicated, along with TRIMD score and transcript size. qRT-PCR amplicon and RNA probe site is shown in red. (**b**) *qRT-PCR analysis of ORF63/64 antisense transcripts.* qRT-PCR was used to amplify a 188 bp amplicon from the ORF63/64 transcript region. DNase-treated RNA was reverse transcribed using either random hexamers or gene- and strand-specific primer (GGCATTGTCCTCATCACCCAG), and real-time PCR was performed using forward (AAAATTGGGCCTCTTATCTCCTGG) and reverse (GTTTGAATAATTGGCCGT CAGC) primers. *Y*-axis indicates raw $C_t$ value. (**c**) *Agarose gel visualization of qRT-PCR amplicons.* Amplicons generated from (**b**) were visualized on a 3% agarose gel. (**d**) *Northern blot analysis of ORF63/64 antisense transcripts.* Northern blot was performed exactly as indicated in the accompanying protocol. Labels indicate putative noncoding RNA transcripts that match the size of northern blot bands

noncoding RNA expression, but is also directly applicable to the design and validation of viral mutants. Below we provide a detailed molecular protocol for the northern blot validation of viral transcripts.

## 2    Materials

To avoid RNA degradation, prepare all buffers, reagents and materials under sterile conditions. Prepare DEPC-treated water by adding 1 mL Diethyl pyrocarbonate (MP Bio) to 1 L of ultrapure deionized water, incubating at room temperature overnight, and autoclaving. This protocol is designed to detect specific murine gammaherpesvirus 68 (MHV68) transcripts, but can be applied to any other host or virus transcripts.

**2.1  RNA Extraction**

1. TRIzol® Reagent (Thermo Fisher Scientific).
2. Chloroform.
3. Isopropanol.
4. 75% EtOH.
5. GlycoBlue (Invitrogen).
6. DEPC-treated water.

**2.2  Formaldehyde Agarose Gel Electrophoresis**

1. Ultrapure Agarose (Invitrogen).
2. 10× MOPS buffer: Dissolve 41.9 g MOPS, 8.2 g sodium acetate anhydrous (13.6 if it is trihydrate), and 3.7 g EDTA in 1 L water. Adjust pH to 7.0 and wrap in aluminum foil to protect from light. Store at room temperature.
3. Formaldehyde 37%.
4. 20× SSC: Dissolve 175.3 g NaCl and 88.2 g Sodium Citrate in 1 L water, autoclave and store at room temperature.
5. 2× RNA loading buffer: 95% formamide, 0.01% SDS, 0.01% Bromophenol Blue, 0.005% xylene cyanol, 0.5 µM EDTA.
6. Millennium RNA Marker (Ambion). This ladder provides excellent resolution for transcripts from 0.5 kb to 9 kb. To avoid freeze-thawing, divide into 2 µL aliquots and store at −80 °C.

**2.3  Transfer, Blotting, Radiolabeling and Hybridization**

1. Amersham Hybond N+ membrane (GE Healthcare).
2. Whatman Blotting paper GB003 (0.8 mm).
3. Whatman blotting paper 3MM.
4. ULTRAhyb hybridization buffer (Ambion).
5. Methylene blue solution: 0.02% methylene blue, 0.3 M sodium acetate.
6. DNA polymerase (NEB Q5 2× MM).
7. MAXIscript T7 Transcription Kit (Invitrogen).
8. CTP ($\alpha$-$^{32}$P) 800 Ci/mmol 10 mCi/mL EasyTide 250 µCi (PerkinElmer BLU508X250UC). Use fresh reagent if possible, as the half-life of $^{32}$P is 14.3 days. If the reagent is nearing 14 days, double the quantity used for the labeling reaction.
9. Agarose gel running system (Thermofisher Owl B3), power supply.
10. UV Crosslinker.
11. Hybridization oven.
12. Autoradiography cassette, film, and developer.

13. Wash buffer 1: $2\times$ SSC and 0.1% SDS.

14. Wash buffer 2: $1\times$ SSC and 0.1% SDS.

15. Wash buffer 3: $0.1\times$ SSC and 0.1% SDS.

## 3 Methods

To avoid RNA degradation, it is important to clean the pipettes and the work area with RNaseZap. If possible, use separate workspace and equipment for RNA work.

### 3.1 RNA Extraction

1. Infect one 10 cm dish ($2 \times 10^6$ cells per dish) or one well of a 6-well plate ($2 \times 10^5$ per well) of NIH 3T12 cells at multiplicity of infection (MOI) of 5 with MHV68.

2. At 6, 12 or 18 h post-infection, remove media and harvest cells in 1 mL TRIzol. Add TRIzol to the cells and transfer the solution into 1.5 mL Eppendorf tubes. If desired, at this stage TRIzol lysates can be stored at $-20$ °C for a few days or at $-80$ °C for up to a year.

3. Add 0.2 mL chloroform to 1 mL TRIzol lysate. Mix by shaking for 15 s, then place on ice for 5 min. Centrifuge at $16{,}000 \times g$ for 15 min at 4 °C.

4. Transfer the top clear aqueous phase into a new 1.5 mL Eppendorf tube and add 0.5 mL isopropanol. Mix by inversion and then let stand at room temperature for 5–10 min. Centrifuge at $16{,}000 \times g$ for 15 min at 4 °C.

5. Add GlycoBlue for visualization of the pelleted RNA.

6. Wash the RNA pellet with 1 mL of 75% ice cold ethanol and transfer it to 1.5 mL Eppendorf tube. Spin at $16{,}000 \times g$ for 10 min at 4 °C.

7. Remove all of the EtOH by air drying, then resuspend the RNA in 50–100μL of DEPC-treated water. At this stage, purified RNA can be stored at $-80$ °C. For NIH 3T12 fibroblasts, this procedure yields approximately 1μg/μL of RNA in a volume of 50μL.

### 3.2 Formaldehyde Gel Electrophoresis

1. Prepare 1.0% agarose gel with formaldehyde: Microwave 73 mL DEPC-treated water and 1 g Ultrapure agarose. Allow the solution to cool to 55 °C, then add 10 mL of $10\times$ MOPS buffer and 16.2 mL of 37% Formaldehyde. Cast the gel in a fume hood by using the thinner side of a 12 well comb (*see* **Note 1**). Percent agarose can be adjusted from 0.8% to 1.5% depending upon the size of the target transcript; however, 1% agarose generally works well for transcripts that range from 0.5 to 9 kb.

2. Mix the RNA samples with 2× RNA loading buffer. 4–5μg total RNA in ~15–20μL final volume generates sharp, nicely visible bands seen by methylene blue staining. Optionally, EtBr can be added into the loading buffer for RNA visualization under UV. Heat the samples at 70 °C for 5 min then chill on ice.

3. Load each sample into one lane of the gel. If extra wells are available, avoid the wells near the edges and use the middle portion of gel to minimize the risk of aberrant migration of RNA.

4. Run the gel at 70–80 V for 3–4 h in 1× MOPS running buffer containing formaldehyde. The bromophenol blue runs around 0.3 kb (300 nts) and xylene cyanol runs around 4.0 kb. Use this indicator to determine how long to run the gel. For example, stopping the gel run when the bromophenol blue is 2–3 cm from the bottom of the gel should provide good resolution for 1.0 to 5.0 kb transcripts (*see* **Note 2**).

5. At this point, ribosomal bands on the gel can be visualized using a UV box or handheld UV light. To optimize fit to transfer membrane, excess gel can be removed using a razor blade.

*3.3 Transfer to Membrane*

1. Wash the gel four times with deionized water for 10 min each. Then wash with 1× SSC buffer for 15 min.

2. Prepare Hybond N+ membrane slightly larger than the size of the gel. Soak in 1× SSC for 2–3 min.

3. Set up the transfer system as shown in Fig. 2: First place 20 layers of dry GB003 Whatman paper, then 1 layer of dry 3MM Whatman paper. Soak one additional layer of 3MM Whatman paper in 1x SSC and then place on top. Next place the soaked Hybond N+ membrane, then place the gel onto the membrane. Remove any air bubbles by carefully rolling over the gel with a sterile pipette. Place two layers of soaked 3MM Whatman paper on top. Finally, place (as shown in the Fig. 2) the soaked final layer of 3MM Whatman paper with larger dimensions to serve as the wick for transfer buffer. 20× SSC will flow through this layer to the dry paper, enabling the transfer of the RNA to the membrane. Cover the transfer system with a lid to protect the transfer buffer from evaporation (do not place additional weight). Transfer without disturbance overnight (*see* **Note 3**).

4. The next morning, disassemble the transfer system. If the transfer worked, 20× SSC will be soaked to the lower layers of Whatman paper and the gel should be almost dry. Carefully remove the membrane, keeping track of which side was adjacent to the gel. Place in a glass container that has been cleaned

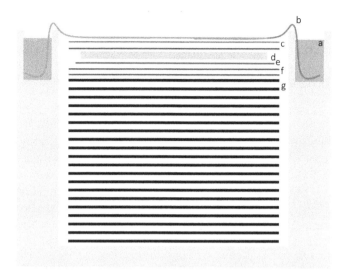

a.  20X SSC

b.  1 layer 20X14 cm 3MM Whatman paper

c.  2 layers 11x14cm 3MM Whatman paper

d.  Gel

e.  Membrane

f.  2 layers 11x14cm 3MM Whatman paper

g.  20 layers 11x14cm GB003 Whatman paper

**Fig. 2** Setup of northern blot downward capillary transfer

with RNaseZap. Use a pencil to carefully mark the side of the membrane to indicate the location of the bromophenol blue (approximately 0.3 kb) and xylene cyanol (approximately 4 kb) bands. Gently soak the membrane in DEPC-treated water to remove running buffer salts.

5. Crosslink the RNA to the membrane using UV light at $1200\mu J/m^2$. Repeat crosslink. Soak the membrane for 5 min in methylene blue solution. Wash the membrane twice with deionized water. At this stage, 18S rRNA (approximately 1.9 kb) and 28S rRNA (approximately 5.0 kb) and the RNA ladder will become visible. Carefully mark the side of the membrane with the positions of the marker and ribosomal bands with a pencil to ensure correct membrane orientation moving forward (*see* **Note 4**).

*3.4 Preparation of the Radiolabeled RNA Probe and Hybridization*

1. Prepare the labeled probe by in vitro transcription by PCR amplifying the target region using primer containing T7 promoter sequence upstream of 5′ primer sequence (if desired, Sp6 promoter sequence can be used upstream of 3′ primer sequence to generate complementary strand probe for strand-specific control. The PCR product can be stored in −20 °C in aliquots for a few weeks. For the best results, the in vitro transcribed RNA probe should be used fresh each time (*see* **Note 5**).

    (a) Prepare the PCR reaction by mixing 1μL of 10μM Forward primer with T7 promoter sequence at the 5′ (TAA TACGACTCACTATA G̲GG...), 1μL of 10μM Reverse primer, 1μL of the DNA template, 22μL of nuclease-free water, and 25μL of Q5 DNA polymerase 2× Mastermix.

    (b) PCR amplify using the following cycling conditions: (1) 98 °C for 2 min (initial denaturation); (2) 98 °C for

15 s (denaturation); (3) 55 °C for 15 s (primer annealing temperature may be optimized for each primer set. However, the T7/Sp6 promoter sequences should not be included while calculating the $T_m$); (4) 72 °C for 60 s/ kb (extension), Repeat **steps 2–4** 30 cycles; and 72 °C for 2 min (final extension).

(c) Run on agarose gel and purify amplicon using gel purification kit.

(d) Prepare in vitro transcription reaction by mixing Gel purified PCR amplicon (at least 300 ng), 1µL from each of ATP, GTP, UTP from the MAXIscript Transcription Kit, 1µL of T7 or SP6 Enzyme mix (depending on the promoter used), 2µL of 10× in vitro transcription buffer, Add up to 19µL with nuclease free water and 1µL of $\alpha$-$^{32}$P CTP.

(e) Incubate at 37 °C for 2–4 h (1 h is generally enough but if the target region is small, increasing the incubation time and enzyme will yield higher activity probe).

(f) Add 1µL of DNase to the reaction, then incubate 20 min at 37 °C.

(g) Add 1µL of 0.5 M EDTA to stop DNase reaction and incubate at 95 °C for 5 min.

2. Prewarm the ULTRAhyb buffer at 60 °C for at least 30 min prior to use. Place the UV cross-linked membrane in the hybridization tube with the side that was adjacent to the gel facing inward. Add 5 mL of the prewarmed hybridization buffer to the tube. Prehybridize the membrane for at least 1 h; this can be accomplished while preparing the radiolabeled probe.

3. Add all of the probe to the hybridization bottle. When using the ULTRAhyb buffer, it is not necessary to change the buffer after prehybridization or remove unincorporated radionucleotides from the in vitro transcription reaction (*see* **Note 6**).

4. Rotate overnight at 60 °C in the hybridization oven. This temperature may be optimized for best results based on the length and GC content etc. of the probe being used (*see* **Note 7**).

5. Wash the membrane with wash buffer 1 for 20 min at 72 °C. Repeat with wash buffer 2, then repeat with wash buffer 3. All of the washes should be disposed in radioactive liquid waste containers (*see* **Note 8**).

6. Drip excess liquid from the membrane and then wrap with Saran Wrap and seal the sides. In a darkroom, place the membrane into an exposure cassette, followed by autoradiography film and intensifying screen. Expose at −80 °C. Depending on the abundance of the RNA, exposure time will need to be

optimized from a few hours to several days. Overnight exposure is a good starting point for many RNAs, but with experience initial exposure times can be adjusted by assessing membrane radioactivity using a Geiger counter.

7. Develop the film in the dark room.

8. In our experience, stripping northern membranes is extremely difficult and generates a large amount of radioactive liquid waste. If a membrane must be reused for control probes, it is advised to begin with probes to expected low abundance targets, followed subsequent use of probes for expected higher abundance transcripts.

## 4    Notes

1. To improve band sharpness, it is best to try to keep the loaded RNA volume to smaller quantities and use thinner combs and spacers when preparing the gel, as the RNA will transfer to the membrane more efficiently when using thinner gels. The addition of formaldehyde and MOPS buffer will cool the gel solution very quickly; therefore, to avoid uneven gel formation it is advisable to pour the gel immediately after adding these reagents.

2. Running the agarose gel for 2 h or longer heats up the buffer and causing the gel to soften. Placing ice packs around the gel tank to keep the buffer chilled will help prevent subsequent gel breaks during wash steps.

3. The Whatman TurboBlotter downward transfer system provides a highly reproducible and efficient system for transfers without the use of additional weights or paper towels. Care should be taken to carefully remove air bubbles at this step as they will interfere with RNA transfer. Unused portions and the wells of the gel can be excised during transfer set up.

4. The 28S rRNA band should be twice the amount of the 18S rRNA band. This can be used to assess the integrity and the quality of both RNA extraction and the transfer. To keep track of which side of the membrane is adjacent to the gel, carefully mark the side of the membrane with pencil when disassembling the transfer apparatus. If the membrane will not be probed immediately after transfer, then it can be wrapped in Saran Wrap or sealed in plastic and stored at −80 °C for several months.

5. One easy method to generate template for in vitro transcription reactions is to add promoter sequences upstream of 5′ PCR primers. We typically use T7 promoter sequence [ TAATAC GACTCACTATA<u>G</u>GG] upstream of the forward primer and

Sp6 promoter sequence [ ATTTAGGTGACACTATA **GAA**] upstream of the reverse primer (the bold underlined nucleotide is the first nucleotide incorporated into the radiolabeled RNA), allowing the complementary strand transcript to be probed using a reverse complement of the same PCR amplicon. If the complementary strand will be probed, use Sp6 Enzyme mix instead of T7 Enzyme mix in the labeling reaction. MAXIscript Sp6/T7 Transcription Kit form Invitrogen should be ordered instead of MAXIscript T7 Transcription Kit. It is important to check the template PCR reaction on an agarose gel for quality; if any other bands are observed, a gel extraction kit must be used to excise the correct amplicon. Our experience is that a 300 nt nucleotide target region provides a reliably size for specific target identification with low background. If the PCR product is stored for long periods, the ends of the DNA amplicon, that contains short promoter sequences for T7 and Sp6, may become compromised. This may result in ineffective transcription initiation. Therefore, it is best to use fresh or only a few weeks old DNA amplicons that are stored in −20 °C. Plasmid may be used as a template for in vitro transcription; however, in this case it is important that the plasmid is linearized prior to transcription. Although the method described here utilizes random incorporation of radiolabel of large probes to identify lower abundance transcripts, the use of end labeling reaction with T4 PNK is an excellent alternative to generate similar or shorter probes for identification of highly abundant transcripts.

6. In our experience, when using ULTRAhyb hybridization buffer, column-based removal of unincorporated nucleotides after in vitro transcription is not necessary as the presence of free nucleotides does alter blot quality or probe hybridization. However, if the probe will be stored for one or two days, it is best to remove unincorporated nucleotides since they may cause radioactive decay in the RNA backbone.

7. In some cases, the 18S and/or 28S rRNA may become visible on the final film due to nonspecific binding of the probe. To improve nonspecific background binding, we advise increasing the hybridization temperature, decreasing the hybridization time from overnight to 4–6 h, and decreasing the quantity of probe used. The hybridization temperature is a key factor and should be carefully optimized for each new probe.

8. Lowering salt content with the later washes helps with background by reducing nonspecific binding, with the lowest salt concentration on the final wash enriching specific RNA–RNA interactions.

## Acknowledgments

S.A.T. was supported by NIH R01AI108407 and NIH P01CA214091. We thank Dr. Erik Flemington and Dr. Rolf Renne and members of the Renne and Flemington labs for helpful discussions and suggestions.

## References

1. Consortium TEP (2012) An integrated encyclopedia of DNA elements in the human genome. Nature 489:57–74

2. Derrien T, Johnson R, Bussotti G et al (2012) The GENCODE v7 catalog of human long noncoding RNAs: analysis of their gene structure, evolution, and expression. Genome Res 22:1775–1789

3. Hangauer MJ, Vaughn IW, McManus MT (2013) Pervasive transcription of the human genome produces thousands of previously unidentified long intergenic noncoding RNAs. PLoS Genet 9:e1003569

4. Djebali S, Davis CA, Merkel A et al (2012) Landscape of transcription in human cells. Nature 489:101–108

5. Arvin A, Campadelli-Fiume G, Mocarski E, Moore PS, Roizman B, Whitley R, Yamanishi K (2007) Human herpesviruses: biology, therapy, and Immunoprophylaxis. Cambridge University Press, Cambridge

6. Tombácz D, Csabai Z, Szűcs A, Balázs Z, Moldován N, Sharon D, Snyder M, Boldogkői Z (2017) Long-read isoform sequencing reveals a hidden complexity of the transcriptional landscape of herpes simplex virus type 1. Front Microbiol 8:1079

7. Chandriani S, Xu Y, Ganem D (2010) The lytic transcriptome of Kaposi's sarcoma-associated herpesvirus reveals extensive transcription of noncoding regions, including regions antisense to important genes. J Virol 84:7934–7942

8. Arias C, Weisburd B, Stern-Ginossar N, Mercier A, Madrid AS, Bellare P, Holdorf M, Weissman JS, Ganem D (2014) KSHV 2.0: a comprehensive annotation of the Kaposi's sarcoma-associated herpesvirus genome using next-generation sequencing reveals novel genomic and functional features. PLoS Pathog 10:e1003847

9. Kara M, O'Grady T, Feldman ER, Feswick A, Wang Y, Flemington EK, Tibbetts SA (2019) Gammaherpesvirus Readthrough transcription generates a long non-coding RNA that is regulated by antisense miRNAs and correlates with enhanced lytic replication in vivo. Noncoding RNA 5:6

10. Tycowski KT, Guo YE, Lee N, Moss WN, Vallery TK, Xie M, Steitz JA (2015) Viral noncoding RNAs: more surprises. Genes Dev 29:567–584

11. O'Grady T, Wang X, Höner Zu Bentrup K, Baddoo M, Concha M, Flemington EK (2016) Global transcript structure resolution of high gene density genomes through multi-platform data integration. Nucleic Acids Res 44(18):e145. https://doi.org/10.1093/nar/gkw629

12. O'Grady T, Feswick A, Hoffman BA, Wang Y, Medina EM, Kara M, van Dyk LF, Flemington EK, Tibbetts SA (2019) Genome-wide transcript structure resolution reveals abundant alternate isoform usage from murine Gammaherpesvirus 68. Cell Rep 27:3988–4002.e5

13. Quinn JJ, Chang HY (2016) Unique features of long non-coding RNA biogenesis and function. Nat Rev Genet 17:47–62

14. Liu W, Ding C (2017) Roles of LncRNAs in viral infections. Front Cell Infect Microbiol 7:205

15. Wang Z, Zhao Y, Zhang Y (2017) Viral lncRNA: a regulatory molecule for controlling virus life cycle. Noncoding RNA Res 2:38–44

16. Elfman J, Li H (2020) Detection and measurement of chimeric RNAs by RT-PCR. In: Li H, Elfman J (eds) Chimeric RNA methods Protoc. Springer US, New York, NY, pp 83–94

17. Shi X, Qin F, Li H (2020) Confirmation of transcriptional read-through events by RT-PCR. Methods Mol Biol 2079:177–186

18. Su W-C, Lai MMC (2018) Quantitative RT-PCR analysis of influenza virus endocytic escape. Methods Mol Biol 1836:185–194

# Part V

## LncRNA Analysis in Liquid Biopsy

# Chapter 18

# Phospho-RNAseq Profiling of Extracellular mRNAs and lncRNAs

## Maria D. Giraldez and Muneesh Tewari

### Abstract

Extracellular RNAs (exRNAs) in biofluids have attracted great interest as potential biomarkers. Although extracellular microRNAs in blood plasma are extensively characterized, extracellular messenger RNA (mRNA) and long noncoding RNA (lncRNA) studies are limited. We have recently reported that human plasma contains fragmented mRNAs and lncRNAs that are missed by standard small RNA-seq protocols due to lack of 5′phosphate or presence of 3′phosphate. Here, we describe a modified protocol for preparation of small RNA libraries for next generation sequencing called "phospho-RNA-seq." This protocol has been optimized for use with low-input exRNA-containing samples, such as plasma or serum, and has modifications introduced to capture extracellular RNA with varied 5′and 3′ends.

**Key words** Extracellular RNA, Liquid biopsy, RNA-seq, lncRNAs, mRNAs

## 1 Introduction

The identification of a variety of extracellular RNA (exRNA) molecules present in the human bloodstream and other biofluids has opened up new avenues for the development of minimally invasive biomarkers for a wide range of diseases [1–4] Characterization of exRNAs in blood has mostly focused on microRNAs because they have been shown to be highly stable in human biofluids as a result of being protected in complexes with Argonaute proteins and extracellular vesicles [5, 6]. However, miRNAs only represent a small fraction of the transcriptome and there are more predominant components, notably mRNAs and lncRNAs, which are still poorly characterized in plasma. Importantly, mRNAs and lncRNAs are highly appealing from the standpoint of biomarkers for monitoring health and disease due to their tissue and disease specificity [7–12]. RNA-seq has transformed transcriptome characterization in a wide range of biological contexts [13, 14] including its application to analyze exRNA in body fluids [15, 16]. Thanks to recent initiatives aimed to characterize human exRNA, we are beginning to

Alfons Navarro (ed.), *Long Non-Coding RNAs in Cancer*, Methods in Molecular Biology, vol. 2348,
https://doi.org/10.1007/978-1-0716-1581-2_18, © Springer Science+Business Media, LLC, part of Springer Nature 2021

elucidate the complex composition of exRNA in blood [1, 3, 4, 17]. There have been studies reporting the present of extracellular mRNA and lncRNA in plasma, but results have been inconsistent, with some profiling studies reporting a variable percentage of them and others not even reporting their presence [1–4, 17–20]. In this sense, it is worth mentioning, that plasma concentration of RNases is high [21] which could prevent or dramatically reduce existence of full-length form mRNAs and lncRNAs. Moreover, standard ligation-based small RNA-seq methods are not suitable to detect such fragments because they are designed to capture microRNAs [22, 23], which by virtue of being products of RNase III class enzymes (e.g., Dicer) consistently present 5′monophosphate (5′P) and 3′hydroxyl (3′OH) ends [24]. In contrast, the 5′ and 3′ends of RNA cleavage products generated by different ribonucleases vary substantially, thus preventing efficient adapter ligation with standard small RNA-seq methods. For example, abundant RNases in human blood circulation, such as those belonging to the ribonuclease A superfamily [25], degrade RNA dinucleotide bonds, leaving a 5′OH and 3′P product [26]. We have recently reported that in order to sequence a broader space of exRNAs beyond microRNAs, it is essential to develop modifications to small RNA-seq protocols to enable capture of RNA fragments that may have these alternate 5′ and 3′phosphorylation states [23]. To do so, we have modified the standard small RNA-seq approach by incorporating an upfront 5′RNA phosphorylation/3′dephosphorylation step using T4 polynucleotide kinase (referred to subsequently as "PNK") (*see* **Note 1**). This approach, which we called "phospho-RNA-seq" (Fig. 1), revealed a large, untapped space of mRNAs and lncRNA fragments present in human plasma [23].

## 2 Materials

### 2.1 Instruments

1. Thermal cycler with heated lid.
2. Single channel manual pipettes, 2, 20, 200, and 1000 μL.
3. Vacuum manifold QIAvac 24 Plus (Qiagen) or equivalent.
4. Benchtop microcentrifuge.
5. Electrophoresis power supply.
6. XCell SureLock Mini-Cell electrophoresis unit (Life Technologies).
7. Room temperature tube shaker or tube rotator.
8. Dark reader Blue Light Transilluminator (Discovery Scientific Solutions).

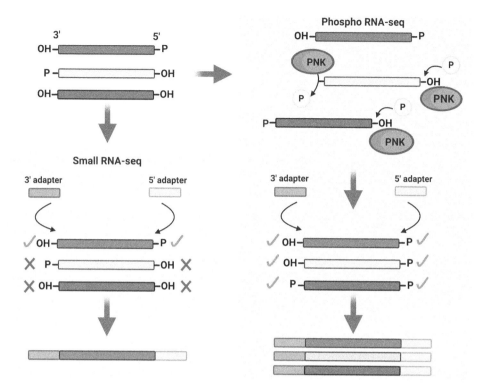

**Fig. 1** Phospho RNA-seq vs. standard small RNA-seq. Standard ligation-based small RNA-seq methods are designed to capture RNA molecules with 5′monophosphate (5′P) and 3′hydroxyl (3′OH) ends. In contrast, Phospho RNA-seq includes an upfront 5′RNA phosphorylation/3′dephosphorylation step using T4 PNK which enable the capture of RNA molecules with varied 5′ and 3′ends

| | |
|---|---|
| **2.2 Reagents for RNA 5′ Phosphorylation and Removal of 3′ Phosphoryl Groups** | 1. T4 Polynucleotide Kinase, T4 PNK, and supplied T4 PNK Ligation buffer (New England BioLabs). |
| | 2. 10 mM adenosine 5′-triphosphate, ATP (New England Bio-Labs). Make small aliquots and store at −20 °C. Aliquots are stable for several freeze-thaw cycles. |
| | 3. 1.7 mL low adhesion microcentrifuge tubes (GeneMate). |
| | 4. 8-strip PCR tubes, 0.2 mL. |
| **2.3 Reagents for RNA Purification** | 1. Isopropanol 100%, molecular biology grade. |
| | 2. 1 M MgCl₂, molecular biology grade. |
| | 3. 1 M CaCl₂, molecular biology grade. |
| | 4. TCEP-HCl. Store at 4 °C. |
| | 5. VacConnectors (Qiagen). |
| | 6. Zymo-Spin I columns (Zymo). |
| | 7. Buffer RWT (Qiagen). |
| | 8. Buffer RPE (Qiagen). |
| | 9. Ethanol, Absolute (200 Proof), molecular biology grade. |

10. 10 mM Tris pH 7.4: Dilute 1 M Tris pH 7.4 1:100 with nuclease-free water. It is recommended to make small aliquots to avoid contamination.

*2.4 Reagents for Library Preparation*

1. TruSeq small RNA library preparation kit (Illumina).
2. T4 RNA ligase 2, truncated KQ and supplied T4 RNA ligase reaction buffer (New England BioLabs).
3. Superscript III reverse transcriptase with supplied 5′ first strand reaction buffer and 100 mM DTT (Invitrogen).
4. DNA Clean and Concentrator 5 columns (Zymo).

*2.5 Reagent for Gel Purification*

1. Novex TBE gels, 6%, 10 well (Life Technologies).
2. Novex TBE running buffer 5× (Invitrogen).
3. 5× Novex TBE sample loading buffer (Invitrogen).
4. Gel breaker tubes (IST Engineering).
5. SYBR Gold (Invitrogen).
6. SpinX columns (Corning).
7. Qiagen EB buffer (Qiagen).

*2.6 Reagents for Library Validation*

1. High sensitivity DNA chip (Agilent).

# 3 Methods

*3.1 Blood Specimen Processing for Plasma and RNA Isolation*

Methods for sample processing and RNA isolation have been described by us elsewhere [27–29]. Briefly, in the latest version of the plasma collection protocol, we collect whole blood samples in K2EDTA tubes and separate the plasma within 2 h using a two-stage centrifugation protocol to ensure that it is free not only of cells but also of significant numbers of contaminating platelets [29]. We discard plasma samples that show visual evidence of hemolysis. Total RNA containing microRNAs is purified from 200 μL of plasma or serum using the miRNeasy kit (Qiagen) with slight modification as previously described [28] although we have also successfully employed an alternative protocol using the miR-Vana PARIS RNA isolation kit (Ambion) [27]. We find that it is not uncommon for the concentration of purified RNA to be too low for quantification using absorption spectrophotometry. We use a fixed volume of RNA eluate rather than a fixed mass of RNA as input into the subsequent reverse transcription reaction.

*3.2 RNA 5′ Phosphorylation and Removal of 3′ Phosphoryl Groups*

All the following steps should be performed on ice, unless otherwise specified. Ensure good laboratory practice for handling RNA (*see* **Note 2**).

**Table 1**
**PNK Master Mix**

|  | 1× |
|---|---|
| RNA | 7 |
| T4 PNK reaction buffer (10×) | 1 |
| ATP (10 mM) | 1 |
| T4 PNK | 1 |
| Total volume | 10 μL |

1. Thaw T4 PNK reaction buffer and 10 mM ATP on ice. Keep T4 PNK enzyme cold on a portable cooler.

2. Vortex T4 PNK reaction buffer and ATP to ensure adequate mixing and spin down briefly. Spin down briefly T4 PNK enzyme.

3. Add the Master Mix components listed in Table 1 to a low-adhesion microcentrifuge tube. Mix well by pipetting up and down several times before adding T4 PNK enzyme. Then mix again by pipetting up and down five times.

4. Add 10 μL of the Master Mix into a 200 μL PCR tube.

5. Incubate at 37 °C for 30 min (*see* **Note 3**).

**3.3 Purification of PNK-Treated Samples**

*3.3.1 Prepare RNA Binding Buffer*

1. Combine the volumes of isopropanol, $MgCl_2$ and $CaCl_2$ solutions shown in Table 2 in a fresh microcentrifuge tube. You can prepare a large volume if planning for several batches of purification. Do not adjust volume.

2. Mix well and store at room temperature.

3. Before use, add 1% 0.5 M TCEP. To prepare TCEP combine 0.72 g TCEP-HCl and 4 mL of nuclease-free water, adjust to 5 mL with nuclease-free water and vortex until you get a homogeneous solution.

*3.3.2 Prepare Vacuum Manifold (See **Note 4**)*

1. Connect a vacuum manifold to your vacuum source (*see* **Note 5**).

2. Place VacConnectors in all the positions of the vacuum manifold that you plan to use (*see* **Note 6**).

3. Insert a Zymo I column on top of each of VacConnector (*see* **Note 7**).

4. Close unused position with caps.

5. Make sure that the vacuum pressure generated is between −700 and −900 mbar using a vacuum regulator connected between the vacuum source and the vacuum manifold (*see* **Note 8**).

**Table 2**
**Composition of RNA binding buffer**

| Isopropanol (100%) | 981 mL |
|---|---|
| 1 M MgCl$_2$ | 6.8 µL |
| 1 M CaCl$_2$ | 2.3 µL |
| 0.5 M TCEP | 9.9 µL |
| Total volume | 1 mL |

*3.3.3  Column Purification Using Vacuum Manifold*

1. Add 0.1 volumes of 0.5 M TCEP-HCl to the total amount of Qiagen wash buffers RWT and RPE that you plan to use (i.e., 900 µL of each per sample) during the purification (optional).

2. Add 2 to 2.5 volumes of binding buffer to each RNA sample and mix well before proceeding with the column purification (*see* **Note 9**).

3. Transfer each sample to a Zymo-Spin I column placed on a vacuum manifold.

4. Switch on the vacuum. Apply vacuum until transfer is complete. Switch off the vacuum and ventilate the vacuum manifold (i.e., close the main vacuum valve and open the screw cap valve to vent the manifold. Close the screw cap valve after the vacuum is released from the manifold) (*see* **Note 10**).

5. Add 900 µL of RWT buffer to each column.

6. Switch on the vacuum. Apply vacuum until transfer is complete. Switch off the vacuum and ventilate the vacuum manifold.

7. Add 900 µL on RPE buffer to each column.

8. Switch on the vacuum. Apply vacuum until transfer is complete. Switch off the vacuum and ventilate the vacuum manifold.

9. Add 900 µL of 200 Proof ethanol.

10. Switch on the vacuum. Apply vacuum until transfer is complete. Switch off the vacuum and ventilate the vacuum manifold.

11. Add 900 µL of 80% ethanol.

12. Switch on the vacuum. Apply vacuum until transfer is complete. Switch off the vacuum and ventilate the vacuum manifold.

13. Transfer columns to 2 mL collection tubes and place them into a microcentrifuge.

14. Spin at full speed at RT for 2 min to dry silica matrix.

15. Transfer columns into prelabeled low-adhesion microcentrifuge tubes.

16. Elute in a small volume of 10 mM Tris pH 7.4. The elution volume can be as small as 6 μL (*see* **Note 11**).

17. Spin at full speed for 1 min at room temperature to elute RNA.

18. Store purified samples at −80 °C until use.

**3.4  Library Preparation (See Note 12)**

*3.4.1  3′ Adapter Ligation*

1. Preheat thermal cycler to 70 °C.

2. Combine the volumes indicated in Table 3 in a PCR tube on ice. The total volume added to the tube should be 6 μL (*see* **Note 13**).

3. Pipet up and down several times to mix, and then centrifuge briefly.

4. Place on preheated thermal cycler.

5. Incubate at 70 °C for 2 min to denature sample.

6. Remove immediately from the thermal cycler after the 2 min incubation and place on ice for at least 2 min.

7. Preheat the thermal cycler to 28 °C.

8. Thaw Illumina ligation buffer (HML) on ice and keep RNase inhibitor and T4 RNA ligase 2, truncated KQ (T4 RNL2 KQ) cold on a portable cooler (*see* **Note 14**).

9. Vortex the ligation buffer to ensure adequate mixing and spin down briefly. Spin down briefly RNase inhibitor and T4 RNL2 KQ.

10. Combine the volumes indicated in Table 4 in a new 200 μL PCR tube on ice:

11. Pipet to mix, and then centrifuge briefly.

12. Add 4 μL to the tube of 3′adapter/PNK treated RNA mixture. The total volume is 10 μL.

13. Place on preheated thermal cycler.

14. Incubate at 28 °C for 1 h (*see* **Note 15**).

15. Add 1 μL stop solution to each of the tubes without removing them from the thermal cycler. Pipet to mix.

16. Continue incubating at 28 °C for 15 min.

17. Remove from the thermal cycler and place on ice.

18. Immediately proceed to 5′ adapter ligation (*see* **Note 16**).

*3.4.2  5′ Adapter Ligation*

1. Preheat the thermal cycler to 70 °C.

2. Thaw 5′ adapter on ice (*see* **Note 17**).

3. Vortex 5′ adapter to ensure adequate mixing and spin down briefly.

**Table 3**
**3' adapter/PNK mixture**

| PNK treated RNA | $x$ µL |
|---|---|
| 3' adapter | 1 µL |
| Nuclease-free water | Up to 6 µL |

**Table 4**
**3' Ligation Master Mix**

| Illumina Ligation Buffer | 2 µL |
|---|---|
| RNase inhibitor | 1 µL |
| T4 RNL2 KQ | 1 µL |
| Total volume | 4 µL |

4. In a separate PCR tube, add $1.1 \times N$ (number of samples being prepared) µL of 5' adapter.

5. Place on the preheated thermal cycler.

6. Incubate at 70 °C for 2 min to denaturate.

7. Remove immediately from the thermal cycler after the 2 min incubation and place on ice for at least 2 min.

8. Thaw 10 mM ATP on ice and keep T4 RNA Ligase cold on a portable cooler.

9. Vortex the 10 mM ATP to ensure adequate mixing and spin down briefly. Spin down briefly T4 RNA Ligase.

10. Add $1.1 \times N$ µL 10 mM ATP to the tube of 5' adapter.

11. Pipet to mix, and then centrifuge briefly.

12. Add $1.1 \times N$ µL T4 RNA Ligase to the mixture.

13. Pipet to mix, and then centrifuge briefly.

14. Add 3 µL of the mixture to each tube of 3' ligated product. The total volume is 14 µL.

15. Pipet to mix.

16. Place on the preheated thermal cycler.

17. Incubate at 28 °C for 1 h.

18. Remove from the thermal cycler and place on ice.

19. Immediately proceed to reverse transcription.

*3.4.3 Reverse Transcription*

1. Preheat the thermal cycler to 70 °C.

2. Thaw on ice Reverse transcription (RT) primer, $5 \times$ First Strand Buffer, dNTP Mix and DTT. Keep RNase inhibitor and

**Table 5**
**Reverse transcription Master Mix**

| | |
|---|---|
| 5× First Strand Buffer | 2 μL |
| 12.5 mM dNTP mix | 0.5 μL |
| 100 mM DTT | 1 μL |
| RNase inhibitor | 1 μL |
| SuperScript III reverse transcriptase | 1 μL |
| Total volume | 5.5 μL |

SuperScript III Reverse Transcriptase T4 RNA cold on a portable cooler.

3. Vortex RT primer to ensure adequate mixing and spin down briefly.

4. Add 6 μL of each adapter-ligated RNA sample to a new 200 μL PCR tube (*see* **Note 18**).

5. Add 1 μL RNA RT Primer to each tube of adapter-ligated RNA sample.

6. Pipet to mix, and then centrifuge briefly.

7. Incubate at 70 °C for 2 min.

8. Remove immediately from the thermal cycler after the 2-min incubation and place on ice for at least 2 min.

9. Preheat the thermal cycler to 50 °C.

10. Vortex 5× First Strand Buffer, dNTP Mix, and DTT to ensure adequate mixing and spin down briefly. Spin down briefly RNase inhibitor and T4 RNL2 KQ.

11. Dilute 1:2 dNTP Mix.

12. Combine the volumes shown in Table 5 in a new 200 μL PCR tube on ice. Multiply each volume by the number of libraries being prepared. Make 10% extra reagent if you are preparing multiple libraries to account for pipetting losses.

13. Pipet to mix, and then centrifuge briefly.

14. Add 5.5 μL to each tube of denatured RNA and RT primer.

15. Pipet to mix, and then centrifuge briefly. The total volume is 12.5 μL.

16. Place on the preheated thermal cycler.

17. Incubate at 55 °C for 1 h.

18. Remove from the thermal cycler and place on ice.

19. Immediately proceed to PCR amplification.

*3.4.4 PCR Amplification*

1. Thaw on ice Illumina PCR Mix (PML), PCR primer (RP1) and the PCR indexes that you plan to use (*see* **Note 19**).

2. Vortex PCR primer to ensure adequate mixing and spin down briefly. Mix PML by pipetting up and down several times and spin down briefly.

3. Prepare in a fresh microcentrifuge tube on ice the master mix shown in Table 6. Multiply each volume by the number of libraries being prepared. Make 10% extra reagent to account for pipetting losses.

4. Add 35.5 μL of the master mix to each library.

5. Vortex PCR indexes to ensure adequate mixing and spin down briefly.

6. Index your libraries by adding 2 μL of a different index to each of them. The total volume is 50 μL.

7. Pipet to mix, and then centrifuge briefly.

8. Place on ice.

9. Incubate using the following program on the thermal cycler (*see* **Note 20**): 98 °C for 30 s; X cycles of (*see* **Note 21**): 98 °C for 10 s, 60 °C for 30 s and 72 °C for 15 s; and finally, 72 °C for 10 min and hold at 4 °C until proceed with next step.

10. Purify PCR product using DNA Clean and Concentrator 5 columns following manufacturer's instructions. Elute in 50 μL (or a smaller amount if desired).

11. Store your libraries at −20 °C for up to 7 days or proceed with the following step.

**3.5 Gel Purification (See Note 22)**

1. Combine 2 μL Custom RNA Ladder (CRL) and 2 μL DNA loading dye in a new 1.5 mL microcentrifuge tube and pipet to mix (*see* **Note 23**).

2. Combine 1 μL High Resolution Ladder (HRL) and 1 μL DNA loading dye in a new 1.5 mL microcentrifuge tube and pipet to mix (*see* **Note 24**).

3. Add 12.5 μL 5× Novex TBE sample loading buffer to PCR product and pipet to mix.

4. Load 2 gel lanes of a 10-well 6% TBE gel with 2 μL CRL/loading dye mixture.

5. Load 1 gel lane with 2 μL HRL–loading dye mixture.

6. Split each library into 3 lanes of the gel (*see* **Note 25**).

7. Run for 80 min at 100 V or until the blue front dye leaves the gel.

8. Warm SYBR Gold to room temperature and then briefly centrifuged in a microfuge to deposit the DMSO solution at the bottom of the vial.

**Table 6**
**PCR Master Mix**

| | |
|---|---|
| Ultrapure water | 8.5 µL |
| PML | 25 µL |
| RP1 | 2 µL |
| Total volume | 35.5 µL |

9. Open the cassette and place the gel in the staining container such as a pipette-tip box.

10. Cover the gel with 50 mL of TBE.

11. Add 5 µL of SYBR Gold to the TBE to stain the gel.

12. Protect the staining solution from light by covering with aluminum foil.

13. Agitate the gel gently at room temperature for 10–15 min.

14. View the gel on a blue-light transilluminator.

15. Cut out desired bands from each library (*see* **Note 26**).

16. Transfer to a gel breaker tube, place into a 2 mL microcentrifuge tube and centrifuge at $16,000 \times g$ for 4–5 min to crush gel slices.

17. Soak gel fragments overnight in 300 µL Qiagen EB buffer at room temperature in a Thermomixer.

18. Spin through SpinX column (Corning 8163) to remove gel fragments and ethanol precipitate DNA.

19. Resuspend in 10–15 µL and run on Bioanalyzer DNA 1000 chip to check library size.

## 4   Notes

1. This chapter focuses on the experimental methodology of Phospho-RNAseq. We have also developed a custom, high-stringency bioinformatic data analysis pipeline to analyze non-microRNA small RNA fragments sequenced with our method. Details about bioinformatics analysis can be found in the original publication and its supplementary materials [23].

2. Working with RNA requires special precautions because of the chemical instability of the RNA and the ubiquitous presence of RNases. Ensure good laboratory practice for handling and storage of RNA to achieve optimal performance of the protocol: (1) always wear disposable gloves, and work in a nuclease-free environment; (2) treat surfaces of benches and glassware with commercially RNase inactivating agents such as

RNaseZap (Life Technologies); (3) reserve a set of pipettes for RNA work. Use sterile RNase-free filter pipette tips to prevent cross-contamination; (4) use nuclease-free, low nucleic acid binding plasticware; (5) always ensure that all reagents and chemicals purchased commercially are guaranteed to be RNase-free; (6) keep tubes capped when possible, always spin tubes before opening; (7) work on ice. It is recommended to hold samples on an aluminum rack to maintain proper temperature and ensure sample integrity; (8) for long-time storage, RNA may be stored at $-80\ °C$; and (9) Avoid repeated freeze–thaw cycles.

3. Do not heat inactive PNK after completing this incubation. PNK will be removed by column purification.

4. Column purification could also be performed using a centrifuge rather than a vacuum manifold, but the latter is likely more convenient, and we optimized our protocol using it.

5. It is advisable to reserve a vacuum manifold for RNA use only in order to avoid potential DNA contamination.

6. The use of VacConnectors is optional but highly recommended as they are helpful to prevent potential cross-contamination. VacConnectors are single use and their price is affordable.

7. You can replace Zymo-Spin I for some other silica-based spin column. We use Zymo-Spin I because they allow eluting in small volume.

8. Using a vacuum regulator is recommended to ensure that the applied vacuum is adequate at all moment. Low pressure can result in RNA losses during the process.

9. Our homemade binding buffer might be replaced with other similar commercial binding buffers or isopropanol alone. Just make sure to mix your samples with an appropriate volume of binding buffer before transferring to the column to avoid RNA losses.

10. Switching off the vacuum and ventilating the vacuum manifold between loading steps is advisable to maintain uniform conditions for each sample.

11. We usually elute in 16–17 µL to have enough volume for preparing triplicate libraries for each sample. You can elute in smaller volume if you do not plan to run replicates.

12. Here we continue the protocol preparing TruSeq small RNA libraries but you could use your PNK treated samples as input for any other ligation based small RNA library preparation protocol.

13. We recommend an input volume of PNK treated RNA of 5 µL.

14. T4 RNL2 KQ contains two mutations, which make it preferable to other truncated T4 RNA ligase 2 variants. The K227Q mutation reduces side products and the R55K mutation increases the rate of ligation compared to the K227Q mutant alone [30, 31].

15. If a thermal cycler with adjustable temperature heated lid is available, disable the heated lid during incubations at 28 °C. If heated lid cannot be disabled, leave the lid open for 28 °C incubations.

16. RNA is labile and easily degradable. Avoid extended pauses in the protocol until the RNA is in the form of double-stranded DNA.

17. 5′ adapter is an RNA oligonucleotide and, therefore, highly susceptible to degradation. Keep it on ice at all times.

18. The remaining ligated RNA may be stored at −80 °C for future use.

19. There are 48 different indexes available for this library preparation kit (RPI1-RPI48).

20. Set lid preheat to 100 °C.

21. Small RNA libraries from biofluids typically require 10–25 total cycles of PCR amplification depending on the type and amount of input RNA. It has been shown that increased amplification does not significantly affect library bias [32, 33]. However, increasing the number of PCR cycles may overamplify the adapter dimer PCR product, causing it to smear in the gel and making it difficult to separate from the desired PCR products.

22. Electrophoretic purification of PCR is necessary due to the large excess of adapters in low-input small RNA libraries. Use of an automated size selection instrument (e.g., PippinPrep, BluePippin, or PippinHT) might reduce variability introduced during gel excision.

23. Illumina custom RNA ladder (CRL) consists of three dsDNA fragments: 145 bp, 160 bp, and 500 bp.

24. Illumina high resolution ladder (HRL) consist of nine dsDNA fragments: 100, 120, 140, 160, 180, 200, 300, 400, and 500 bp.

25. If you run two different libraries in the same gel leave one empty well between them to avoid cross-contamination.

26. Size selection parameters have to be determined by the user based on the size of the desired inserts.

## Acknowledgments

M.D.G. acknowledges support from a Juan Rodes contract (JR18/00026) funded by the Spanish Institute of Health Carlos III from the Ministry of Economy and Competitiveness (cofunded by European Social Fund (ESF)). M. Tewari acknowledges funding support from the United States National Institutes of Health (NIH) Extracellular RNA Communication Common Fund U01 grant HL126499 and from an A. Alfred Taubman Medical Research Institute Grand Challenge Award.

## References

1. Freedman JE, Gerstein M, Mick E, Rozowsky J, Levy D, Kitchen R, Das S, Shah R, Danielson K, Beaulieu L et al (2016) Diverse human extracellular RNAs are widely detected in human plasma. Nat Commun 7:11106

2. Yuan T, Huang X, Woodcock M, Du M, Dittmar R, Wang Y, Tsai S, Kohli M, Boardman L, Patel T et al (2016) Plasma extracellular RNA profiles in healthy and cancer patients. Sci Rep 6:19413

3. Godoy PM, Bhakta NR, Barczak AJ, Cakmak H, Fisher S, MacKenzie TC, Patel T, Price RW, Smith JF, Woodruff PG et al (2018) Large differences in small RNA composition between human biofluids. Cell Rep 25:1346–1358

4. Max KEA, Bertram K, Akat KM, Bogardus KA, Li J, Morozov P, Ben-Dov IZ, Li X, Weiss ZR, Azizian A et al (2018) Human plasma and serum extracellular small RNA reference profiles and their clinical utility. Proc Natl Acad Sci U S A 115:E5334–E5343

5. Hunter MP, Ismail N, Zhang X, Aguda BD, Lee EJ, Yu L, Xiao T, Schafer J, Lee M-LT, Schmittgen TD et al (2008) Detection of microRNA expression in human peripheral blood microvesicles. PLoS One 3:e3694

6. Arroyo JD, Chevillet JR, Kroh EM, Ruf IK, Pritchard CC, Gibson DF, Mitchell PS, Bennett CF, Pogosova-Agadjanyan EL, Stirewalt DL et al (2011) Argonaute2 complexes carry a population of circulating microRNAs independent of vesicles in human plasma. Proc Natl Acad Sci U S A 108:5003–5008

7. Perou CM, Sørlie T, Eisen MB, van de Rijn M, Jeffrey SS, Rees CA, Pollack JR, Ross DT, Johnsen H, Akslen LA et al (2000) Molecular portraits of human breast tumours. Nature 406:747–752

8. Potti A, Mukherjee S, Petersen R, Dressman HK, Bild A, Koontz J, Kratzke R, Watson MA, Kelley M, Ginsburg GS et al (2006) A genomic strategy to refine prognosis in early-stage non-small-cell lung cancer. N Engl J Med 355:570–580

9. Chen H-Y, Yu S-L, Chen C-H, Chang G-C, Chen C-Y, Yuan A, Cheng C-L, Wang C-H, Terng H-J, Kao S-F et al (2007) A five-gene signature and clinical outcome in non-small-cell lung cancer. N Engl J Med 356:11–20

10. Ben-Porath I, Thomson MW, Carey VJ, Ge R, Bell GW, Regev A, Weinberg RA (2008) An embryonic stem cell-like gene expression signature in poorly differentiated aggressive human tumors. Nat Genet 40:499–507

11. Liu X, Yu X, Zack DJ, Zhu H, Qian J (2008) TiGER: a database for tissue specific gene expression and regulation. BMC Bioinformatics 9:271

12. Iyer MK, Niknafs YS, Malik R, Singhal U, Sahu A, Hosono Y, Barrette TR, Prensner JR, Evans JR, Zhao S et al (2015) The landscape of long noncoding RNAs in the human transcriptome. Nat Genet 47:199–208

13. Mortazavi A, Williams BA, McCue K, Schaeffer L, Wold B (2008) Mapping and quantifying mammalian transcriptomes by RNA-Seq. Nat Methods 5:621–628

14. Wang Z, Gerstein M, Snyder M (2009) RNA-Seq: a revolutionary tool for transcriptomics. Nat Rev Genet 10:57–63

15. Adiconis X, Borges-Rivera D, Satija R, DeLuca DS, Busby MA, Berlin AM, Sivachenko A, Thompson DA, Wysoker A, Fennell T et al (2013) Comparative analysis of RNA sequencing methods for degraded or low input samples. Nat Methods 10:623–629

16. Giraldez MD, Spengler RM, Etheridge A, Godoy PM, Barczak AJ, Srinivasan S, De Hoff PL, Tanriverdi K, Courtright A, Lu S et al (2018) Comprehensive multi-center assessment of small RNA-seq methods for

quantitative miRNA profiling. Nat Biotechnol 36:746–757

17. Yeri A, Courtright A, Reiman R, Carlson E, Beecroft T, Janss A, Siniard A, Richholt R, Balak C, Rozowsky J et al (2017) Total extracellular small RNA profiles from plasma, saliva, and urine of healthy subjects. Sci Rep 7:44061

18. Huang X, Yuan T, Tschannen M, Sun Z, Jacob H, Du M, Liang M, Dittmar RL, Liu Y, Liang M et al (2013) Characterization of human plasma-derived exosomal RNAs by deep sequencing. BMC Genomics 14:319

19. Koh W, Pan W, Gawad C, Fan HC, Kerchner GA, Wyss-Coray T, Blumenfeld YJ, El-Sayed YY, Quake SR (2014) Noninvasive in vivo monitoring of tissue specific global gene expression in humans. Proc Natl Acad Sci U S A 111:7361–7366

20. Danielson KM, Rubio R, Abderazzaq F, Das S, Wang YE (2017) High throughput sequencing of extracellular RNA from human plasma. PLoS One 12:e0164644

21. Kamm RC, Smith AG (1972) Ribonuclease activity in human plasma. Clin Biochem 5:198–200

22. Hafner M, Landgraf P, Ludwig J, Rice A, Ojo T, Lin C, Holoch D, Lim C, Tuschl T (2008) Identification of microRNAs and other small regulatory RNAs using cDNA library sequencing. Methods 44:3–12

23. Giraldez MD, Spengler RM, Etheridge A, Goicochea AJ, Tuck M, Choi SW, Galas DJ, Tewari M (2019) Phospho-RNA-seq: a modified small RNA-seq method that reveals circulating mRNA and lncRNA fragments as potential biomarkers in human plasma. EMBO J 38(11): e101695

24. Lee Y, Ahn C, Han J, Choi H, Kim J, Yim J, Lee J, Provost P, Rådmark O, Kim S et al (2003) The nuclear RNase III Drosha initiates microRNA processing. Nature 425:415–419

25. Lu L, Li J, Moussaoui M, Boix E (2018) Immune modulation by human secreted RNases at the extracellular space. Front Immunol 9:1012

26. Cuchillo CM, Nogués MV, Raines RT (2011) Bovine pancreatic Ribonuclease: fifty years of the first enzymatic reaction mechanism. Biochemistry 50:7835–7841

27. Mitchell PS, Parkin RK, Kroh EM, Fritz BR, Wyman SK, Pogosova-Agadjanyan EL, Peterson A, Noteboom J, O'Briant KC, Allen A et al (2008) Circulating microRNAs as stable blood-based markers for cancer detection. Proc Natl Acad Sci U S A 105:10513–10518

28. Kroh EM, Parkin RK, Mitchell PS, Tewari M (2010) Analysis of circulating microRNA biomarkers in plasma and serum using quantitative reverse transcription-PCR (qRT-PCR). Methods 50(4):298–301

29. Cheng HH, Yi HS, Kim Y, Kroh EM, Chien JW, Eaton KD, Goodman MT, Tait JF, Tewari M, Pritchard CC (2013) Plasma processing conditions substantially influence circulating microRNA biomarker levels. PLoS One 8: e64795

30. Viollet S, Fuchs RT, Munafo DB, Zhuang F, Robb GB (2011) T4 RNA ligase 2 truncated active site mutants: improved tools for RNA analysis. BMC Biotechnol 11:72

31. Song Y, Liu KJ, Wang TH (2014) Elimination of ligation dependent artifacts in T4 RNA ligase to achieve high efficiency and low bias microRNA capture. PLoS One 9(4):e94619

32. Jayaprakash AD, Jabado O, Brown BD, Sachidanandam R (2011) Identification and remediation of biases in the activity of RNA ligases in small-RNA deep sequencing. Nucleic Acids Res 39(21):e141

33. Hafner M, Renwick N, Brown M, Mihailovic A, Holoch D, Lin C, Pena JT, Nusbaum JD, Morozov P, Ludwig J, Ojo T, Luo S, Schroth G, Tuschl T (2011) RNA-ligase-dependent biases in miRNA representation in deep sequenced small RNA cDNA libraries. RNA 7(9):1697–1712

# Chapter 19

# Detection of Circulating RNA Using Nanopore Sequencing

## Jennifer Lindemann, Irene K. Yan, and Tushar Patel

## Abstract

RNA sequencing using nanopore sequencing is a powerful method for transcriptome analysis. The approach is appropriate for comprehensive profiling of the wide range of long noncoding RNAs. Use of nanopore-based sequencing can provide information on novel transcripts, sequence polymorphisms, and splicing variants, and thus has advantages over other gene expression profiling methods such as microarrays. Circulating extracellular long noncoding RNAs are of particular interest because of their potential use as biomarkers. Here, we describe a protocol for cDNA-PCR sequencing of circulating RNA for biomarker discovery in whole blood samples using commercially available kits and nanopore sequencing.

**Keywords** Long noncoding RNA, RNA sequencing, Biofluids, Biomarker discovery, Nanopore sequencing

## 1 Introduction

Sequencing of long noncoding and other RNA is feasible using Nanopore sequencing technologies. Nanopore sequencing enables the detection, quantification, and complete full-length characterization of native RNA or cDNA [1, 2]. This technology is based on the application of a nanoscale pore with a voltage bias that is used to measure the passage of a single-stranded RNA or DNA molecule as it passes through a pore [3]. Translocation through the pore occurs enzymatically one nucleotide at a time. As the molecule passes through the pore, there is a disruption in the ionic current that is specific to the nucleotide occupying the pore at the time. These can be detected by a sensor, and thus can be used to perform base calling in real time (a schematic overview of the technique is shown in Fig. 1). In one commercial application, a single RNA or DNA strand is drawn by an electric potential through parallel 512 protein nanopores that are embedded in a polymer rich membrane surrounded by an electrophysiological solution. This allows for massively parallel sequencing for long reads that are limited only by the length of input nucleotide [4].

Alfons Navarro (ed.), *Long Non-Coding RNAs in Cancer*, Methods in Molecular Biology, vol. 2348,
https://doi.org/10.1007/978-1-0716-1581-2_19, © Springer Science+Business Media, LLC, part of Springer Nature 2021

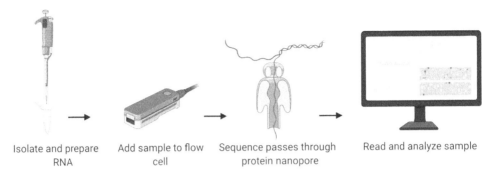

Isolate and prepare RNA    Add sample to flow cell    Sequence passes through protein nanopore    Read and analyze sample

**Fig. 1** Schematic overview of RNA nanopore sequencing. RNA is isolated from samples of interest. Library preparation is performed, and involves ligation of samples with an adaptor. The sample preparations are added to a flow cell in which a single stranded RNA molecule passes through a protein nanopore. Base calling and sequence determination occur in real time

Using just low sample input, a highly informative gene sequence profile can be determined. Short-read next-generation RNA sequencing is limited by the steps of fragmentation of the messenger RNA molecules followed by computational reassembly of the sequences detected. Unlike traditional second-generation transcript analysis technologies, nanopore sequencing offers real-time analysis and a quicker turnaround as amplification is not required. Nanopore-based RNA sequencing provides the potential ability to discover and quantitate isoforms or fusion transcripts, and to directly sequence full-length transcripts without fragmentation or significant sequence bias [5]. The methods can be modified to enable detection of epigenetically derived base modifications in high yields. The use of massively parallel nanopore sequencing of single strands will further allow for comprehensive sequencing of long reads of RNA. Furthermore, the presence of transcription start sites, splice sites, poly(A)-sites and posttranscriptional events or DNA/RNA modifications can be determined, as these are detected simultaneously as the nucleotides pass through the pore [6, 7].

Herein, we describe a detailed method for the use of nanopore sequencing for the identification of circulating RNA from blood. This method utilizes a cDNA-PCR based sequencing method to demonstrate the utility of transcriptomic sequencing technology for biomarker discovery studies, but can be readily used for other applications to perform sequencing of long noncoding or other RNA.

## 2    Materials

Prepare all solutions using nuclease-free water and prepare all buffer concentrates with appropriate volumes of (96–100%) ethanol at room temperature before starting. Store reagents at room temperature unless otherwise noted by the manufacturers. Make sure all pipettes and equipment have been maintained, calibrated, and cleaned before use. Make sure all methods are performed in an RNase-free environment. Follow all waste disposal regulations and wear proper safety equipment.

**2.1  RNA Extraction**

1. PAXgene Blood RNA Tubes (PreAnalytix) (*see* **Note 1**).
2. Paxgene Blood RNA Kit (PreAnalytix) (*see* **Note 2**).
3. RNase-free DNase I.
4. RDD Buffer.
5. RNase-free water. Store at −20 °C.
6. Ethanol (96–100%, purity grade).
7. Isopropanol (100%, purity grade).
8. Pipettors (1 µl – 4 ml) and RNase-free pipette tips.
9. Sterile, aerosol-barrier.
10. Vortex mixer.
11. Test tube rack and microcentrifuge tube rack.
12. Permanent marking pen.
13. Small lab bench ice bucket with crushed ice.
14. Microcentrifuge capable of 1000–8000 × $g$ and equipped with swing out rotor and round bottom tube adaptors.
15. Shaker-incubator to reach incubation temperatures of 55–65 °C and shaking at 400 rpm but not above 1400 rpm (3 × $g$).
16. NanoDrop.

**2.2  RNA Poly-A Tailing**

1. RNA sample(s): purified prior to use and suspended in nuclease-free water (*see* **Note 3**).
2. *E. coli* Poly(A) Polymerase: 1 µl needed per 1–10 µg of RNA in 15 µl nuclease-free water sample.
3. 10× *E. coli* Poly(A) Polymerase Reaction Buffer: 2 µl needed per 1–10 µg of RNA in 15 µl nuclease-free water sample.
4. ATP (10 mM): 2 µl needed per 1–10 µg of RNA in 15 µl nuclease-free water sample.
5. Pipettes: 2–20 µl and RNase-free pipette tips.
6. Small lab bench ice bucket with crushed ice.
7. Permanent marking pen.
8. Incubator capable of reaching incubation temperature of 37 °C.

| | |
|---|---|
| ***2.3 RNA Clean and Concentrator*** | 1. Clean and Concentrator Kit-5 (Zymo) (*see* **Note 4**). |
| | 2. Centrifuge capable of speeds between 10,000 and 16,000 × *g*. |
| | 3. Pipettes: 1 μl – 1 ml and RNase-free pipette tips. |
| | 4. 1.5 ml microcentrifuge tubes. |
| | 5. Permanent marking pen. |
| | 6. NanoDrop. |

| | |
|---|---|
| ***2.4 cDNA-PCR Sequencing*** | 1. cDNA-PCR Sequencing Kit (Oxford Nanopore Technologies). |
| | 2. 10 mM dNTP Solution (New England Biolabs). |
| | 3. Maxima H Minus Reverse Transcriptase (ThermoFisher). |
| | 4. RNaseOUT (Life Technologies). |
| | 5. Exonuclease 1 (New England Biolabs). |
| | 6. LongAmp Taq 2× Master Mix (New England Biolabs). |
| | 7. Agencourt AMPure XP Beads (Beckman Coulter). |
| | 8. Magnetic Separator, suitable for 1.5 ml microtubes. |
| | 9. Gentle rotator mixer. |
| | 10. Flow Cell Priming Kit (Oxford Nanopore Technologies). |
| | 11. MinION SpotON flow cell (Oxford Nanopore Technologies). |
| | 12. Thermal cycler. |

## 3    Methods

Prepare all reactions using nuclease-free water and filtered pipette tips in an RNase-free workstation. Prepare all Buffer concentrates with appropriate volumes of 100% ethanol as instructed by the manufacturer. All procedures can be performed at room temperature except during incubations or unless noted otherwise.

***3.1 RNA Extraction from PAXgene Blood RNA Tubes***

Important: Before proceeding, confirm blood sample has been incubated at least 2 h at room temperature (15–25 °C) in PAXgene Blood RNA Tubes for total lysis of blood cells. An overall schematic is presented in Fig. 2.

1. Prepare kit reagents as instructed. Thaw PAXgene Blood RNA Tube samples to room temperature for 2 h if frozen.

2. Using a swing-out rotor with tube adaptors, centrifuge PAXgene Blood RNA tubes for 10 min at 3000–5000 × *g* (*see* **Note 5**).

3. Decant or pipet supernatant carefully not to disturb pellet. Wipe away any residual supernatant on end of tube and add

Thaw Blood for 2 hours

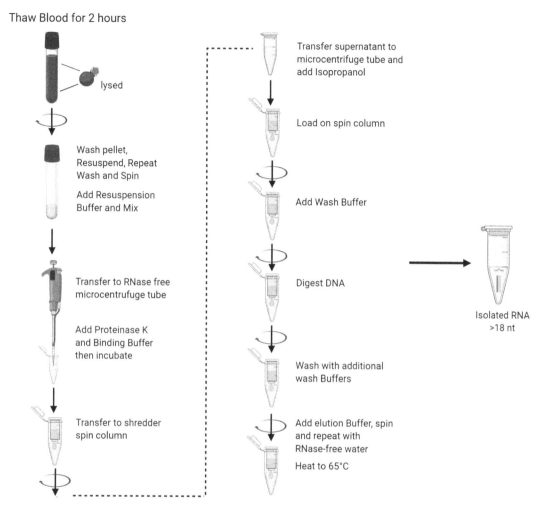

lysed

Wash pellet,
Resuspend, Repeat
Wash and Spin

Add Resuspension
Buffer and Mix

Transfer to RNase free
microcentrufuge tube

Add Proteinase K
and Binding Buffer
then incubate

Transfer to shredder
spin column

Transfer supernatant to
microcentrifuge tube and
add Isopropanol

Load on spin column

Add Wash Buffer

Digest DNA

Wash with additional
wash Buffers

Add elution Buffer, spin
and repeat with
RNase-free water

Heat to 65°C

Isolated RNA
>18 nt

**Fig. 2** Isolation of RNA from whole blood samples using PAXgene RNA collection tubes and RNA isolation kit

4 ml RNase-free water to the pellet. Discard original closure
and use a fresh Hemoguard closure.

4. Vortex until the pellet is dissolved. Using a swing-out rotor,
   centrifuge PAXgene Blood RNA Tubes for 10 min at
   $3000\text{--}5000 \times g$. Decant or pipet entire supernatant and discard appropriately (*see* **Note 6**).

5. Add 350 μl of Buffer BM1, and vortex until pellet is fully
   dissolved.

6. Perform a short spin of samples to eliminate any residual sample on cap.

7. Pipet sample into 1.5 microcentrifuge tube. To the tube, add
   300 μl of Buffer BM2, and 40 μl proteinase K. Vortex for 5 s
   and incubate tube in a shaker-incubator at 400 rpm for 10 min
   at 65 °C (*see* **Note 7**).

8. Pipet 700 μl of sample into a PAXgene Shredder spin column placed in a 2 ml processing tube and centrifuge at $14,000 \times g$ at room temperature for 3 mins.

9. Transfer entire supernatant from flow through to a new 1.5 ml RNase-free microcentrifuge tube without disturbing the pellet.

10. Add 700 μl of 100% purity grade isopropanol, vortex, and spin down.

11. Pipet 700 μl of sample into PAXgene RNA spin column placed in a 2 ml processing tube. Close lid gently and centrifuge at $14,000 \times g$ at room temperature for 1 min. Place the spin column into a new processing tube and discard old processing tube.

12. Pipet the remaining sample into PAXgene RNA spin column placed in the new 2 ml processing tube. Place the spin column into a new processing tube and discard old processing tube.

13. Add 300 μl of manufacturer's Buffer, BM3, to PAXgene RNA spin column. Close lid gently and centrifuge at $14,000 \times g$ at room temperature for 30 s. Place the spin column into a new processing tube and discard old processing tube.

14. Add 10 μl DNase I stock solution to 70 μl of Buffer RDD in a 1.5 ml microcentrifuge tube for each sample (i.e., for eight samples, prepare a master mix 85 μl DNase I + 595 μl Buffer RD, including a .5 sample error correction) (*see* **Note 8**).

15. Pipet 80 μl of DNase I master mix directly onto the PAXgene RNA spin column membrane. Careful not to puncture membrane with pipette tip. Incubate sample at room temperature on benchtop for 15 min.

16. Add 300 μl of manufacturer's Buffer, BM3, to PAXgene RNA spin column. Close the lid gently and centrifuge at $14,000 \times g$ at room temperature for 1 min. Place the spin column into a new processing tube and discard old processing tube.

17. Add 500 μl of Buffer, BM4 to PAXgene RNA spin column. Close the lid gently and centrifuge at $14,000 \times g$ at room temperature for 1 min. Place the spin column into a new processing tube and discard old processing tube.

18. Add another 500 μl of BM4 to PAXgene spin column. Close the lid gently and centrifuge at $14,000 \times g$ at room temperature for 2 min.

19. Discard the processing tube and place PAXgene spin column in a new 2 ml processing tube. Centrifuge at $14,000 \times g$ at room temperature for 1 min.

20. Discard the processing tube containing flow through and place the PAXgene spin column in an RNase-free 1.5 ml microcentrifuge tube. Add 40 μl of Buffer, BM5, directly to the spin

column membrane. Careful not to puncture membrane with pipette tip. Close lid gently and centrifuge at 14,000 × *g* at room temperature for 1 min to elute RNA.

21. Repeat the elution step (**step 20**) using 40 μl of RNase-free water into the same PAXgene spin column.

22. Incubate 80 μl of RNA elute for 5 min at 65 °C. Place samples on ice immediately after incubation.

23. Measure RNA concentration by NanoDrop before proceeding to next procedures.

*3.2 RNA Poly-A Tailing*

Keep reagents on ice during sample preparations.

1. Prepare 0.75 μg of sample RNA in 15 μl nuclease-free water in a 1.5 ml RNase-free tube.

2. Add the following reagents to each sample in the following order.

   • 2 μl of 10× *E. coli* Poly(A) Polymerase Reaction Buffer.

   • 2 μl of ATP (10 mM).

   • 1 μl of *E. coli* Poly(A) Polymerase.

3. Incubate the 20 μl of contents in the tube at 37 °C for 30 min.

4. Directly proceed to RNA cleaning and concentration steps.

*3.3 RNA Clean and Concentrator*

Prepare all Buffer concentrates with appropriate columns of 100% ethanol as instructed by the manufacturer (Zymo). All procedures can be performed at room temperature and final RNA product can be stored at −70 °C or used for cDNA-PCR seq library prep.

1. Adjust RNA poly-A tail sample volume to a minimum of 50 μl using RNase-free water.

2. Add 100 μl of RNA Binder Buffer to each 50 μl sample and mix (*see* **Note 9**).

3. Add 150 μl of ethanol (95–100%) to each sample and mix (*see* **Note 10**).

4. Transfer the sample to the IC Column in a collection tube and centrifuge at 10,000–16,000 × *g* at room temperature for 30 s. Discard the flow-through (*see* **Note 11**).

5. Add 400 μl of manufacturer's Prep Buffer to the column and centrifuge at 10,000–16,000 × *g* at room temperature for 30 s. Discard the flow-through.

6. Add 700 μl of manufacturer's RNA Wash Buffer to the column and centrifuge at 10,000–16,000 × *g* at room temperature for 2 min. Check to make sure wash buffer is completely removed.

7. Carefully transfer the IC Column to an RNase-free tube.

8. Add 10 μl of DNase/RNase-free water directly to the column matrix. Careful not to puncture membrane with pipette tip. Centrifuge at 10,000–16,000 × *g* at room temperature for 30 s (*see* **Note 12**).

9. NanoDrop RNA elute. Use RNase/DNase-free water as your blank (*see* **Note 13**).

10. RNA elute is ready for cDNA-PCR seq library prep or can be stored immediately at −70 ° C (*see* **Note 14**).

### 3.4  cDNA-PCR Sequencing

#### 3.4.1  Library Preparation

1. Prepare 20 ng PolyA+ RNA into 9 μl of nuclease-free water into 0.2 ml PCR tube.

2. Mix gently by flicking then spin down in microfuge.

3. Add 1 μl VNP and 1 μl dNTPs.

4. Gently mix the 11 μl and spin down in microfuge.

5. Incubate at 65 °C for 5 min, then snap cool on ice immediately after.

6. In a separate 0.2 ml PCR tube, prepare strand switching mix: 4 μl 5× RT buffer, 1 μl RNaseOUT, 1 μl nuclease-free water, and 2 μl Strand-Switching Primer.

7. Add strand switching mix (8 μl) to annealed mRNA (11 μl), mix gently and spin down.

8. Incubate at 42 °C for 2 min.

9. Add 1 μl Maxima H Minus Reverse Transcriptase.

10. Gently mix and spin down and incubate at 42 °C for 90 min, 85 °C for 5 min, then 4 °C on hold.

#### 3.4.2  Selecting for Full-Length Transcripts

1. Prepare four separate PCR reactions from cDNA.

2. In PCR tube, prepare the following: 25 μl 2× LongAmp Taq Master Mix, 1.5 μl cDNA Primer, 18.5 μl nuclease-free water, and 5 μl of reverse transcribed RNA from the previous section.

3. Mix gently and spin down.

4. Place into thermal cycler with the protocol indicated in Table 1.

5. Add 1 μl Exonuclease to each PCR reaction.

6. Incubate at 37 °C for 15 min and then 80 °C for 15 min.

7. Combine the 4 PCR reactions into a 1.5 ml microtube.

8. Add 160 μl AMPure beads to microtube and mix gently (*see* **Note 15**).

9. Incubate tube on rotator mixer for 5 min at room temperature.

10. Gently spin down sample and place onto magnetic rack.

11. Once pellet forms, keep tube on rack and gently remove supernatant (*see* **Note 16**).

**Table 1**
**PCR protocol**

| Cycle step | Temperature °C | Time | Cycles |
|---|---|---|---|
| 1. Initial denaturing | 95 | 30 s | 1 |
| 2. Denaturing | 95 | 15 s | 14 |
| Annealing | 62 | 15 s | 14 |
| Extension | 65 | 50 s | 14 |
| 3. Final extension | 65 | 6 min | 1 |
| 4. Hold | 4 | Hold | 1 |

12. Add 200 µl of fresh 70% ethanol without disturbing pellet. Remove 70% ethanol and discard.

13. Repeat the previous step.

14. Dry pellet for 30 s to remove residual ethanol (*see* **Note 17**).

15. Remove tube from magnetic rack and add 12 µl elution buffer. Mix gently by pipetting.

16. Incubate at room temperature for 10 min.

17. Place tube on magnetic rack and pellet beads until supernatant is clear.

18. Transfer 12 µl of eluate to fresh 1.5 ml microtube.

19. Use immediately or store at −80 °C.

*3.4.3 Adapter Addition*

1. Add 1 µl of Rapid Adapter to 11 µl of amplified cDNA library from the previous step.

2. Mix gently and spin down.

3. Incubate for 5 min at room temperature.

*3.4.4 Priming and Loading SpotON Flow Cell*

1. Perform flow cell check on SpotON to make sure pores are sufficient.

2. Prepare SpotON by removing air bubble from priming port (*see* **Note 18**).

3. Add 30 µl Flush Tether to a tube of Flush buffer. Mix gently and spin down.

4. Add 800 µl of prepared flush buffer to priming port of SpotON (*see* **Note 19**).

5. Incubate at room temperature for 5 min.

6. Prepare library by adding 37.5 µl Sequencing buffer and 25.5 µl Loading Beads with 12 µl of DNA library.

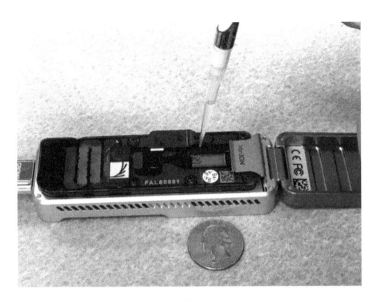

**Fig. 3** Loading of sample onto flow cell

7. Open SpotON cover, and add 200 μl Flush Buffer to priming port.

8. Dropwise add 75 μl of sample on to SpotON port (*see* **Note 20**, Fig. 3).

9. Close SpotON port and then close priming port.

*3.4.5 Sequencing and Data Analysis*

1. Open MinKNOW software and enter in metadata details of new experiment for sample.

2. Start sequencing run and perform data acquisition and base calling in real time or skip base calling to perform at a later time (*see* **Note 21**).

3. Downstream analysis can be used on Oxford Nanopore's EPI2ME platform (*see* **Note 22**).

## 4    Notes

1. Tube for blood collection, transport, and storage that stabilizes and preserves intracellular RNA for gene expression profiling. RNA must be stabilized immediately after blood draw as degradation of RNA and downregulation and upregulation of transcripts can occur immediately if not preserved.

2. Nucleic acid purification kit containing spin columns, Shredder spin columns, processing tubes, RNase-Free DNase I, RNase-free reagents, microcentrifuge tubes, Proteinase K, and proprietary buffers: BM1 resuspension buffer, BM2 binding buffer containing guanidine salt, BM3 and BM4 wash buffer

concentrates, BR5 elution buffer. **Warning**: Guanidine salts form highly reactive compounds in the presence of bleach. If these buffers are spilled, use laboratory detergent and water instead.

3. Purified RNA should not be in the presence of either EDTA or salts. RNase inhibitor can be added to stabilize RNA and the volume of inhibitor can be subtracted from the total volume of nuclease-free water used for the Poly(A) tailing reaction.

4. Proprietary kit includes RNA Binding Buffer, IC Columns, Collection Tubes, RNA Prep Buffer, RNA Wash Buffer concentrate, DNase/RNase-Free Wash Buffer RNA. Wash Buffer Concentrate must be diluted with 100% ethanol.

5. The rotor must contain tube adapters for round bottom tubes. Otherwise, tubes may break.

6. If entire supernatant is not removed, lysis will be inhibited, and lysate will be diluted. Conditions for RNA binding to the PAXgene membrane could be affected.

7. Do not mix Buffer BM2 with proteinase K together prior to adding to the sample.

8. DNase I is sensitive to physical denaturation. Do not vortex and only flick tube to mix contents.

9. Two volumes of RNA Binding Buffer should be added to the volume sample with poly-A tailing.

10. An equal volume of ethanol should be added to your total volume from step 1.

11. If sample volume is >800 μl, spin columns can be reloaded according to the manufacturer.

12. To obtain highly concentrated RNA, use ≥6 μl elution as recommended by the manufacturer.

13. Using RNase-free water only as your blank may cause inaccurate concentration readings.

14. RNA ≥ 18 nt will be recovered.

15. Prepare AMPure XP beads according to the manufacturer's protocol prior to use.

16. Make sure beads adhere to wall of magnet and supernatant is clear.

17. Do not dry the pellet to the point of cracking.

18. Be sure to avoid introducing air bubbles to flow cell, this causes irreversible damage to sensors.

19. Pipet sample to mix gently prior to adding. Add sample dropwise to ensure each drop enters port before adding more.

20. Using a P1000 pipette, insert tip into priming port and turn pipette dial until a small volume of buffer enters the tip (20–30 µl). This ensures continuous buffer across the sensor array.

21. Base calling can be done after sequencing run using guppy stand-alone.

22. Continuous raw current traces and read decisions can be recorded by enabling this output option when configuring a sequencing run to start in MinKNOW.

## References

1. Bayega A, Wang YC, Oikonomopoulos S, Djambazian H, Fahiminiya S, Ragoussis J (2018) Transcript profiling using long-read sequencing technologies. Methods Mol Biol 1783:121–147. https://doi.org/10.1007/978-1-4939-7834-2_6

2. Marinov GK (2017) On the design and prospects of direct RNA sequencing. Brief Funct Genomics 16(6):326–335. https://doi.org/10.1093/bfgp/elw043

3. Kono N, Arakawa K (2019) Nanopore sequencing: review of potential applications in functional genomics. Develop Growth Differ 61 (5):316–326. https://doi.org/10.1111/dgd.12608

4. Garalde DR, Snell EA, Jachimowicz D, Sipos B, Lloyd JH, Bruce M, Pantic N, Admassu T, James P, Warland A, Jordan M, Ciccone J, Serra S, Keenan J, Martin S, McNeill L, Wallace EJ, Jayasinghe L, Wright C, Blasco J, Young S, Brocklebank D, Juul S, Clarke J, Heron AJ, Turner DJ (2018) Highly parallel direct RNA sequencing on an array of nanopores. Nat Methods 15(3):201–206. https://doi.org/10.1038/nmeth.4577

5. Goodwin S, McPherson JD, McCombie WR (2016) Coming of age: ten years of next-generation sequencing technologies. Nat Rev Genet 17(6):333–351. https://doi.org/10.1038/nrg.2016.49

6. Jonkhout N, Tran J, Smith MA, Schonrock N, Mattick JS, Novoa EM (2017) The RNA modification landscape in human disease. RNA 23 (12):1754–1769. https://doi.org/10.1261/rna.063503.117

7. Depledge DP, Srinivas KP, Sadaoka T, Bready D, Mori Y, Placantonakis DG, Mohr I, Wilson AC (2019) Direct RNA sequencing on nanopore arrays redefines the transcriptional complexity of a viral pathogen. Nat Commun 10(1):754. https://doi.org/10.1038/s41467-019-08734-9

# Chapter 20

# LncRNA Quantification from Extracellular Vesicles Isolated from Blood Plasma or Conditioned Media

## Joan J. Castellano, Jordi Canals, Bing Han, Tania Díaz, Mariano Monzo, and Alfons Navarro

## Abstract

During the last years, the study of extracellular vesicles (EVs) and its cargo has gained interest in the scientific media. EVs have been found in all biofluids and it is postulated that all cells are capable to secrete a wide variety of these vesicles, which play a key role in different cell-to-cell communication processes as well as in the microenvironment modulation. In the EV cargo, DNA, protein, and RNA molecules can be found, including long noncoding RNAs (lncRNAs). Several authors consider the study of EV lncRNAs an ideal source of biomarkers due to the easy sampling of EVs in different biofluids and the high specificity of the lncRNA expression pattern.

In the present chapter, a detailed explanation of the EV isolation workflow followed by RNA isolation and lncRNA gene expression study is provided for two sample sources: blood plasma and cell culture conditioned media. EVs from both plasma samples and cell cultured media are isolated using sequential ultracentrifugation method (UC), which has been reported as one of the best methods available to date in terms of purity. UC is followed by RNA extraction based on the combination of phenol/guanidine-based lysis of samples with silica-membrane–based purification of total RNA. LncRNA quantification is performed by qRT-PCR. This chapter includes detailed discussion on lncRNA quantification using hydrolysis probes, recommended housekeeping genes and evaluation of methods for comparing lncRNA levels between EVs and its parental cells. In summary, we describe here the main steps for a successful isolation of the EVs-lncRNA cargo, paying attention to how overcome the different challenges found in the experimental procedure and in the data analysis of lncRNA expression from this source.

Key words Extracellular vesicles, Exosomes, Biofluids, Liquid Biopsy, lncRNA, Plasma, Conditioned media

## 1 Introduction

It is considered that the vast majority of cell types are able to produce and secrete a myriad of different extracellular vesicles (EVs) [1], which is the generic term for cellular released particles delimited by a lipid bilayer not containing a functional nucleus [2]. EVs include exosomes, which are small extracellular vesicles from endosomal origin; microvesicles, formed by direct budding of

Alfons Navarro (ed.), *Long Non-Coding RNAs in Cancer*, Methods in Molecular Biology, vol. 2348,
https://doi.org/10.1007/978-1-0716-1581-2_20, © Springer Science+Business Media, LLC, part of Springer Nature 2021

the cell plasmatic membrane; and apoptotic bodies, which are by-products of the cell death [3]. For the last years, many authors have referred to the smallest-size EV fraction as exosomes (those with less than 150 nm) [4, 5]. However, the International Society for Extracellular Vesicles (ISEV) established that, unless a specific endosomal origin can be determined in the EVs, it is recommended to use the term small EVs instead of exosomes [2].

EVs play a role in cell-to-cell communication, arising as a key mechanism to regulate the cell behavior in the local microenvironment as well as in distant parts in complex organisms [6, 7]. Their utility as biomarkers, especially the analysis of their cargo (DNA, RNA, proteins, etc.), and their biocompatibility for drug delivery are some of the most promising areas of current research [8, 9]. Among the EV cargo, noncoding RNAs are overrepresented. Although small noncoding RNAs such as microRNAs or piwiRNAs account for 80% of the content, long noncoding RNAs, found in a smaller proportion (2.4%) [10, 11], seem to show an EV characteristic expression pattern that differs from its parental cell. This points to a specific loading of these lncRNAs in the EVs, most of them overrepresented in the EVs in comparison to the secreting cells [12]. Therefore, the study of the lncRNAs content in EVs has been postulated as one of the most promising sources of biomarkers due to its possible isolation from different biofluids and to the high specificity of the lncRNAs expression pattern [13]. Furthermore, the EV lncRNA content might help to decipher the mechanisms of microenvironment modulation shown in different diseases such as cancer [14, 15] by studying the transfer of lncRNAs from EVs-secreting cells to the vicinity cells [7, 16, 17].

EV isolation from different sources can be achieved using a variety of procedures. Each of the developed procedures shows differences in the amount, integrity, and purity of the isolated EVs. Every method relies in different EV properties for its isolation, including affinity purification based on EV surface markers, size exclusion chromatography, or precipitation. The vast majority of this methods has been recently reviewed by ISEV, showing that ultracentrifugation (UC) is the most reliable, and also cost-effective method, to isolate EVs, especially in terms of purity (78% [UC] vs 15.8% [Average of: polymer precipitation, size exclusion and membrane filtration]) [18].

In the following, we will describe the workflow, methodology, required materials and highlight the most commonly found challenges during lncRNAs isolation from EVs derived from either human blood plasma or conditioned media from cultured human cell lines samples using UC. We will comment the different challenges that might be found due to the sample availability or the differences between EV sources.

## 2  Materials

### 2.1  Blood Plasma Collection

1. EDTA tube for blood plasma collection.
2. Centrifuge with a rotor for EDTA tubes that allows 1500–2000 × $g$ centrifugation.
3. 1.5 mL microcentrifuge tubes.
4. Micropipette.

### 2.2  Cell Lines, Cell Culture, and Conditioned Medium Collection

1. NCI-H23 cell line (American Type Culture Collection).
2. HCC-44 (DSMZ).
3. 75 cm$^2$ T-Flasks.
4. RPMI-1640.
5. 10% Fetal Bovine Serum, exosome depleted (Thermo Fisher Scientific).
6. Gibco penicillin–streptomycin–glutamine (100×) (Thermo Fisher Scientific).
7. Trypsin.
8. Sterile pipettes.
9. Pipette filler (Pipetus/Pipetman/Pipetboy type).
10. Cell counter.
11. Cell incubator.
12. Class II biological safety cabinet for cell culture.

### 2.3  Preprocessing and Ultracentrifugation

1. 1.5 mL microcentrifuge tubes.
2. 15 mL conical centrifuge tubes.
3. Refrigerated centrifuge that allows up to 10,000 × $g$ centrifugation.
4. Centrifuge rotor up to 10,000 × $g$ for 1.5 mL microcentrifuge tubes.
5. Centrifuge rotor up to 10,000 × $g$ for 15 mL conical centrifuge tubes.
6. Ultracentrifuge with fixed angle rotors that that allows up to 100,000 × $g$ centrifugation. For small volume samples (plasma) Sorvall MX plus micro-ultracentrifuge with a rotor S140-AT or similar is adequate. For big volume samples (conditioned medium) Beckman Coulter Optima L-100 XP ultracentrifuge with rotor 70.1 ti or similar is adequate.
7. Ultracentrifuge polycarbonate tubes of 1 mL. In our system we use Thermo Scientific Tube PC Thickwall 1 mL PK/100 (Fisher Scientific).

8. Ultracentrifuge Polycarbonate tubes of 10 mL. In our system we use 10 mL, Open-Top Thickwall Polycarbonate Tube, 16 × 76 mm (Beckman Coulter) which has a maximum capacity of 13.5 mL.

9. Dulbecco's phosphate buffered saline (DPBS).

10. 50 mL syringe.

11. 18G needle.

12. 0.2 µM syringe filter.

13. Micropipettes and Sterile Filter pipette tips.

**2.4  RNA Isolation**

1. miRNAeasy mini kit (Qiagen). Store at room temperature.

2. RNA MS2 from bacteriophage MS2 (Merck). Store at −20 °C.

3. Ethanol absolute (100%). Store at room temperature.

4. Chloroform. Store at room temperature.

5. Fume hood.

6. Tabletop centrifuge up to $16,000 \times g$.

7. NanoDrop-type spectrophotometer.

**2.5  LncRNA Quantification Using Hydrolysis Probes**

1. High Capacity cDNA reverse transcription kit with RNase Inhibitor (Thermo Fisher Scientific). Store at −20 °C.

2. 96-well PCR plates or individual PCR microtubes of 0.2 mL.

3. Flat PCR caps, strips of 8, compatible with our 96-well PCR plates.

4. Centrifuge up to $2000 \times g$ with a rotor for 96-well plates.

5. PCR Thermocycler.

6. Specific hydrolysis probes for our lncRNA of interest and for the selected endogenous control.

7. TaqMan Universal PCR Master Mix 2×. Store at 4 °C.

8. Nuclease-free water.

9. MicroAmp Optical Adhesive Film or Microamp optical 8-cap strips (Thermo Fisher Scientific).

10. Applied Biosystems 7500 Real time PCR (Thermo Fisher Scientific) or similar.

# 3  Methods

**3.1  Collection of Blood Plasma and Preprocessing**

1. Collect 5 ml of venous blood in an EDTA tube.

2. Centrifuge the tube at $1500 \times g$ for 15 min at room temperature.

3. Transfer the supernatant (plasma) in fractions of 250 μL to 1.5 mL tubes (*see* **Note 1**).

4. Go to **step 5** or save it a −80 °C if you are not proceeding to EV purification immediately (Stopping point).

5. Use 1 tube with 250 μL of fresh or frozen (*see* **Note 2**) plasma for preprocessing (consecutive centrifugations steps to eliminate all cell debris and other components that might interfere in EV isolation and/or RNA extraction).

6. Centrifuge 250 μL of fresh plasma at $300 \times g$ for 5 min at 4 °C.

7. Collect the supernatant gently using a micropipette (*see* **Note 3**) and transfer to a new 1.5 mL tube.

8. Centrifuge the tube at $2500 \times g$ for 20 min at 4 °C.

9. Collect the supernatant gently using a micropipette and transfer to a new 1.5 mL tube.

10. Centrifuge the tube at $10,000 \times g$ for 30 min at 4 °C.

11. Collect the supernatant gently using a micropipette and transfer to a new 1.5 mL tube.

12. Go to Subheading 3.3.

### 3.2 Collection of Conditioned Media and Preprocessing

1. Prepare the experimental design for your own in vitro study (*see* **Note 4**). For a typical transfection experiment with a siRNA in NCI-H23 or HCC44 cells we used to prepare three 75 cm² T-Flask with $3 \times 10^6$ cells/flask cultured with 15 mL of EV-free medium (RPMI-1640 supplemented with 10% Fetal Bovine Serum, exosome depleted) per flask.

2. After 96 h of cell culture (*see* **Note 5**), collect all the conditioned media from each flask and transfer it to a 15 mL conical tube.

3. Go to **step 4** or save it a −80 °C if you are not proceeding to EV purification immediately (Stopping point).

4. Centrifuge the tubes at $2500 \times g$ for 20 min at 4 °C.

5. Collect the supernatant gently using a pipette (try not to disturb the pellet) and transfer to a new 15 mL tube.

6. Centrifuge the tube at $10,000 \times g$ for 30 min at 4 °C.

7. Collect the supernatant gently using pipette (try not to disturb the pellet) and transfer to a new 15 mL tube.

8. Go to Subheading 3.3.

### 3.3 Ultra-centrifugation

The ultracentrifugation protocol in our laboratory for plasma samples was performed in a Sorvall MX Plus Micro-Ultracentrifuge with a rotor S140AT (Maximum volume per sample of 1 mL) and for conditioned medium we used the Beckman Coulter Optima

**A** **B**

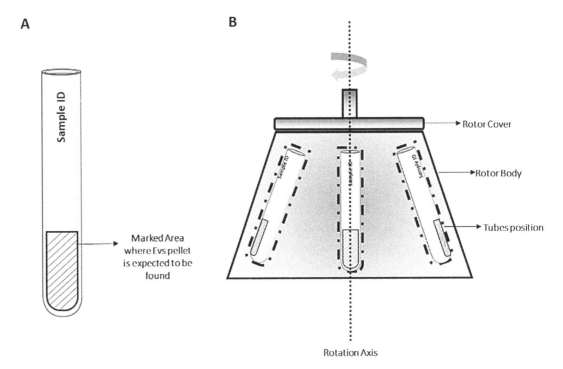

**Fig. 1** (a) Representation of the ultracentrifuge labeled tube. (b) Schematic representation of the tubes positions after being loaded in the rotor

L-100 XP ultracentrifuge with a rotor 70.1 ti (Maximum volume per sample of 10 mL).

1. Open the ultracentrifuge and precool it and also the rotor to be used to 4 °C at least 20 min prior to sample loading (*see* **Note 6**).

2. Prepare the ultracentrifuge tubes: mark the sample of each tube and draw a circle in the bottom-side of the tube where the sample will be expected to precipitate since in many cases EV pellet is hardly visible (Fig. 1a).

3. Transfer the samples gently to the ultracentrifuge tubes (use as many tubes as necessary to collect all sample according to your ultracentrifuge tube maximum loading volume). In the case of plasma samples (initial volume was 250 μL) dilute the sample using filtered DPBS to a final volume of 1 mL.

4. Once all tubes have been filled, it is extremely necessary to carefully calibrate the tubes weight (ultracentrifuges are really sensitive to unbalanced rotors). Use a precision scale to set up all tubes with a difference weight below decagrams (0.00XX grams). Calibrate using the heaviest tube as reference by gently adding filtered DPBS drop by drop until acceptable weight difference has been reached.

5. Load the tubes gently into the precooled ultracentrifuge rotor with a plastic tweezers (*see* **Note 7**). It is important to put the tube in the rotor with the circle located as shown in Fig. 1b.

6. Close the rotor cover and insert the rotor in the centrifuge.

7. Set up the run indicating the rotor (in some centrifuges is automatically detected), the centrifugation speed, the time, the temperature, and the acceleration and braking ramp. For the present procedure the acceleration and braking ramp have to be the shortest as possible (in our ultracentrifuges ramp 9 represents the shortest).

8. Close the centrifuge cover and activate the vacuum system. Wait until a minimum vacuum have been reached (2 of 3 vacuums in our centrifuge) before starting the run.

9. Start the run to centrifuge the tubes at $100,000 \times g$ for 2 h at $4\,^\circ$C.

10. Once the run is finished, stop the vacuum, open the centrifuge cover and extract the rotor with the samples. Open the rotor cover with care to avoid sample disturbing (sometimes this could be difficult since the vacuum system produced a hermetic closing of the rotor).

11. Discard the supernatant carefully, paying attention to not disturb any pellet (probably not visible) formed in the marked area of the tube.

12. Fill the tube with the initial sample volume of fresh filtered DPBS (1 mL for plasma samples and 8 mL for conditioned media samples) and calibrate the tubes weight as described in **step 4** again. Repeat **steps 5–8**.

13. Start the run to centrifuge the tubes at $100,000 \times g$ for 1 h at $4\,^\circ$C.

14. Once the run is finished, stop the vacuum, open the centrifuge cover and extract the rotor with the samples. Open the rotor cover with care to avoid sample disturbing.

15. Discard the supernatant carefully, paying attention to not disturb any pellet (probably not visible) formed in the marked area of the tube.

16. If all sample will be used for RNA isolation proceed to Subheading 3.4. Alternatively, all the sample or part of it can be used for EV characterization using western blot, nanoparticle tracking analysis or electron microscopy (*see* **Note 8**).

*3.4* **RNA Isolation**

1. Prepare an RNA isolation master mix containing 800 μL of QIAzol +1.25 μL of MS2 RNA (package of 10 $A_{260}$ units) (*see* **Note 9**) per sample (*see* **Note 10**).

2. Resuspend the EV pellet obtained after ultracentrifugation with 750 μL of RNA isolation master mix by pipetting. If more than one ultracentrifugation tube was used per sample, then resuspend the first sample with 750 μL of RNA isolation master mix and after resuspension transfer the liquid to next tube and repeat the resuspension process. Do this as many times as tubes you have of the same sample.

3. Transfer all tube content to a 1.5 mL tube.

4. Add 200 μL of chloroform and vortex vigorously the tube.

5. Let the mix rest for 10–15 min at room temperature.

6. Centrifugate the samples at $12,000 \times g$ for 15 min at 4 °C in a refrigerated centrifuge.

7. After centrifugation two separated phases would be clearly visible separated by a slightly visible interphase. Collect the upper aqueous and noncolored phase by pipetting and transfer to a new 1.5 mL tube.

8. Add 1.5 volumes (in relation to the volume obtained of sample in the previous step) of absolute ethanol and mix thoroughly by inverting the tube.

9. Transfer 700 μL of the mixed content to the RNeasy® Mini column located in a 2 mL tube.

10. Centrifugate in a tabletop centrifuge at $15,600 \times g$ for 1 min and discard the flow-through.

11. Repeat the **steps 9–10** until all sample volume has passed through the column.

12. Add 700 μL of buffer RWT and centrifuge at $15,600 \times g$ for 1 min and discard the flow-through.

13. Add 500 μL of buffer RPE and centrifuge at $15,600 \times g$ for 1 min and discard the flow-through.

14. Repeat **step 13**.

15. Centrifuge the empty column at $15,600 \times g$ for 1 min to eliminate any residual buffer bonded to the column surface.

16. Transfer the column to a new RNase-free 1.5 mL tube properly labeled with the sample id.

17. Add 20–30 μL of sterile RNase-free water directly to the center of the column.

18. Let it rest for 5–10 min with the column sealed.

19. Elute the RNA by centrifugation at $15,600 \times g$ for 1 min.

20. Quantify RNA using desired method (usually spectrophotometer) and the RNA is ready for downstream applications.

**3.5 Expected Recovery Yield of EVs and EVs-Derived RNA**

During these procedures one of the key steps is to establish the initial amount of sample required for a successful EV isolation. Table 1 summarizes the amount of EVs (quantified using Nano-Sight, Fig. 2) and RNA recovered from three biological replicates of two different non–small-cell lung cancer cell lines, NCI-H23 and HCC44, using $9 \times 10^6$ cells cultured during 96 h [19]; and from 3 samples of human plasma (250 μL per sample) obtained from peripheral vein [20] using the methodology previously described.

**Table 1**
**Expected extracellular vesicles and EVs-derived RNA yield recovered**

| Sample | Replicate[a] | Average EVs/mL[b] | Mean size (nm) | Size mode (nm) | Total EVs recovered | [RNA] ng/μL | Total RNA recovered (ng)[c] |
|---|---|---|---|---|---|---|---|
| NCI-H23 | 1 | $9.02 \times 10^9$ | 184 | 136 | $2.26 \times 10^9$ | 28.5 | 712.5 |
| | 2 | $7.15 \times 10^9$ | 176 | 149 | $1.79 \times 10^9$ | 29.6 | 740 |
| | 3 | $5.51 \times 10^9$ | 191 | 128 | $1.38 \times 10^9$ | 34.8 | 870 |
| | Average | $7.23 \times 10^9$ | 183.67 | 137.67 | $1.81 \times 10^9$ | 31 | 774.2 |
| HCC44 | 1 | $9.85 \times 10^{10}$ | 217 | 157 | $2.46 \times 10^{10}$ | 31.7 | 792.5 |
| | 2 | $7.34 \times 10^{10}$ | 224 | 161 | $1.84 \times 10^{10}$ | 27.6 | 690 |
| | 3 | $3.75 \times 10^{11}$ | 210 | 151 | $9.38 \times 10^{10}$ | 37.1 | 927.5 |
| | Average | $1.82 \times 10^{11}$ | 217.00 | 156.33 | $4.56 \times 10^{10}$ | 32.1 | 803.3 |
| Patient's plasma | 1 | $2.72 \times 10^9$ | 152.9 | 114.1 | $6.80 \times 10^8$ | 26.1 | 652.5 |
| | 2 | $2.00 \times 10^9$ | 156.2 | 106.5 | $5.00 \times 10^8$ | 25.1 | 627.5 |
| | 3 | $1.02 \times 10^{10}$ | 152.2 | 108.1 | $2.55 \times 10^9$ | 27.6 | 690 |
| | Average | $4.97 \times 10^9$ | 153.8 | 109.6 | $1.24 \times 10^9$ | 26.3 | 675.7 |

[a]Indicates the number of biological replicates. Each replicate data is the result of three technical replicate measures
[b]Analyzed by Nano-Tracking Analysis (NTA) using NanoSight NS300. For cell culture conditioned media, a total volume of 45 mL of EV-free medium (15 mL/flask) was conditioned by $9 \times 10^6$ cells ($3 \times 10^6$ cells/flask) for 96 h. For EVs derived from patient's plasma a total of 250 μL of plasma per sample were used
[c]Total number of nanograms obtained using a final RNA elution volume of 25 μL

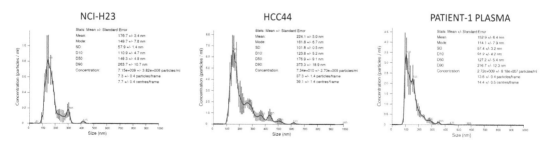

**Fig. 2** Representatives reports obtained by nanoparticle tracking analysis (NTA) using NanoSight 3000 device for (**a**) H23 cells (**b**) HCC44 cells (**c**) Plasma samples

**Table 2**
**RT reaction master mix**

| RT master mix components[a] | Volume per sample (μL) |
|---|---|
| RT buffer (10×) | 2 |
| RT random primers (10×) | 2 |
| dNTP mix (100 mM, 25×) | 0.8 |
| MultiScribe reverse transcriptase (50 U/μL) | 1 |
| RNase inhibitor | 1 |
| Nuclease-free water | 0.7 |
| Total | 7.5 |

[a]All components are part of the High-Capacity cDNA Reverse Transcription Kit with RNase Inhibitor

**3.6 EVs-Derived lncRNA Quantification Using Hydrolysis Probes**

For single lncRNA expression quantification qRT-PCR with hydrolysis probes (sequence-specific, double-labeled probes; commonly known as "TaqMan" probes) are used and described in this section. However, other systems such as SYBR green can be used in this step to quantify single lncRNA expression (*see* Chapter 6).

*3.6.1 Reverse Transcription*

cDNA is obtained using an RNA input of 250 ng (*see* **Note 11**) and the "*High Capacity cDNA reverse transcription kit*" (ThermoFisher Scientific).

1. Thaw on ice all components provided in the High Capacity cDNA reverse transcription kit except for MultiScribe Reverse Transcriptase, which will be kept in the freezer until you are ready to use it.

2. Prepare the RT reaction Master mix according to Table 2 for the total number of samples including at least two additional reactions in the calculations to provide excess volume.

3. In a 96-well plate (or individual PCR tubes depending on the number of samples), add 7.5 μL of RT reaction master mix per well according experimental design.

4. Add 12.5 μL of RNA (20 ng/ μL) into the wells containing the RT reaction master mix.

5. Seal the 96-well plate with flat-cap strips.

6. Centrifuge the 96 well plate *772 × g (1200 rpm)* for 2 min.

7. Load the thermal cycler with the 96-well plate and run the following program: (1) Hold 10 min at 25 °C; (2) hold 120 min at 37 °C; (3) hold 5 min at 85 °C; and (4) hold ∞ at 4 °C.

8. If you are not performing the quantification by real-time PCR immediately, you can save it at 4 °C maximum 24 h or at −20 °C for long-term storage (Stopping point).

<table>
<tr><td>3.6.2 Hydrolysis Probes<br>Design</td><td>For the most common lncRNAs commercial predesigned TaqMan probes are available. However, when no predesigned TaqMan probe are available we need to design it and adequate TaqMan probe design is crucial for a successful determination. The TaqMan assay design can be performed using the free online software Primer3 (https://primer3.ut.ee) [21, 22] as follows.</td></tr>
</table>

1. Search for the cDNA sequence of the lncRNA of interest (*see* **Note 12**) and select the desired amplification region.

2. Paste the sequence fragment in the box indicated in the Primer3web tool to paste the source sequence.

3. Check the option *Pick hybridization probe (internal oligo) or use oligo below.*

4. Modify in the *General Primer Picking Conditions* the *Primer Tm* as follows (*see* **Note 13**):
   • Min: 59.0.
   • Opt: 60.0.
   • Max:62.0.

5. Modify in the *General Primer Picking Conditions* the *Primer GC%* as follows (*see* **Note 14**):
   • Min: 35.
   • Opt: 50.
   • Max:65.

6. Erase in the *General Primer Picking Conditions* the *Product Size Ranges* included by defect and use the range 50–150.

7. Modify in the *Internal Oligo (Hyb Oligo) General Conditions* the Internal Oligo Tm as follows (*see* **Note 15**):
   • Min: 66.
   • Opt: 68.
   • Max:70.

8. Star calculations pushing the button *Pick Primers.*

9. Once you have obtained your potential pair of primers and probe check the specificity of your primer set. It is always necessary to check that your amplification is specific when using custom hydrolysis designed primer sets after running the firsts RTqPCR. The adequate strategies would include running and agarose gel to evaluate the band size and potential presence of different bands, cloning the PCR product, and perform and standard curve (last will be further explained in Subheading 3.8).

**Table 3**
**Real-time PCR reaction master mix**

| Components | Volume per sample (μL) |
|---|---|
| TaqMan universal PCR master mix 2× | 5 |
| TaqMan assay 20× | 0.5 |
| Nuclease-free water | 3.5 |
| Total | 9 |

*3.6.3  Real-Time PCR Assay*

1. Thaw on ice the frozen TaqMan assay (hydrolysis probes) to be used and the cDNA (if it was frozen). Mix by vortexing and centrifuge briefly.

2. Prepare the Real time PCR Master mix according to Table 3 for the total number of samples including at least two additional reactions in the calculations to provide excess volume.

3. In a 96-well plate, add 9 μL of the Real time PCR reaction Master mix per well according experimental design.

4. Add 1 μL of cDNA into the wells containing the Real time PCR reaction master mix.

5. Seal the 96-well plate with an optical adhesive cover or with optical-cap strips.

6. Centrifuge the 96-well plate *772 × g (1200 rpm)* for 2 min.

7. Load the 7500 Real Time PCR System (*see* **Note 16**) with the 96-well plate and run the standard program for Relative quantification: (1) Hold 2 min at 50 °C; (2) Hold 10 min at 95 °C; and (3) 40 cycles of: 15 s at 95 °C followed of 1 min at 60 °C.

8. Once the run is finished, export the raw Ct from the analyzed lncRNA and the endogenous control used (*see* Subheading 3.6.4 for endogenous control selection) and proceed to calculate the relative quantification levels of each samples using the $2^{-\Delta\Delta Ct}$ method.

*3.6.4  Housekeeping Genes for EV lncRNA Expression Assessment*

To date, remains challenging the establishment of an adequate housekeeping gene that serves as endogenous control for gene expression normalization in EV samples [23]. Several authors have explored the suitability of several classical housekeeping genes obtaining different results depending on the source or type of EVs used, quite often, microRNAs arise as good candidates for gene expression normalization [24, 25]. Table 4 summarizes some of the housekeeping genes used in the literature for EVs-related lncRNA quantification.

**Table 4**
**Housekeeping genes used for lncRNA quantification in extracellular vesicles**

| Housekeeping gene | Suitable for mRNA | Suitable for lncRNAs | Suitable for small ncRNAs | Sample source of EVs | Reference |
|---|---|---|---|---|---|
| U6 | Yes | NA | No | Cardiosphere derived cells | [23] |
| | NA | NA | Yes | Astrocytes | [26] |
| | NA | NA | Yes | Bronchoalveolar lavage | [27] |
| | NA | Yes | NA | Hepatocellular carcinoma | [28] |
| miR-23a-3p | No | NA | Yes | Cardiosphere derived cells | [23] |
| miR-101-3p, miR-23a-3p, miR-26a-5p (arithmetic combination) | No | NA | Yes | Cardiosphere derived cells | [23] |
| miR-99a-5p, miR-30a-5p and miR-221-3p | No | NA | Yes | Healthy and cancer donor plasma | [29] |
| GAPDH | Yes | NA | NA | Mesenchymal stem cells | [30] |
| | Yes | NA | NA | Urine | [31] |
| | Yes | NA | NA | Endothelial cells | [32] |
| | NA | Yes | NA | Breast cancer | [33] |
| | NA | Yes | NA | Esophageal squamous cell carcinoma | [34] |
| Cyclophilin A | Yes | NA | NA | Astrocytes | [26] |
| β-Actin | Yes | NA | NA | Bronchoalveolar lavage | [27] |
| | NA | Yes | NA | Human embryonic kidney cells 293 (HEK293) | [35] |
| B2M | Yes | NA | NA | Endothelial cells | [32] |
| RPLP0 | Yes | NA | NA | Endothelial cells | [32] |
| 18S | No | Yes | NA | Chondrocytes | [36] |

It has also shown that the addition of spike-ins RNAs during isolation process may help for the gene expression determination. However, ISEV guidelines recommends the use of spike-in RNAs for the calculation of RTqPCR efficiency, but not as normalization tool [23].

Selecting an adequate housekeeping gene is not complicated when a uniform set of samples is being analyzed. In this case, the most recommended strategy is to test the gene expression of a battery of different commonly used housekeeping genes based on bibliography, and use any available tool such as Normfinder [37] or Genorm [38] to found the most adequate gene or gene combination that shows the most consistent expression across all samples. However, the gene expression comparison between EVs and their secreting cells becomes more complex (*see* Subheading 3.7).

*3.7 Comparing lncRNA Expression Between EVs and Secreting Cells*

As we have mentioned above, the comparison of lncRNA expression between different samples types used to be challenging. This mainly to possible bias when housekeeping genes with different expression between samples are used for normalization. The most common comparison in this line appears when we want to assess whether our lncRNA of interest is enriched in the EVs compared to the EV secreting cells. Many lncRNAs has been reported to be enriched in EVs when compared to their secreting cell when compared using housekeeping normalization, which might indicate and specific loading and possible function of this lncRNAs in the receptor cells [12].

For this comparison, the use of a housekeeping is specially challenging since the expression of many housekeeping genes might differ significantly between cells and EVs. Consequently, when gene expression is calculated normalizing using housekeeping, most of the effect shown can be due to the difference in housekeeping gene expression introducing a significant bias in the expression of our lncRNA of interest.

In our laboratory, we have used a strategy based on the normalization in the RNA input and normalized based on the raw Ct (Cycle threshold) reported on the RTqPCR procedure. This strategy is not accurate but might serve to detect a trend on the enrichment of our lncRNA of interest in the EVs. In the following, we will explain this procedure and which considerations must be taken in order to use this methodology.

This procedure is based on Eq. 1:

$$N_{Ct} = n \times E^{Ct} \qquad (1)$$

where the variables are $N_{Ct}$: Number of copies generated by the RTqPCR reaction when cycle threshold is reached; $n$: the number of copies in the original sample (RTqPCR input); $E$: Efficiency of the RTqPCR reaction; $Ct$: the number of cycles required to override the RTqPCR threshold. It is important, in order to apply this calculation, that the RNA input used for the cDNA generation was the same between the two samples studied.

This equation defines the basis of the RTqPCR calculation and will allow us to compare the variable $n$ between two different samples. In order to be able to apply this equation, we need first to assess the reaction efficiency ($E$) between the different samples (See box 2 for more information about RTqPCR efficiency calculation). If there are no significant differences in the efficiency of the RTqPCR reaction between both samples we can assume that, when both samples override the cycle threshold, the number of copies generated by the RTqPCR will be similar. This is due to the hydrolysis probe technology basis, where each new copy generated produces a new fluorochrome molecule available for excitation. Consequently, the number of required free fluorophore molecules for detection must be the same between two samples where reaction efficiency is the same and the same threshold is used.

Based on the above mentioned, we can consider, that for samples one (1) and two (2).

$$N_{Ct1} = n_1 \times E^{Ct1}$$

$$N_{Ct2} = n_2 \times E^{Ct2}$$

As previously mentioned, we can consider that $N_{Ct1}$ and $N_{Ct2}$ will be the same between two samples, so we can consider one equation equal to the other one and proceed as follows.

$$n_1 \times E^{Ct1} = n_2 \times E^{Ct2}$$

Since we want to know the relationship between the $n_1$ and $n_2$, we can group the variables as follows.

$$\frac{n_1}{n_2} = \frac{E^{Ct2}}{E^{Ct1}}$$

In this equation we the value of $E$ and the values of $Ct1$ and $Ct2$ will be known, so we will be able to determine the relationship between $n_1$ and $n_2$.

It is important to remark that this is not an accurate method due to some technical reasons related to the RTqPCR itself. However, we consider it is a reliable approach for the exploration of enrichment trends in EV-lncRNA expression.

Using this method, we studied the expression of lincRNA-p21 in EVs derived from non–small-cell lung cancer cell lines and compared with the expression in the cell lines itself [19]. Our results were concordant with previous studies in this regard [12], and also, this method and the use of a housekeeping genes reported results in the same line.

### 3.8 Performing an RTqPCR Standard Curve for Efficiency Calculation

Standard curve will allow us to calculate the RTqPCR reaction efficiency and also serve as control for the reaction specificity. This process will require the following steps:

1. Generate a serial dilution battery from cDNA. Using a nonrelevant sample generate dilutions 1:1, 1:10, 1:100, 1:1000, 1:10,000, and 1:100,000.

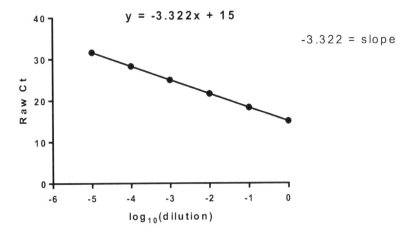

**Fig. 3** This is the representation of a perfect RTqPCR standard curve graph with efficiency = 2 (meaning that each copy in the sample generates two copies at the end of each RT-qPCR cycle). The values on y-axis were arbitrary chosen to plot this graph. Dilution values on the x-axis are the result of the log10 of each dilution, that is, dilution 1:10 = 0.1, $\log_{10}(0.1) = 1$; dilution 1:100 = 0.01, $\log^{10}(0.01) = -2$

2. Run RTqPCR using technical triplicates per sample: Use the mean value of all triplicates to perform the standard curve. If values differ more than one Ct, repeat the procedure.

3. Collect the results and prepare a scatter plot with the $\log_{10}[$dilution$]$ in the x-axis; and with the raw Ct value in the y-axis. When the trend line is added a similar graph to the one shown in Fig. 3 should be obtained.

4. Perform the efficiency calculation (*see* **Note 17**). To determine the efficiency of the reaction we need to apply the following equation: $E = 10^{\left(-1/\text{Slope}\right)}$.

# 4   Notes

1. Usually 2–3 mL of plasma are obtained from 5 mL of blood. Save it a −80 °C if you are not proceeding to EV purification immediately (Stopping point).

2. If you are working with frozen plasma be sure to do an extensive vortexing after thawing the plasma sample.

3. Do not transfer the liquid by direct decantation. Always use micropipette to gently collect and transfer the supernatant to a new sterile tube between each centrifugation step to not disturb any pellet formed during the centrifugation.

4. One of the key steps of the experimental design is to establish the initial number of cells, amount of medium, and minimum

culture time required for a successful EV isolation, which can depend on the cell line used and the treatment or transfection performed. In our laboratory we established that for cell culture conditioned medium downstream application, at least three 75 cm$^2$ T-flask with 15 mL of medium conditioned by $3 \times 10^6$ cells/flask (NCI-H23 or HCC44 cells) where necessary to collect enough amount of EVs. In our experimental procedure, EV-free medium is recovered after 96 h of cell culture; however, this time-point might be modified due to experimental requirements.

5. The minimum culture time to recover enough EVs for further analysis (NanoSight quantification, exosome characterization, and RNA purification) is 96 h, but this time-point might be modified due to experimental requirements or depending on the number of analysis needed to perform. The time elongation is directly related to an increment on the number of EV recovered. However, depending on the cell line used, modifications of this time can be required since EV production depends also on the cell line used.

6. Ultracentrifuge rotors used to be stored at 4 °C. In case rotor was stored at room temperature and need to be precooled inside the ultracentrifuge, do not seal completely the rotor cover to avoid vacuum make it difficult to open at sample-loading time.

7. Ideally, plastic tweezers must be used to handle the tubes in order to avoid damaging the polycarbonate surface of the rotor.

8. For EV characterization using nanoparticle tracking analysis (NTA) we recommend resuspend the EV pellet in a volume range of 150–200 μL of 0.22 μm filtered DPBS. For western blot purposes the EV pellet can be resuspended directly in western blot loading buffer at a final volume of 30–40 μL and charge all the volume in the acrylamide gel. If protein quantification is required prior western blot running, resuspend the pellet in 50–100 μL of filtered DPBS.

9. The use of MS2 RNA carrier have been showed increase the total RNA obtained from samples with low RNA quantities such as plasma [39]. However, depending on the downstream analysis performed the presence of the MS2 RNA could affect the results. We do not recommend including it if we are planning to use the RNA for RNAseq experiments.

10. We are going to use only 750 μL of RNA isolation master mix per sample but we are preparing it in excess taking in account potential pipetting problems when handling several samples.

11. We can use up to 2 μg of RNA in a 20 μL volume reaction, but we are always using 250 ng of RNA per reaction, which

according our experience will allow us to repeat the reverse transcription procedure 2–3 times per sample. Moreover, the increment of the initial RNA quantity will require to concentrate the samples using a Vacuum concentrator centrifuge according the expected recovery yields of RNA.

12. Use reliable genomic sequence information. Most lncRNAs has uncertain annotation and different sequences can be found when different databases are used. Make sure to use the most reliable genomic sequence found in order to design your probes. In our laboratory, we commonly use the transcript information from UCSC genome browser database (https://genome.ucsc.edu), but there are several specific lncRNA databases available (*see* Chapter 1). Try to use exons junction for design. Just as mRNA, lncRNA genomic structure is divided in exons and introns that undergoes to splicing processing. Using exon junction as amplification target (the amplicon should also span at least one intron) to prevent amplification of the target gene in genomic DNA.

13. Select primers with adequate melting temperature (Tm) and annealing temperature (Ta): Adequate Tm for primers used to range between 60 and 62 °C but can be slightly modified. Make sure that primers have a Ta which is no more than 5 °C below Tm.

14. Check GC content and avoid G-5′ ends. As general rule primers and probe GC content should range between 35% and 65%. Try to avoid 5′ terminal G since might quench the fluorophore signal.

15. It is important that probes Tm is 6–10 °C higher than primers Tm for an optimal hybridization.

16. If you are using a different real time PCR system from the 7500 Real time PCR system (Thermo Fisher Scientific), please check if are required to modify the amplification protocol to adapt to your system characteristics.

17. Ideal RTqPCR efficiency reaction should be close to 2. In case low efficiency values are obtained it is convenient to optimize the RTqPCR procedure for a reliable amplification.

## Acknowledgments

This work was supported by grants from the Ministry of Economy, Industry, and Competition, Agencia Estatal de Investigación cofinanced with the European Union FEDER funds SAF2017-88606-P (AEI/FEDER, UE).

## References

1. Kalluri R, LeBleu VS (2020) The biology, function, and biomedical applications of exosomes. Science 367(6478):eaau6977

2. Théry C, Witwer KW, Aikawa E, Alcaraz MJ, Anderson JD, Andriantsitohaina R, Antoniou A, Arab T, Archer F, Atkin-Smith GK (2018) Minimal information for studies of extracellular vesicles 2018 (MISEV2018): a position statement of the International Society for Extracellular Vesicles and update of the MISEV2014 guidelines. J Extracell Vesicles 7 (1):1535750

3. Raposo G, Stoorvogel W (2013) Extracellular vesicles: exosomes, microvesicles, and friends. J Cell Biol 200(4):373–383

4. Keller S, Sanderson MP, Stoeck A, Altevogt P (2006) Exosomes: from biogenesis and secretion to biological function. Immunol Lett 107 (2):102–108

5. Théry C, Zitvogel L, Amigorena S (2002) Exosomes: composition, biogenesis and function. Nat Rev Immunol 2(8):569–579

6. Tetta C, Ghigo E, Silengo L, Deregibus MC, Camussi G (2013) Extracellular vesicles as an emerging mechanism of cell-to-cell communication. Endocrine 44(1):11–19

7. Mathieu M, Martin-Jaular L, Lavieu G, Thery C (2019) Specificities of secretion and uptake of exosomes and other extracellular vesicles for cell-to-cell communication. Nat Cell Biol 21 (1):9–17

8. Rak J (2013) Extracellular vesicles–biomarkers and effectors of the cellular interactome in cancer. Front Pharmacol 4:21

9. Vader P, Mol EA, Pasterkamp G, Schiffelers RM (2016) Extracellular vesicles for drug delivery. Adv Drug Deliv Rev 106:148–156

10. Turchinovich A, Drapkina O, Tonevitsky A (2019) Transcriptome of extracellular vesicles: state-of-the-art. Front Immunol 10:202

11. Huang X, Yuan T, Tschannen M, Sun Z, Jacob H, Du M, Liang M, Dittmar RL, Liu Y, Liang M (2013) Characterization of human plasma-derived exosomal RNAs by deep sequencing. BMC Genomics 14(1):319

12. Gezer U, Özgür E, Cetinkaya M, Isin M, Dalay N (2014) Long non-coding RNAs with low expression levels in cells are enriched in secreted exosomes. Cell Biol Int 38 (9):1076–1079

13. Dragomir M, Chen B, Calin GA (2018) Exosomal lncRNAs as new players in cell-to-cell communication. Transl Cancer Res 7(Suppl 2):S243

14. Webber J, Yeung V, Clayton A (2015) Extracellular vesicles as modulators of the cancer microenvironment. Semin Cell Dev Biol 40:27–34

15. Wendler F, Favicchio R, Simon T, Alifrangis C, Stebbing J, Giamas G (2017) Extracellular vesicles swarm the cancer microenvironment: from tumor–stroma communication to drug intervention. Oncogene 36(7):877–884

16. Bouvy C, Wannez A, Laloy J, Chatelain C, Dogné J-M (2017) Transfer of multidrug resistance among acute myeloid leukemia cells via extracellular vesicles and their microRNA cargo. Leuk Res 62:70–76

17. Sousa D, Lima RT, Vasconcelos MH (2015) Intercellular transfer of cancer drug resistance traits by extracellular vesicles. Trends Mol Med 21(10):595–608

18. Tian Y, Gong M, Hu Y, Liu H, Zhang W, Zhang M, Hu X, Aubert D, Zhu S, Wu L (2020) Quality and efficiency assessment of six extracellular vesicle isolation methods by nano-flow cytometry. J Extracell Vesicles 9 (1):1697028

19. Castellano JJ, Marrades RM, Molins L, Viñolas N, Moises J, Canals J, Han B, Li Y, Martinez D, Monzó M (2020) Extracellular vesicle lincRNA-p21 expression in tumor-draining pulmonary vein defines prognosis in NSCLC and modulates endothelial cell behavior. Cancers 12(3):734

20. Navarro A, Molins L, Marrades RM, Moises J, Viñolas N, Morales S, Canals J, Castellano JJ, Ramírez J, Monzo M (2019) Exosome analysis in tumor-draining pulmonary vein identifies NSCLC patients with higher risk of relapse after curative surgery. Cancers 11(2):249

21. Thornton B, Basu C (2011) Real-time PCR (qPCR) primer design using free online software. Biochem Mol Biol Educ 39(2):145–154

22. Untergasser A, Cutcutache I, Koressaar T, Ye J, Faircloth BC, Remm M, Rozen SG (2012) Primer3—new capabilities and interfaces. Nucleic Acids Res 40(15):e115–e115

23. Gouin K, Peck K, Antes T, Johnson JL, Li C, Vaturi SD, Middleton R, de Couto G, Walravens A-S, Rodriguez-Borlado L (2017) A comprehensive method for identification of suitable reference genes in extracellular vesicles. J Extracell Vesicles 6(1):1347019

24. Moldovan L, Batte K, Wang Y, Wisler J, Piper M (2013) Analyzing the circulating microRNAs in exosomes/extracellular vesicles from serum or plasma by qRT-PCR. Methods Mol Biol 1024:129–145

25. Crossland RE, Norden J, Bibby LA, Davis J, Dickinson AM (2016) Evaluation of optimal extracellular vesicle small RNA isolation and qRT-PCR normalisation for serum and urine. J Immunol Methods 429:39–49

26. Ibáñez F, Montesinos J, Ureña-Peralta JR, Guerri C, Pascual M (2019) TLR4 participates in the transmission of ethanol-induced neuroinflammation via astrocyte-derived extracellular vesicles. J Neuroinflammation 16(1):136

27. Lee H, Groot M, Pinilla-Vera M, Fredenburgh LE, Jin Y (2019) Identification of miRNA-rich vesicles in bronchoalveolar lavage fluid: insights into the function and heterogeneity of extracellular vesicles. J Control Release 294:43–52

28. Takahashi K, Yan IK, Kogure T, Haga H, Patel T (2014) Extracellular vesicle-mediated transfer of long non-coding RNA ROR modulates chemosensitivity in human hepatocellular cancer. FEBS Open Bio 4:458–467

29. Yuan T, Huang X, Woodcock M, Du M, Dittmar R, Wang Y, Tsai S, Kohli M, Boardman L, Patel T (2016) Plasma extracellular RNA profiles in healthy and cancer patients. Sci Rep 6:19413

30. Ragni E, Banfi F, Barilani M, Cherubini A, Parazzi V, Larghi P, Dolo V, Bollati V, Lazzari L (2017) Extracellular vesicle-shuttled mRNA in mesenchymal stem cell communication. Stem Cells 35(4):1093–1105

31. Royo F, Zuñiga-Garcia P, Torrano V, Loizaga A, Sanchez-Mosquera P, Ugalde-Olano A, González E, Cortazar AR, Palomo L, Fernández-Ruiz S (2016) Transcriptomic profiling of urine extracellular vesicles reveals alterations of CDH3 in prostate cancer. Oncotarget 7(6):6835

32. de Jong OG, Verhaar MC, Chen Y, Vader P, Gremmels H, Posthuma G, Schiffelers RM, Gucek M, van Balkom BW (2012) Cellular stress conditions are reflected in the protein and RNA content of endothelial cell-derived exosomes. J Extracell Vesicles 1(1):18396

33. Dong H, Wang W, Chen R, Zhang Y, Zou K, Ye M, He X, Zhang F, Han J (2018) Exosome-mediated transfer of lncRNA-SNHG14 promotes trastuzumab chemoresistance in breast cancer. Int J Oncol 53(3):1013–1026

34. Kang M, Ren M, Li Y, Fu Y, Deng M, Li C (2018) Exosome-mediated transfer of lncRNA PART1 induces gefitinib resistance in esophageal squamous cell carcinoma via functioning as a competing endogenous RNA. J Exp Clin Cancer Res 37(1):171

35. Tao S-C, Rui B-Y, Wang Q-Y, Zhou D, Zhang Y, Guo S-C (2018) Extracellular vesicle-mimetic nanovesicles transport LncRNA-H19 as competing endogenous RNA for the treatment of diabetic wounds. Drug Deliv 25(1):241–255

36. Bai J, Zhang Y, Zheng X, Huang M, Cheng W, Shan H, Gao X, Zhang M, Sheng L, Dai J (2020) LncRNA MM2P-induced, exosome-mediated transfer of Sox9 from monocyte-derived cells modulates primary chondrocytes. Cell Death Dis 11(9):1–13

37. Jensen J, Ørntoft T (2004) Normalization of real-time quantitative RT-PCR data: a model based variance estimation approach to identify genes suited for normalization-applied to bladder-and colon-cancer data-sets. Cancer Res 64(5245):50

38. Vandesompele J, De Preter K, Pattyn F, Poppe B, Van Roy N, De Paepe A, Speleman F (2002) Accurate normalization of real-time quantitative RT-PCR data by geometric averaging of multiple internal control genes. Genome Biol 3(7):research0034

39. Ramón-Núñez LA, Martos L, Fernández-Pardo Á, Oto J, Medina P, España F, Navarro S (2017) Comparison of protocols and RNA carriers for plasma miRNA isolation. Unraveling RNA carrier influence on miRNA isolation. PLoS One 12(10):e0187005

# Part VI

## Circular RNAs

# Chapter 21

## The Use of circRNAs as Biomarkers of Cancer

### Carla Solé, Gartze Mentxaka, and Charles H. Lawrie

## Abstract

CircRNAs are a subclass of lncRNAs that have been found to be abundantly present in a wide range of species, including humans. CircRNAs are generally produced by a noncanonical splicing event called backsplicing that is dependent on the canonical splicing machinery, giving rise to circRNAs classified into three main categories: exonic circRNA, circular intronic RNA, and exon–intron circular RNA. Notably, circRNAs possess functional importance and display their functions through different mechanisms of action including sponging miRNAs, or even being translated into functional proteins. In addition, circRNAs also have great potential as biomarkers, particularly in cancer, thanks to their high stability, tissue type and developmental stage specificity, and their presence in biological fluids, which make them promising candidates as noninvasive biomarkers. In this chapter, we describe the most commonly used techniques for the study of circRNAs as cancer biomarkers, including high-throughput techniques such as RNA-Seq and microarrays, and other methods to analyze the presence of specific circRNAs in patient samples.

**Key words** circRNA, Cancer, Biogenesis, Functions, Methodology, Biomarkers

## 1 Introduction

Although more than 90% of the human genome is transcribed, less than 1% of it encodes for proteins, with the vast majority of RNA being noncoding (ncRNA) [1–4]. NcRNA can be divided into small noncoding RNA (sncRNA) and long noncoding RNA (lncRNA), based in the length. Within the heterogeneous group of lncRNA are circRNAs, which are 5′ and 3′-end covalently linked RNA molecules [5]. CircRNAs were identified for first time by Sanger and colleagues in 1976, who identified circular RNA molecules in plant viruses [6]. Afterward, circular RNA genomes were also identified in other viruses, such as hepatitis virus [7, 8], and later in eukaryotes, with the circular transcripts of human *DCC* gene and *ETS1* gene [9, 10] and murine *Sry* gene [11]. Since this time, more than 10,000 circRNAs have been identified in a range of animals including humans [12–17].

The functional significance of circRNAs were demonstrated for first time by Salzman and colleagues who discovered that a

Alfons Navarro (ed.), *Long Non-Coding RNAs in Cancer*, Methods in Molecular Biology, vol. 2348,
https://doi.org/10.1007/978-1-0716-1581-2_21, © Springer Science+Business Media, LLC, part of Springer Nature 2021

substantial fraction of spliced transcripts identified by next-generation sequencing (NGS) of RNA (RNA-Seq) in acute lymphoblastic leukemia (ALL) cell lines were in fact circRNAs [18]. This study found similar results in other tissues and cells, and suggested that circRNAs were not uncommon oddities but rather much more abundant than first realized. Indeed, subsequent studies have shown that cirRNAs are both highly evolutionarily conserved, and in at least some cases even more abundant than their linear counterparts [19–21].

In this book chapter, we will consider the current state of knowledge of circRNA biosynthesis, functions, and methods used for their detection.

## 2    CircRNA Classification and Biogenesis

CircRNAs can be classified into three main categories according to their origin; exonic circRNA (ecircRNA) [19, 21, 22], circular intronic RNA (ciRNA) [21, 23, 24], and exon–intron circular RNA (EIcircRNA) [22, 25]. EcircRNA is by far the most abundant circRNA class accounting for 85% of all human circRNAs [21]. EcircRNAs are synthesized from one to five exons and are generally localized cytoplasmically [26]. In contrast, both EIcircRNAs and ciRNAs are predominantly found in the nucleus, and both classes of circRNAs can promote transcription of their parental genes via interaction with U1 or by regulation of RNA polymerase II [24, 27]. The nuclear export of circRNAs has been described to be dependent on the length of the circRNA and is regulated by URH49/UAP56 [28], while ciRNAs appear to be exported from the nucleus via the NXF1/NXT1 pathway [23].

CircRNAs are generally produced by a noncanonical splicing event called backsplicing that is dependent on the canonical splicing machinery [29]. Backsplicing is produced when a downstream 5′ donor site is ligated to an upstream 3′ acceptor site, resulting in a closed circular structure ligated by a 3′-5′ phosphodiester bound, a process opposite to canonical splicing (Fig. 1) [21, 26]. However, backsplicing and canonical splicing compete against each other as they are regulated by the same elements but with opposite functions [30].

Jeck and colleagues described two different models for ecircRNA formation, one known as lariat-driven circularization or exon skipping, where circularization is a result of connection between two distant donor and acceptor site with formation of intermediate lariat structure than undergo exon skipping [19]. The other termed intron pairing–driven circularization or direct backsplicing, occurs where the circular structure is formed by direct base-pairing of flanking introns with reverse complementary sequences, such as ALU repeats, followed by excision of

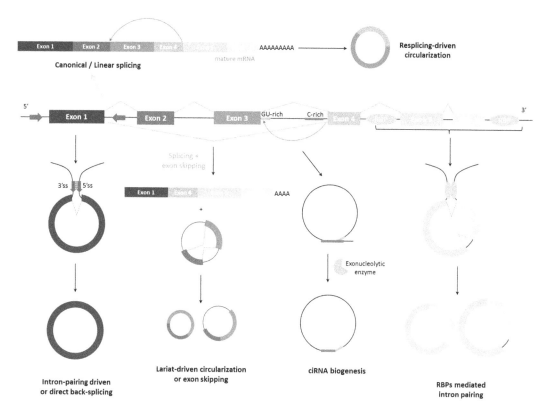

**Fig. 1** Biogenesis of circRNAs. Four different models of backsplicing have been described to explain the formation of circRNAs (ecircRNA and ElcircRNA), these are lariat-driven circularization or exon skipping; intron-pairing driven or direct backsplicing; resplicing-driven circularization; and RBPs mediated intron pairing. In addition to the model described to explain the ciRNA formation. RBP, RNA binding protein

internal introns [19, 31]. The biogenesis of ElcircRNAs can result from the same mechanisms described for ecircRNAs but in this case introns are only partially removed [27]. In addition to models proposed by Jeck, another model for ecircRNAs has been proposed, called resplicing-driven circularization, where backsplicing occurs after mature mRNA synthesis through canonical pre-mRNA splicing [32].

Unlike exon-containing circRNAs, ciRNA biogenesis depends on consensus motifs in introns, a 7 nt GU-rich sequence near to 5′ splice site and a 11 nt C-rich sequence near the branch-point site. Therefore, ciRNAs are 2′-5′ phospholipid-linked molecules instead of 3′-5′ [24].

Additionally, researchers have identified that some trans-acting RBPs (RNA binding proteins) can play an important role in the backsplicing process. The RBPs that have been described to promote circularization of exons include Quaking (QKI) [33], FUS [34], NF90/NF100 [35], the DEAD-box RNA helicase Prp5 [36] and muscleblind protein (MLB) [30]. However, some RBPs have been found to prevent circRNA biogenesis by destabilizing intron pairing interactions, such as is the case for ADAR (adenosine deaminase acting on RNA1) and DHX9 (ATP-dependent RNA helicase A) [37, 38]. Interestingly, HNRNPL (heterogeneous nuclear ribonucleoprotein L) has been described to regulate both positively or negatively backsplicing in prostate cancer [39].

## 3    Biological Function/Mechanisms of Action

In recent years numerous studies have demonstrated that circRNAs are not only splicing by-products of little functional importance but rather are important regulators of gene expression and, more recently, key modulators of protein function. Until recently, circRNA functions were believed to be restricted to their RNA moiety [40, 41]; however, several recent studies suggest that at least some circRNAs can also be translated into proteins to realize their function [42–45].

### 3.1    miRNA sponges

The majority of studies to date have focused on the ability of circRNA to act as *sponges* of miRNAs, thereby indirectly regulating gene expression. Some circRNAs contain miRNA response elements (MREs) that bind to specific miRNAs, thereby sequestering them and diminishing miRNA binding capacity to its target mRNAs acting as competing endogenous RNAs (ceRNAs) otherwise known as miRNA sponges [21, 42]. Multiple characteristics can affect the effectiveness of this regulatory mechanism including the number of binding sites in the circRNA for the same miRNA [41, 46], the abundance of the circRNA [47], the number of target genes of the sponged miRNA [48] or the affinity of the miRNA for the circRNA compared to the affinity for its target gene [21].

*CiRS-7*, *circ-SRY*, and *circHIPK3* are some of the best characterized circRNAs that act as ceRNAs, sponging *miR-7*, *miR-138*, and *miR-124* respectively, inhibiting their activity and consequently upregulating their cognate target mRNAs [21, 41, 46, 47]. Subsequently, many more circRNAs have been demonstrated to display miRNA sponge activity [49–53]. However, it is important to note that the vast majority of circRNAs do not contain MREs, suggesting that whilst miRNA sponging is the most commonly studied function it may not be the most prevalent in this class of ncRNAs [41, 46, 54].

### 3.2    Effect on alternative splicing

The production of circRNAs derived from exons can lead to an impaired splicing of the precursor mRNA, leading to changes in gene expression of different isoforms [30, 31, 55]. In fact, a negative correlation between splicing efficiency and circRNA biogenesis has been demonstrated suggesting competition between circRNA biogenesis and canonical splicing [30, 56]. In some cases, high levels of circRNA can completely displace the linear form of their mRNA [26, 57]. This competition takes place at least in part through RNA Pol II activity. It has been demonstrated that a mutation in RNA Pol II that increases splicing efficiency also significantly reduces the numbers of circRNAs [30, 56]. Moreover, RNA Pol II elongation rate and efficiency of linear splicing are inversely correlated [58], and circRNA-producing genes were found to be transcribed at a faster-than-average rate [59]. These observations indicate that backsplicing is dependent on mechanisms that delay or otherwise compromise linear splicing at circRNA loci [54]. However, it is unclear how RNA Pol II is modulated for the production of circRNAs [60]. In addition, circRNA-forming exons are often surrounded by unusually long introns in which splicing is thought to be less efficient [30, 54, 56].

### 3.3  Effect on Protein Translation/mRNA Tramps

In the case where an ecircRNA contains an initiation codon and instead of translation results in circularization of the noncoding transcript this can result in a reduction in the expression level of the corresponding protein [57]. This for example has been shown to be the case for the *Fmn* transcript [57]. A study of circRNA in patients with a dystrophinopathy showed that ecircRNA arising from the *DMD* gene may lead to inactive transcripts thereby reducing the pool of mRNAs that can be translated and enhancing the disease phenotype in these patients [61]. Indeed, it has been observed in human fibroblasts that 34% of ecircRNAs contain a translation start, suggesting widespread prevalence of this mechanism [26, 57].

### 3.4  circRNAs as regulators of transcription

Unlike ecircRNAs, which are mostly located in the cytoplasm, intron-containing circRNAs (i.e., EIciRNAs and ciRNAs) are mainly distributed in the nucleus and play a crucial role as regulators of transcription through direct modulation of gene expression. EIciRNAs such as *circ-EIF3J* and *circ-PAIP2*, can bind to U1 snRNP in the nucleus to form EIciRNA-U1 snRNP complexes. The complexes can interact with RNA Pol II in the promoter region of genes, therefore enhancing the transcription of their parental genes [27, 62, 63]. Similar to EIciRNA, ciRNAs such as *ci-ankrd52* and *ci-sirt7* also can stimulate the transcription of their parental genes, *ANKRD52* and *SIRT7* respectively, by upregulating the activity of RNA polymerase II [24]. Recently, analysis of differentially expressed circRNAs and their parental genes using an Alzheimer's disease mouse model suggested that abundant circRNAs could regulate parental gene transcription, although the mechanism remains unclear [64].

CircRNAs can also modulate gene expression through epigenetic mechanisms. For example, *circFECR1*, an *FLI1* ecircRNA, utilizes a positive feedback mechanism to activate FLI1 by recruiting *TET1* demethylase to induce DNA demethylation in the CpG islands [65]. Concurrently, circFECR1 also binds to and downregulates in trans DNMT1, a methyltransferase that is essential for the maintenance of DNA methylation.

**3.5 Interaction with proteins**

CircRNAs can also directly bind to several RNA binding proteins (RBPs), and these interactions have been reported to influence protein expression, location, and pathophysiological processes [66, 67].

It has been shown that circRNA can competitively bind to RBPs and effectively act as protein sponges. For example, *circ-Foxo3* can bind and sequester the antisenescence proteins ID-1 and E2F1 as well as antistress proteins FAK and HIF-1α, preventing their nuclear translocation and therefore inhibiting their function [21, 30, 68, 69]. In addition, *CircANRIL* binds to PES1, an essential 60S-preribosomal assembly factor, thereby impairing pre-rRNA processing and ribosome biogenesis [70]. Moreover, *circ-PABPN1* has been reported to bind to HuR protein, which prevents HuR binding to PABPN1 mRNA and lowers PABPN1 translation [71]. This study provides an example of competition between a circRNA and its cognate mRNA for an RBP that affects translation.

CircRNAs have also shown protein decoy functions, cooperating with the target protein to change the protein's routine physiological function [60, 72]. These interactions usually involve protein translocations, thereby changing the protein transporter characteristics of the circRNA. For instance, *circ-Amotl1* is able to bind and translocate c-Myc, Akt1, and Stat3 to the nucleus, causing the upregulation of its target genes [73, 74]. Another example is *circ-DNMT1*, which promotes P53 and AUF1 nuclear translocation in breast cancer cells. Nuclear translocation of p53 induced cellular autophagy while AUF1 nuclear translocation reduced Dnmt1 mRNA instability, resulting in increased Dnmt1 translation [75]. Additionally, *circMYBL2* regulates FLT3 translation by recruiting PTBP1 to promote internal tandem duplication of the FLT3 gene during acute myeloid leukemia progression [76]. Subsequent studies have shown the widespread nature of circRNA-protein interactions [77–87].

**3.6 Protein Production**

Due to the absence of 5′ and 3′ ends, circRNAs were initially considered as noncoding RNAs. However, recently evidence has been mounting that at least some circRNAs can be translated in a cap-independent manner, producing functional proteins [26, 43, 44, 66, 88–91].

It was initially reported that circRNAs with an internal ribosome entry site (IRES) were able to synthesized polypeptides in a cap-independent manner [88]. Some of the IRES containing-circRNAs that have been found to be translated are *circ-ZNF609*, *circ-MBL* and circ-*FBXW7* [43, 45, 89]. It has been demonstrated that *circ-ZNF609* depends on N6-methyladenosine (m6A) modification to be translated [92]. Through recognition of m6A, YTHDF3 and eIF4G2 physically associate with the endogenous *circ-ZNF609* and enable its translation. Interestingly, researchers have found that a variety of sequences can function as IRESs to drive circRNA translation and that a single m6A site is sufficient to drive translation initiation, requiring eIF4G2 and YTHDF3 factors [26, 43, 44, 66, 88–91]. High-throughput m6A-seq indicates that at least 13% of circRNAs carry m6A modification, and 250 circRNAs have been found to be associated with polysomes, indicating that at least a fraction of circRNAs may have actively translation potential [26, 43, 44, 66, 88–91].

Recent studies indicate that proteins produced by circRNAs are functional and play important roles in physiological and pathological processes. CircRNA derived peptides are often truncated versions of the canonical proteins that may act as dominant-negative protein variants, decoys, or modulators of alternative protein complexes [43, 45, 89, 93]. For example, the protein produced by *circ-FBXW7* (FBXW7-185aa) competes with FBXW7 protein to bind USP28, an inhibitor of c-myc degradation, inhibiting proliferation and cell cycle acceleration in glioblastoma [43, 45, 89]. More examples of functional peptides translated form circRNA can be found in the literature [94–98].

## 4    circRNAs as cancer biomarkers

In addition to the different biological functions described above, circRNAs also have great potential as biomarkers, particularly in cancer, as they have many advantageous characteristics when compared to other RNA species. Firstly, they are dysregulated in cancerous tissues compared to noncancerous tissues [21]. Moreover, circRNAs display cell type and developmental stage-specific expression pattern [21, 22, 27]. Secondly circRNAs are very stable, with a higher half-life than linear transcripts, exceeding 48h compared with <20h for linear transcripts [19]. This stability, due to lack of free 5′ and 3′ ends, makes them resistant to RNA exonucleases [99], and furthermore makes them particularly promising candidates as noninvasive biomarkers. In blood, the biological fluid most studied, circRNAs have been described to have 15-fold higher expression than liver tissue, with expression levels comparable to circRNA-rich cerebellum [100]. Li Y and colleagues were first to describe the presence of circRNAs in serum exosomes and its usefulness as a biomarker to distinguish cancer patients [101]. Recently, several reports are focused in circulating circRNAs, and they found that changes in expression in biofluids could serve as potential noninvasive biomarkers in hepatocellular, bladder, lung, gastric, and colorectal cancer, among others [102–106].

Nowadays many studies have been focused on the role of circRNAs in cancer and their potential use as biomarkers. It has been described that deregulated circRNAs in cancer have effect on tumor cell proliferation [107, 108], inhibition of cell apoptosis [109, 110], promoting migration, invasion, and angiogenesis [111, 112]. CircRNAs regulates these cancer hallmarks through regulation of important signaling pathways, such as Wnt/beta-catenin [113, 114], MAPK/ERK [115], and PI3K/AKT pathways [116].

### 4.1 Commonly Dysregulated Cancer-Associated circRNAs

Many of the circRNAs studied to date are found to be dysregulated in multiple cancer types (Table 1). At this stage in the field it is not clear whether this is because they are the circRNAs most studied or whether those circRNAs are truly the most commonly dysregulated in cancer.

One of most studied deregulated circRNA in cancer is *CDR1as*, also known as *ciRS-7*, arises from the antisense sequence of cerebellar degeneration related protein 1 (*CDR1as*) gene. Until recently the linear counterpart of this circRNA was elusive with various studies suggesting that it only existed as a circular molecule [21, 42]. However, recently it has been described that *CDR1as* is embedded in an upstream lncRNA (*LINC00632*) and linear splicing products of this gene also contains *CDR1as* [117, 118]. *CDR1as* contain multiple sites of binding for *miR-7* [21, 42], and this circRNA has been shown to regulate levels of *miR-7* in many cancers including gastric, breast, and lung cancers [115, 119–130].

*CDR1as* is generally found to be upregulated in tumor cells compared to nontumor cells as can be seen is Table 1. Meta-analysis of many of these studies have demonstrated that *CDR1as* has great potential as a diagnostic biomarker for many solid tumors including esophageal squamous cell carcinoma (ESCC), non–small-cell lung cancer (NSCLC), osteosarcoma, laryngeal squamous cell carcinoma (LSCC), cervical squamous cell carcinoma (CESC), cholangiocarcinoma, colorectal cancer (CRC), digestive system cancer, hepatocellular cancer (HCC), and triple-negative breast cancer (TNBC) [131]. The authors of this study further found that patients with higher expression of CDR1as had worse overall survival (OS), and demonstrated the usefulness of this circRNA as a prognostic biomarker in ESCC, NSCLC, LSCC, cholangiocarcinoma, CRC, digestive system cancer, HCC, and gastric cancer (GC). Another meta-analysis study reached similar conclusions for NSCLC, CRC, and GC, and extended the analysis to show a correlation between higher expression of *CDR1as* with increasing tumor stage and OS [132]. Other studies demonstrated that higher *CDR1as* expression is associated with higher tumor stage, lymph node metastasis, and poor OS for patients with GC, NSCLC, and CRC [115, 121, 122, 133, 134], and also with the presence of

**Table 1**
CircRNAs that are dysregulated in multiple cancer types

| circRNA | Cancer type | Biomarker type | Tumor expression | Biopsy source | Cohort size | Diag. power (AUC) | Detect. method | Ref |
|---|---|---|---|---|---|---|---|---|
| CDR1as/ ciRS-7 | CRC | Prog. | Up | T | 500 | | RT | [132] |
| | | Diag./Prog. | Up | T | 80/500 | 0.68 | RT | [131] |
| | | Diag./Prog. | Up | T | 40/318 | | RT | [122] |
| | | Diag./Prog. | Up | T | 40/182 | | RT | [134] |
| | ESCC | Prog. | Up | T | 209 | | RT | [132] |
| | | Diag./Prog. | Up | T | 337 vs. 319 / 173 | 0.66 | RT | [131] |
| | GC | Prog. | Up | T | 256 | | RT | [131, 132] |
| | | Diag./Prog. | Up | T | 102 / 154 | | RT | [115] |
| | NSCLC | Prog. | Up | T | 320 | | RT | [132] |
| | | Diag./Prog. | Up | T | 192 vs. 152 / 320 | 0.83 | RT | [131] |
| | | Diag./Prog. | Up | T | 128 | | RT | [133] |
| | | Diag./Prog. | Up | T | 60 | | RT | [121] |
| | CHOL | Diag./Prog. | Up | T | 54 | 0.86 | RT | [131, 230] |
| | TNBC | Diag. | Up | T | 32 | 0.98 | RT | [131, 231] |
| | CESC | Diag. | Up | T | 40 | 0.8 | RT | [131] |
| | HCC | Diag./Prog. | Up | T | 81 / 95 | 0.71 | RT | [131, 232] |
| | LSCC | Diag./Prog. | Up | T | 30 | 0.98 | RT | [131, 233] |
| | Melanoma | Prog. | Down | T | 105 | | RT | [118] |
| | Osteosarcoma | Diag. | Up | T | 38 vs. 18 | 0.86 | RT | [131, 234] |
| | OVC | Diag./Pred. | Down | S (exo) | 66 vs. 60 | | MC, RT | [135] |
| | | Pred. | Down | | 66 | | MC, RT | [135] |
| | NPC | Diag./Prog. | Up | T | 44 vs. 20 | | RT | [125] |
| HIPK3 | Glioma | Diag./Prog. | Up | T | 48 | | RT | [137] |
| | GC | Diag./Prog. | Up | T | 30 | 0.74 | MC, RT | [138] |
| | PA | Diag./Prog. | Up | T | 63 | | MC, RT | [139] |
| | | Diag./Prog./ Pred. | Up | T | 28 | | RT | [140] |
| | EOC | Diag./Prog. | Up | T | 69 | | RT | [141] |
| | CRC | Diag./Prog. | Up | T | 178 vs. 40 | | RT | [142] |
| | | Prog./Pred. | Up | T | 179 / 49 | | RT | [143] |
| | Prostate cancer | Diag./Prog. | Up | T | 26 | | RT | [144] |

(continued)

**Table 1**
**(continued)**

| circRNA | Cancer type | Biomarker type | Tumor expression | Biopsy source | Cohort size | Diag. power (AUC) | Detect. method | Ref |
|---|---|---|---|---|---|---|---|---|
| | Bladder cancer | Diag./Prog. | Down | T | 47 | | RNAseq, RT | [145] |
| | | Diag./Prog./Pred. | Down | T | 68 | | MC, RT | [146] |
| | Osteosarcoma | Diag./Prog. | Down | T | 82 | | RT | [147] |
| | | Diag. | Down | P | 50 vs. 10 | 0.783 | RT | [147] |
| CircITCH | OVC | Diag./Prog. | Down | T | 250 | | RT | [148] |
| | | Diag./Prog. | Down | T | 45 | | RT | [149] |
| | Bladder cancer | Diag./Prog. | Down | T | 72/70 | | RT | [151] |
| | Glioma | Diag./Prog. | Down | T | 60 | 0.757 | RT | [151] |
| | OSCC | Diag./Prog. | Down | T | 103 | | RT | [152] |
| | Prostate cancer | Diag./Prog. | Down | T | 52 | | RT | [153] |
| | PTC | Diag./Prog. | Down | T | 51 vs. 28 | | RT | [154] |
| | CRC | Diag. | Down | T | 45 | | RT | [113] |
| | Cervical cancer | Diag. | Down | T | 28 | | RT | [235] |
| | Osteosarcoma | Diag. | Down | T | 22 | | RT | [236] |
| | RCC | Diag. | Up | T | 25 | | RT | [157] |
| | CRC | Diag. | Down | T | 20 | | RT | [155] |
| | Colon cancer | Diag./Prog. | Down | T | 87 | | RT | [98] |
| | Bladder cancer | Diag./Prog. | Down | T | 56 / 82 | | RT | [156] |
| | PTC | Diag./Prog. | Up | T | 42 | | RT | [159] |
| | | Diag. | Up | S (exo) | 42 vs.40 | 0.891 | RT | [159] |
| | GC | Diag./Prog. | Down | T | 50 | | MC, RT | [160] |
| | NSCLC | Diag./Prog. | Down | T | 50 | | RT | [161] |
| | Retinoblastoma | Diag./Prog. | Down | T | 60 vs. 6 | | RT | [162] |

| | | | | Cohort size | AUC | Detect. | Ref. |
|---|---|---|---|---|---|---|---|
| HCC | Diag./Prog. | Down | T | 84 | | RT | [163] |
| | Diag./Prog. | Down | T | 89 | 0.63 | RT | [164] |
| CHOL | Diag./Prog. | Down | T | 76 | | RT | [165] |
| PA | Diag./Prog. | Up | T | 60 | | RT | [166] |
| Glioma | Diag./Prog. | Up | T | 35 vs. 35 | | RT | [167] |
| Osteosarcoma | Diag./Prog. | Up | T | 57 | | RT | [168] |
| CRC | Diag./Prog. | Up | T | 60 | | RT | [169] |
| | Diag./Prog | Up | T | 33 | | MC, RT | [237] |
| Cervical cancer | Diag. | Up | T | 45 | | RT | [238] |
| Breast cancer | Diag. | Up | T | 40 | | RT | [239] |

Cohort size, for tissue biopsies numbers reflect paired sample from cancer and control tissues; and for liquid biopsies numbers refer to cancer samples. Bars are used to separate Diag./Prog./Pred. cohort sizes. When only one number is shown the same sample size was used for the different analyses

Abbreviations: T: Tissue, S: Serum, Exo: Exosomes, Diag.: Diagnostic, Prog.: Prognostic, Pred.: Predictive, AUC: Area Under the Curve, Detect.: Detection, MA: Microarray, RT: qRT-PCR. CRC: Colorectal cancer, ESCC: esophageal squamous cell carcinoma, GC: gastric cancer, NSCLC: non-small-cell lung cancer, CHOL: cholangiocarcinoma, TNBC: triple-negative breast cancer, CESC: cervical squamous cell carcinoma, HCC: hepatocellular carcinoma, LSCC: laryngeal squamous cell carcinoma, OVC: ovarian cancer, NPC: nasopharyngeal carcinoma, PA: pancreatic cancer; EOC: epithelial ovarian cancer. OSCC: Oral squamous cell carcinoma, PTC: papillary thyroid carcinoma, RCC: Renal cell carcinoma

distant metastasis in GC and CRC cases [115, 122]. In contrast, a low abundance of *CDR1as* was associated with shorter progression-free survival (PFS) and OS in melanoma and with OS in low-grade glioma [118]. Similarly in ovarian cancer downregulation of *CDR1as* was observed and *CDR1as* levels in serum-derived exosomes were found to be lower in cisplatin-resistant patients [135].

*CircHIPK3* is another circRNA widely studied and present in different types of cancer, which derived from chromosomal region 11p13 and originating from exon 2 of the *HIPK3* gene [47]. A recent meta-analysis found that abnormal expression (high or low) of *circHIPK2* was significantly correlated with unfavorable OS and disease-free survival (DFS)/progression-free survival (PFS) in cancer patients, and its expression was related to distal metastasis [136].

*CircHIPK3* has been described to be mostly upregulated as is the cases in cancers including glioma, gastric, pancreatic, ovarian, colorectal, and prostate cancer [137–144]. *CircHIPK3* expression in gastric and prostate cancer has been related with tumor stage [138, 139, 144], and in glioma and pancreatic cancer high expression of circHIPK3 was linked to poor prognosis [137, 140]. High expression of *HIPK3* is an independent prognostic marker un ovarian cancer and colorectal cancer [141, 142]. Moreover, in colorectal cancer level of circHIPK3 also correlated with tumor size, lymph node metastasis, distant metastasis, and recurrence [143], and it has been described to discriminate between responders and nonresponders to oxiplatin-based chemotherapy and also is an independent factor for DFS and OS in patients that received oxiplatin-based chemotherapy after surgery [143].

However, similar to *CDR1a*, in cancers including bladder cancer and osteosarcoma, *circHIPK3* is downregulated [145–147]. In bladder cancer expression was correlated with grade, invasion, lymph node metastasis, gemcitabine insensitivity and OS [145, 146]. In osteosarcoma its expression was correlated with stage, age, gender, tumor location, and the presence of lung metastasis. The authors also showed that plasma *circHIPK3* could be used as an indicator for diagnosis [147].

*Circ-ITCH* is a circRNA located on human chromosome 20 that originates from the protein-coding gene I*TCH* that spans 1-5 exons [21]. Most commonly, it is found to be downregulated in cancer and is proposed to act as a tumor suppressor For example, in ovarian cancer levels of circ-ITCH were lower in tumor cells and s positively correlated with OS in patients [148, 149]. A similar correlation has been observed in bladder cancer, glioma, oral squamous cell carcinoma, and prostate cancer [150–153], and in glioma papillary thyroid cancer this circRNA has been identified as an independent prognostic marker [151, 154].

Like *circ-ITCH, circFNDC3B* is commonly found to be down-regulated in cancer including in tissue of colon, colorectal, and bladder cancers [98, 155, 156]. *CircFNDC3B* originates from exons 5 and 6 of FNDC3B gene located in chromosome 3 [156–158]. Expression levels of *circFNDC3B* correlated with stage in bladder cancer and papillary thyroid cancer [156, 159], while correlated with lymph node metastasis and survival in colon cancer, bladder cancer, and papillary thyroid cancer [98, 156, 159]. Specifically, in gastric cancer low expression of *circFNDC3B* correlated with lymph node metastasis, nerve invasion, tumor recurrence, and death of patients, and also to low PFS and OS [160]. In colon cancer *circFNDC3B* has been defined as an independent prognostic factor [98].

*Circ_0001649* is another circRNAs that is down-regulated in multiple cancer types [161–165]. Expression of this circRNA was correlated with advanced stage in NSCLC and retinoblastoma [161, 162], with grade of differentiation in hepatocellular carcinoma and cholangiocarcinoma [163, 165], with tumor size in hepatocellular carcinoma and cholangiocarcinoma [164, 165], and with lymph node metastasis in NSCLC [161]. Patients with low levels of *circ_0001649* have shorter OS in NSCLC and retinoblastoma, and in both cases expression was found to be an independent prognostic factor [161, 162]. In addition, *circ_0007534* has been shown to be upregulated in several cancers including pancreatic cancer and glioma [166, 167], and the grade of differentiation in osteosarcoma [168], tumor size in osteosarcoma and colorectal cancer [168, 169], and lymph node metastasis in pancreatic cancer and colorectal cancer [166, 169]. Moreover, patients with high expression of *circ_0007534* showed lower survival (OS) in pancreatic cancer, osteosarcoma, and colorectal cancer [166, 168, 169], specifically in pancreatic cancer and osteosarcoma *circ_0007534* has been defined as an independent prognostic marker after surgery [166, 168].

## 5    Discovering and analyzing circRNAs

Increasing interest in the study of circRNAs associated with cancer has equally led to the increasing development of specific tools for circRNA analysis to determine the sequence, expression, subcellular localization, and biological function in pathological and physiological conditions. Below we describe the most commonly used techniques for the study of circRNAs and the advantages and disadvantages of each of them (Fig. 2).

### 5.1    RNA-Seq

At present, the most widely used method for large-scale identification of circRNAs is massive RNA sequencing, also known as RNA-Seq. This technique, based on next-generation sequencing

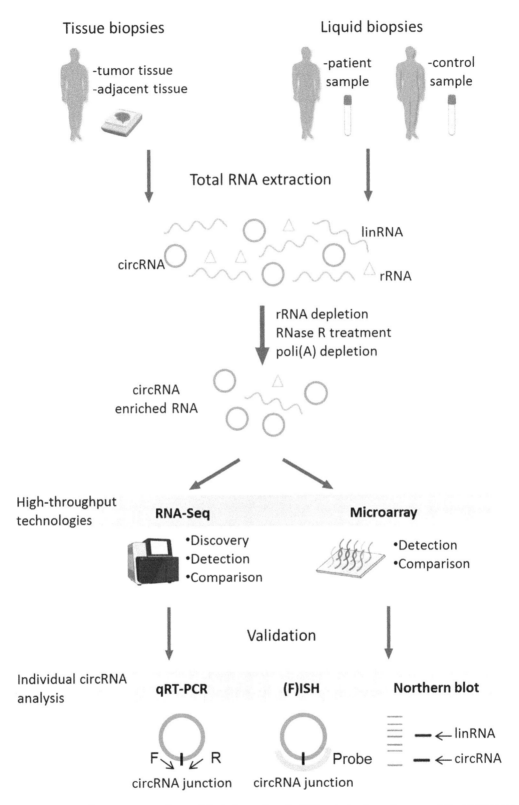

**Fig. 2** Summary of most commonly used techniques for circRNAs study, from tissue and liquid biopsies. Workflow starts with a circRNA enrichment of the sample and then high-throughput technologies, such as RNAseq or circ-Microarray, followed by individual circRNAs analysis, such as qRT-PCR, (F)ISH, and northern blot analysis, among others.

(NGS), has the advantage of potentially identifying novel circRNAs as it requires no a priori sequence information unlike hybridization-based techniques (e.g., microarrays and qRT-PCR). The first step is to perform total RNA extraction, as opposed to mRNA or miRNA extraction, and is usually performed using the TRIzol reagent or similar. In the case of liquid biopsies such as blood, saliva or urine generally a specialized total RNA purification kit such as those available from Norgen or Qiagen are used.

In order to prepare the library for circRNA-Seq a number of modifications are required to the general protocols used for RNA-Seq as these protocols usually contain enrichment steps for either the removal of non-poly(A) RNA or contain a size selection and linearization step that would preclude the inclusion of circRNAs. RNase R treatment is frequently used in circRNA-Seq library preparation as this RNase is specific to linear RNA [19, 22, 26, 31, 41, 170]. Caution should be used when treating RNA with RNase R as some circRNAs can be degraded and conversely some linear RNAs with secondary structures are resistant to treatment [19, 26, 31, 41, 170, 171]. Specifically, it has been found that RNase R is unable to fully digest protein-coding mRNAs with G-quadruplex (G4) structures, as the enzyme stalls within these sections of the transcripts [171]. This problem has been partially overcome by replacing $K^+$ (which stabilizes G4s) with $Li^+$ in the reaction buffer, enabling RNase R to proceed through these sequences and fully degrade the mRNAs [171]. It is also important to bear in mind that RNase treatment can introduce biochemical variability resulting in important differences between RNase R-treated replicates [172]. An improvement to the standard treatment has been developed with circRNA-Seq in mind, "RNase R treatment followed Poly(A) tailing and poly(A) Depletion" (RPAD). RPAD consists of a combination of techniques, starting with the treatment of total RNA with RNase R to remove linear RNA, followed by artificial polyadenylation to detect resistant linear RNA from the previous treatment, and finally by removal of the polyadenylated RNA using beads [173, 174].

After RNA extraction and library preparation followed by NGS the resulting data needs to be analyzed bioinformatically. The obtained reads, usually in fastq format, are first QC-ed and trimmed to remove adaptor sequences and the resulting reads are aligned against the reference transcriptome, firstly to remove non-circRNA sequences but also to identify potential circRNAs from the data most commonly on the basis of the splice junction. Consequently, a number of specialist pipelines have been developed specifically for the identification of circRNAs from NGS data including find_circ [21], circRNA_finder [170], CIRCexplorer [31], CIRI [175], and NCLscan [176], among others [177, 178]. Most of these algorithms and analysis pipelines can detect exonic, intronic, and intergenic circRNAs, whereas CIRCfinder is a pipeline designed to exclusively detect intronic circRNAs [24]. All of these tools work at different efficiencies to balance false positives and false negatives and as a result can be defined as stringent or flexible and the choice of either approach depends on the nature of the original hypothesis [179]. A stringent detection approach, such as NCLScan, reduces the amount of false-positives but can also overlook novel circRNA identification [176]. A flexible detection approach, such as CIRI2 [180] and CIRCexplorer [31], are useful for discovery of novel circRNAs but can also generate false positives.

Although RNA-Seq has the advantage of allowing for de novo identification of circRNAs it has several drawbacks, not least of all the high cost and necessity for high-level, high maintenance infrastructure and equipment that is beyond the means of many. Moreover, even when RNA-Seq data is readily available to the researcher, often the bottleneck is the bioinformatic analysis for which there are not yet standardized methods. Indeed, although several specific circRNA-Seq algorithms do exist, they were developed using distinct alignment methodologies and heuristic, leading to highly different and divergent results [172, 181–183]. Hansen and colleagues compared different algorithms with the same RNA-Seq datasets and obtained dramatic differences between the algorithms; specifically for highly expressed circRNAs and circRNAs derived from proximal splice sites, they proposed that the best approach is to combine different algorithms to achieve reliable predictions [182].

**5.2  Microarrays**

After circRNA-Seq, the use of specialized microarrays is the most common discovery tool used in circRNA studies, and one that is gaining popularity as more platforms become commercially available. Such microarrays contain predesigned probes based around circRNAs junction sequences. As with RNA-Seq, samples of total RNA used in microarrays are generally previously treated with RNase R in combination with enzymatic linear RNA removal to reduce the presence of linear RNA and enhance circRNA detection [71, 107, 184]. Then the RNA is retrotranscribed and labeled in a random primer-based system. RNA samples are incubated on the microarray support, which provides information about which circRNAs are present in the sample and at what level of expression [185–187]. Some of the microarray platforms available that are being used for circRNA analysis include those from Arraystar Technologies [188, 189], KangChen Bio-tech [52, 190], and Capital-Bio Technology [191–193].

Microarray technology has the advantage that it does not require complex bioinformatic analyses as is the case with RNA-Seq. On the other hand, to perform a microarray assay requires the knowledge of the junction sequence a priori; therefore, the technique does not identify novel circRNAs. Moreover, as microarrays are based on splice-junction sequence they do not reveal information about full sequence of circRNAs detected, nor about the number of circRNA transcripts with the same junction [172].

**5.3  qRT-PCR**

This approach is probably one of the most widely used methods to validate the presence of specific circRNAs in cancer samples or cell lines (Table 1). Primarily due to the fact that is a technique that can easily be incorporated in the current workflow of most molecular laboratories. qRT-PCR for circRNAs is performed using divergent primers, unlike primers used for linear RNA, spanning the circRNA junction, so only circRNA will be detected. For this propose, CircInteractome and circPrimer, online resources, could be used to design divergent primers [194, 195]. However, some linear RNA could contain the same sequence as backsplice junctions, generating false positives; these linear RNAs are derived from uncommon events such as trans-splicing, tandem duplications, and reverse transcriptase template switching [26, 196].

Use of RT-qPCR allows for a quantitative estimation of circRNA levels present in the sample [101, 197, 198]. Typically qRT-PCR is performed using SYBR Green approach to detect circRNAs in most of studies carried out to date [198, 199], although Taqman assays have also been used [200, 201]. Roschow H. and colleagues showed that integrity of total RNA affected the accuracy of RT-qPCR expression analysis of circRNAs, similar to mRNA in degraded RNA samples, so they proposed that RNA integrity has to be assessed to obtain reliable circRNA expression data [202]. In addition, the choice of which endogenous control for use in circRNA qRT-PCR remains controversial. Although *β-actin*, *GAPDH*, or *18S* are frequently used as reference genes to normalize circRNA expression between samples [198], when RNase R treatment is used to treat samples prior to qRT-PCR these linear RNAs could/should be removed from the total RNA and if present are unlikely to be stable between samples. Recently, there have been attempts to define a stably expressed circRNA that could serve as a control gene for circRNA expression. The authors of this study found that *circ_0000471* and *circ_0000284* were the most stably expressed circRNA between various cancer and normal tissues and cell lines [203]. However, these results have yet to be independently verified and this remains a contentious issue for the use of qRT-PCR when studying circRNA expression.

In addition to measuring the relative expression levels by qRT-PCR the resulting amplicon can be directly sequenced to verify the presence of backsplicing sequence and to reveal the complete sequence of circRNA [204].

For RT-qPCR analysis is important to avoid potential technical artifacts such as differences in size exclusion protocols and sensitivity of circRNAs to RNase R [19, 22, 170], presence of backsplice sequences that are wrongly identified as circRNAs [205–207], rolling circle amplification or ligation of two independent cDNAs [208, 209], and assessment of RNA integrity and choice of stable and reliable endogenous controls for samples [198, 202, 203].

Similar to qRT-PCR, some authors have used digital droplet PCR (ddPCR) as an alternative technique that has the advantage of providing absolute quantification (i.e., copy number) without the need for a control gene [210, 211]. Moreover, ddPCR is more accurate and has a higher sensitivity than qRT-PCR, although associated reagent and equipment costs are much higher than traditional qRT-PCR [204, 212].

## 5.4 Northern blot

The northern blot technique consists of the size separation of RNA by gel electrophoresis followed by the transfer of RNA to a membrane through capillarity or electrical force. The transferred RNA is immobilized through covalent linkage by UV light or baking and then a (radio)labeled probe against specific RNA sequence is hybridized to the membrane and detected according to the probe type [27, 213]. Several studies have used this technique for circRNA detection [214, 215]. Northern blot analysis for circRNA detection is based on short probes the span the circular splice junction or longer probes complementary to entire circRNA, such as the probe that was used for *circHIPK3* detection [47]. This last option is particularly useful if the backsplice junction sequence is not specific only for circRNA as previously mentioned [26, 196]. In some cases, northern blot analysis can be used to distinguish between circRNA and its normal counterpart as circRNA tend to run more slowly relative to linear markers in denaturing polyacrylamide gels. However, polyacrylamide gels are only suitable for only circRNAs of up to 1 kb, while agarose gels can be used for circRNAs from 0.2 kb to several kilobases, but in the latter case cannot distinguish between circular and linear RNA forms [216]. Unlike the other techniques mentioned above northern blotting has poor sensitivity and requires large (μg) amounts of RNA so may not be suitable for studies where material is limited. Another disadvantage of the northern blot is that only one or a few circRNAs can be analyzed at any one time and this technique is not valid for medium or high-throughput analysis.

## 5.5 FISH

Fluorescence in situ hybridization (FISH) coupled to high-resolution microscopy is a powerful method for detecting specific circRNAs and analyzing their subcellular localization. The detection of circRNAs using FISH relies on the high stability of RNA–DNA hybrid molecules that form in the presence of formamide, and in an appropriate probe design against the circRNA junction sequence. Ideally, there should be 22–24 nucleotides complementary to either sides of the junction in order to avoid off-target hybridization, and the GC content of the probe needs to fall between 40% and 60% [217]. The major drawback of this technique is that it relies on the limited options for probe design, which necessarily has to span the circRNA junction, making sometimes difficult to fulfil probe design requirements. Even so, several circRNAs have been successfully analyzed by FISH, such as *circLARP4* [218], *circYAP1* [219], circDLST [220], or *circ_001783* [221]. Recent advances in RNA FISH have increased the specificity and sensitivity of the method to enable the detection of individual RNA molecules (single-molecule FISH). This technique has been used to visualize circRNA *CDR1as* [222]. Apart from fluorescent probes, circRNAs can also be biotin-labeled and detected via colorimetric assays [97, 223].

## 5.6 Assessing the value of circRNAs as cancer biomarkers

In addition to validating whether or not a particular circRNA is dysregulated in cancer, its suitability as a diagnostic biomarker needs to be assessed. To determine the diagnostic predictive value of a particular circRNA for a specific cancer, the receiver operating characteristic (ROC) curve has to be analyzed [224, 225]. The ROC curve is created by plotting the true positive rate (or sensitivity), against the false positive rate (or specificity) at various threshold settings. Then, the area under the curve (AUC) is calculated to obtain a value between 0.5 and 1. The higher the AUC value, the better the model is at discriminating between patients with a disease and healthy controls [224].

In addition to diagnostic biomarkers, circRNAs can also act as prognostic biomarkers. To assess the prognostic value of a particular circRNA, a cohort of patients is divided in two groups based on their level of the circRNA expression, and the Kaplan–Meier curves regarding their overall survival and/or recurrence-free survival (RFS) and/or disease-free survival (DFS) are drawn [226]. To determine if the curve of patients with high circRNA expression and the curve of patients with low circRNA expression are significantly different, the log-rank test is used [227]. To further demonstrate that the level of expression of a specific circRNA constitutes an independent prognostic factor for the survival of patients, a multivariate analysis is performed. In this analysis, other relevant clinical variables that may be affecting the patients' survival, apart from the expression level of the circRNA, need to be included [228].

# 6    Summary and Future Perspectives

The identification of circRNAs and their association with cancer continues growing as do the number of publications in this field, demonstrating the potential usefulness of circRNAs as both regulators and biomarkers. CircRNAs with biomarker potential have been readily found in tumor tissue but also in liquid biopsies (serum, plasma, saliva, etc.), which represents a great opportunity to use circRNAs as noninvasive biomarkers for cancer. Some cir-cRNAs where found to be deregulated in several types of cancer, such *CDR1as* or *Circ-ITCH,* among others (Table 1), suggesting that these circRNAs are important factors in cancer development. However, this does make them any less interesting than those circRNAs that are only found in one type of cancer, which after all increases their potential discriminatory powers as biomarkers. An example is serum *circ_104075,* which is upregulated in hepatocellular carcinoma (HCC) patients compared with healthy patients, patients with hepatitis and patients with lung, gastric, colon, and breast cancer [102], making this circRNA a serum marker specific for HCC. Several techniques used for other RNAs and ncRNAs have been adapted for the study of circRNAs, such as RNA-seq and qRT-PCR. Specifically Circ-Seq has not yet standardized methods; researchers used different algorithms that are developed using distinct alignment methodologies that lead to divergent results [172, 181, 182]. Moreover, most of techniques are based on detection of splice junction of circRNA which results in a loss of information about circRNA, as not only is splice junction important, but also what circRNA contains is.

Techniques and methods used in the different studies vary greatly at many levels, including use of starting material, purification, detection techniques, and bioinformatics approaches taken. Another important problem for circRNA study is the lack of standardization in the nomenclature of these molecules. Several groups have developed circRNAs databases to act as a central repository for these molecules, but each of them has used their own nomenclature and rules for inclusion in the respective databases have yet to be harmonized. The lack of uniformity can lead to replication of results or even complicate finding information about certain cir-cRNAs that are restricted to only one or few databases [229].

Studies that suggested that circRNAs could be useful biomarkers for cancer, although promising are nearly always performed on retrospective samples, underpowered and are single-center based. Moreover, despite the large number of studies that have been carried out on the use of circRNAs as diagnostic biomarkers, much fewer studies exist of their prognostic power and very few studies on their potential as predictive biomarkers of treatment effectiveness. Although the easiest to study, the clinical need for new diagnostic biomarkers is low, followed by prognostic and there is most clinical interest in predictive biomarkers in cancer. Despite these caveats, circRNAs have great potential as both novel therapeutics and as biomarker molecules and is therefore a topic that will surely increase in the future leading to new and improved protocols for their study.

# References

1. Birney E, Stamatoyannopoulos JA, Dutta A, Guigó R, Gingeras TR, Margulies EH, Weng Z, Snyder M, Dermitzakis ET, Thurman RE, Kuehn MS, Taylor CM, Neph S, Koch CM, Asthana S, Malhotra A, Adzhubei I, Greenbaum JA, Andrews RM, Flicek P, Boyle PJ, Cao H, Carter NP, Clelland GK, Davis S, Day N, Dhami P, Dillon SC, Dorschner MO, Fiegler H, Giresi PG, Goldy J, Hawrylycz M, Haydock A, Humbert R, James KD, Johnson BE, Johnson EM, Frum TT, Rosenzweig ER, Karnani N, Lee K, Lefebvre GC, Navas PA, Neri F, Parker SC, Sabo PJ, Sandstrom R, Shafer A, Vetrie D, Weaver M, Wilcox S, Yu M, Collins FS, Dekker J, Lieb JD, Tullius TD, Crawford GE, Sunyaev S, Noble WS, Dunham I, Denoeud F, Reymond A, Kapranov P, Rozowsky J, Zheng D, Castelo R, Frankish A, Harrow J, Ghosh S, Sandelin A, Hofacker IL, Baertsch R, Keefe D, Dike S, Cheng J, Hirsch HA, Sekinger EA, Lagarde J, Abril JF, Shahab A, Flamm C, Fried C, Hackermüller J, Hertel J, Lindemeyer M, Missal K, Tanzer A, Washietl S, Korbel J, Emanuelsson O, Pedersen JS, Holroyd N, Taylor R, Swarbreck D, Matthews N, Dickson MC, Thomas DJ, Weirauch MT, Gilbert J, Drenkow J, Bell I, Zhao X, Srinivasan KG, Sung WK, Ooi HS, Chiu KP, Foissac S, Alioto T, Brent M, Pachter L, Tress ML, Valencia A, Choo SW, Choo CY, Ucla C, Manzano C, Wyss C, Cheung E, Clark TG, Brown JB, Ganesh M, Patel S, Tammana H, Chrast J, Henrichsen CN, Kai C, Kawai J, Nagalakshmi U, Wu J, Lian Z, Lian J, Newburger P, Zhang X, Bickel P, Mattick JS, Carninci P, Hayashizaki Y, Weissman S, Hubbard T, Myers RM, Rogers J, Stadler PF, Lowe TM, Wei CL, Ruan Y, Struhl K, Gerstein M, Antonarakis SE, Fu Y, Green ED, Karaöz U, Siepel A, Taylor J, Liefer LA, Wetterstrand KA, Good PJ, Feingold EA, Guyer MS, Cooper GM, Asimenos G, Dewey CN, Hou M, Nikolaev S, Montoya-Burgos JI, Löytynoja A, Whelan S, Pardi F, Massingham T, Huang H, Zhang NR, Holmes I, Mullikin JC, Ureta-Vidal A, Paten B, Seringhaus M, Church D, Rosenbloom K, Kent WJ, Stone EA, Batzoglou S, Goldman N, Hardison RC, Haussler D, Miller W, Sidow A, Trinklein ND, Zhang ZD, Barrera L, Stuart R, King DC, Ameur A, Enroth S, Bieda MC, Kim J, Bhinge AA, Jiang N, Liu J, Yao F, Vega VB, Lee CW, Ng P, Shahab A, Yang A, Moqtaderi Z, Zhu Z, Xu X, Squazzo S, Oberley MJ, Inman D, Singer MA, Richmond TA, Munn KJ, Rada-Iglesias A, Wallerman O, Komorowski J, Fowler JC, Couttet P, Bruce AW, Dovey OM, Ellis PD, Langford CF, Nix DA, Euskirchen G, Hartman S, Urban AE, Kraus P, Van Calcar S, Heintzman N, Kim TH, Wang K, Qu C, Hon G, Luna R, Glass CK, Rosenfeld MG, Aldred SF, Cooper SJ, Halees A, Lin JM, Shulha HP, Zhang X, Xu M, Haidar JN, Yu Y, Ruan Y, Iyer VR, Green RD, Wadelius C, Farnham PJ, Ren B, Harte RA, Hinrichs AS, Trumbower H, Clawson H, Hillman-Jackson J, Zweig AS, Smith K, Thakkapallayil A, Barber G, Kuhn RM, Karolchik D, Armengol L, Bird CP, de Bakker PI, Kern AD, Lopez-Bigas N, Martin JD, Stranger BE, Woodroffe A, Davydov E, Dimas A, Eyras E, Hallgrímsdóttir IB, Huppert J, Zody MC, Abecasis GR, Estivill X, Bouffard GG, Guan X, Hansen NF, Idol JR, Maduro VV, Maskeri B, McDowell JC, Park M, Thomas PJ, Young AC, Blakesley RW, Muzny DM, Sodergren E, Wheeler DA, Worley KC, Jiang H, Weinstock GM, Gibbs RA, Graves T, Fulton R, Mardis ER, Wilson RK, Clamp M, Cuff J, Gnerre S, Jaffe DB, Chang JL, Lindblad-Toh K, Lander ES, Koriabine M, Nefedov M, Osoegawa K, Yoshinaga Y, Zhu B, de Jong PJ (2007) Identification and analysis of functional elements in 1% of the human genome by the ENCODE pilot project. Nature 447(7146):799–816. https://doi.org/10.1038/nature05874

2. Carninci P, Yasuda J, Hayashizaki Y (2008) Multifaceted mammalian transcriptome. Curr Opin Cell Biol 20(3):274–280. https://doi.org/10.1016/j.ceb.2008.03.008

3. Pertea M (2012) The human transcriptome: an unfinished story. Genes 3(3):344–360. https://doi.org/10.3390/genes3030344

4. Palazzo AF, Lee ES (2015) Non-coding RNA: what is functional and what is junk? Front Genet 6:2. https://doi.org/10.3389/fgene.2015.00002

5. Chen LL, Yang L (2015) Regulation of circRNA biogenesis. RNA Biol 12(4):381–388. https://doi.org/10.1080/15476286.2015.1020271

6. Sanger HL, Klotz G, Riesner D, Gross HJ, Kleinschmidt AK (1976) Viroids are single-stranded covalently closed circular RNA molecules existing as highly base-paired rod--like structures. Proc Natl Acad Sci U S A 73(11):3852–3856. https://doi.org/10.1073/pnas.73.11.3852

7. Gross HJ, Domdey H, Lossow C, Jank P, Raba M, Alberty H, Sanger HL (1978) Nucleotide sequence and secondary structure

of potato spindle tuber viroid. Nature 273 (5659):203–208

8. Kos A, Dijkema R, Arnberg AC, van der Meide PH, Schellekens H (1986) The hepatitis delta (delta) virus possesses a circular RNA. Nature 323(6088):558–560. https://doi.org/10.1038/323558a0

9. Nigro JM, Cho KR, Fearon ER, Kern SE, Ruppert JM, Oliner JD, Kinzler KW, Vogelstein B (1991) Scrambled exons. Cell 64(3):607–613

10. Cocquerelle C, Daubersies P, Majerus MA, Kerckaert JP, Bailleul B (1992) Splicing with inverted order of exons occurs proximal to large introns. EMBO J 11(3):1095–1098

11. Capel B, Swain A, Nicolis S, Hacker A, Walter M, Koopman P, Goodfellow P, Lovell-Badge R (1993) Circular transcripts of the testis-determining gene Sry in adult mouse testis. Cell 73(5):1019–1030

12. Zaphiropoulos PG (1996) Circular RNAs from transcripts of the rat cytochrome P450 2C24 gene: correlation with exon skipping. Proc Natl Acad Sci U S A 93(13):6536–6541

13. Zaphiropoulos PG (1997) Exon skipping and circular RNA formation in transcripts of the human cytochrome P-450 2C18 gene in epidermis and of the rat androgen binding protein gene in testis. Mol Cell Biol 17(6):2985–2993

14. Li XF, Lytton J (1999) A circularized sodium-calcium exchanger exon 2 transcript. J Biol Chem 274(12):8153–8160

15. Surono A, Van Khanh T, Takeshima Y, Wada H, Yagi M, Takagi M, Koizumi M, Matsuo M (2004) Chimeric RNA/ethylene-bridged nucleic acids promote dystrophin expression in myocytes of duchenne muscular dystrophy by inducing skipping of the nonsense mutation-encoding exon. Hum Gene Ther 15(8):749–757. https://doi.org/10.1089/1043034041648444

16. Houseley JM, Garcia-Casado Z, Pascual M, Paricio N, O'Dell KM, Monckton DG, Artero RD (2006) Noncanonical RNAs from transcripts of the Drosophila muscleblind gene. J Hered 97(3):253–260. https://doi.org/10.1093/jhered/esj037

17. Wu W, Ji P, Zhao F (2020) CircAtlas: an integrated resource of one million highly accurate circular RNAs from 1070 vertebrate transcriptomes. Genome Biol 21(1):101. https://doi.org/10.1186/s13059-020-02018-y

18. Salzman J, Gawad C, Wang PL, Lacayo N, Brown PO (2012) Circular RNAs are the predominant transcript isoform from hundreds of human genes in diverse cell types. PloS One 7(2):e30733. https://doi.org/10.1371/journal.pone.0030733

19. Jeck WR, Sorrentino JA, Wang K, Slevin MK, Burd CE, Liu J, Marzluff WF, Sharpless NE (2013) Circular RNAs are abundant, conserved, and associated with ALU repeats. RNA 19(2):141–157. https://doi.org/10.1261/rna.035667.112

20. Rybak-Wolf A, Stottmeister C, Glazar P, Jens M, Pino N, Giusti S, Hanan M, Behm M, Bartok O, Ashwal-Fluss R, Herzog M, Schreyer L, Papavasileiou P, Ivanov A, Ohman M, Refojo D, Kadener S, Rajewsky N (2015) Circular RNAs in the mammalian brain are highly abundant, conserved, and dynamically expressed. Mol Cell 58(5):870–885. https://doi.org/10.1016/j.molcel.2015.03.027

21. Memczak S, Jens M, Elefsinioti A, Torti F, Krueger J, Rybak A, Maier L, Mackowiak SD, Gregersen LH, Munschauer M, Loewer A, Ziebold U, Landthaler M, Kocks C, le Noble F, Rajewsky N (2013) Circular RNAs are a large class of animal RNAs with regulatory potency. Nature 495(7441):333–338. https://doi.org/10.1038/nature11928

22. Salzman J, Chen RE, Olsen MN, Wang PL, Brown PO (2013) Cell-type specific features of circular RNA expression. PLoS Genet 9(9):e1003777. https://doi.org/10.1371/journal.pgen.1003777

23. Talhouarne GJS, Gall JG (2018) Lariat intronic RNAs in the cytoplasm of vertebrate cells. Proc Natl Acad Sci U S A 115(34):E7970–E7977. https://doi.org/10.1073/pnas.1808816115

24. Zhang Y, Zhang XO, Chen T, Xiang JF, Yin QF, Xing YH, Zhu S, Yang L, Chen LL (2013) Circular intronic long noncoding RNAs. Mol Cell 51(6):792–806. https://doi.org/10.1016/j.molcel.2013.08.017

25. Meng X, Li X, Zhang P, Wang J, Zhou Y, Chen M (2017) Circular RNA: an emerging key player in RNA world. Brief Bioinform 18(4):547–557. https://doi.org/10.1093/bib/bbw045

26. Jeck WR, Sharpless NE (2014) Detecting and characterizing circular RNAs. Nat Biotechnol 32(5):453–461. https://doi.org/10.1038/nbt.2890

27. Li Z, Huang C, Bao C, Chen L, Lin M, Wang X, Zhong G, Yu B, Hu W, Dai L, Zhu P, Chang Z, Wu Q, Zhao Y, Jia Y, Xu P,

Liu H, Shan G (2015) Exon-intron circular RNAs regulate transcription in the nucleus. Nat Struct Mol Biol 22(3):256–264. https://doi.org/10.1038/nsmb.2959

28. Huang C, Liang D, Tatomer DC, Wilusz JE (2018) A length-dependent evolutionarily conserved pathway controls nuclear export of circular RNAs. Genes Dev 32 (9-10):639–644. https://doi.org/10.1101/gad.314856.118

29. Huang G, Li S, Yang N, Zou Y, Zheng D, Xiao T (2017) Recent progress in circular RNAs in human cancers. Cancer Lett 404:8–18. https://doi.org/10.1016/j.canlet.2017.07.002

30. Ashwal-Fluss R, Meyer M, Pamudurti NR, Ivanov A, Bartok O, Hanan M, Evantal N, Memczak S, Rajewsky N, Kadener S (2014) circRNA biogenesis competes with pre-mRNA splicing. Mol Cell 56(1):55–66. https://doi.org/10.1016/j.molcel.2014.08.019

31. Zhang XO, Wang HB, Zhang Y, Lu X, Chen LL, Yang L (2014) Complementary sequence-mediated exon circularization. Cell 159(1):134–147. https://doi.org/10.1016/j.cell.2014.09.001

32. Kramer MC, Liang D, Tatomer DC, Gold B, March ZM, Cherry S, Wilusz JE (2015) Combinatorial control of Drosophila circular RNA expression by intronic repeats, hnRNPs, and SR proteins. Genes Dev 29 (20):2168–2182. https://doi.org/10.1101/gad.270421.115

33. Conn SJ, Pillman KA, Toubia J, Conn VM, Salmanidis M, Phillips CA, Roslan S, Schreiber AW, Gregory PA, Goodall GJ (2015) The RNA binding protein quaking regulates formation of circRNAs. Cell 160(6):1125–1134. https://doi.org/10.1016/j.cell.2015.02.014

34. Errichelli L, Dini Modigliani S, Laneve P, Colantoni A, Legnini I, Capauto D, Rosa A, De Santis R, Scarfo R, Peruzzi G, Lu L, Caffarelli E, Shneider NA, Morlando M, Bozzoni I (2017) FUS affects circular RNA expression in murine embryonic stem cell-derived motor neurons. Nat Commun 8:14741. https://doi.org/10.1038/ncomms14741

35. Li X, Liu CX, Xue W, Zhang Y, Jiang S, Yin QF, Wei J, Yao RW, Yang L, Chen LL (2017) Coordinated circRNA biogenesis and function with NF90/NF110 in viral infection. Mol Cell 67(2):214–227. e217. https://doi.org/10.1016/j.molcel.2017.05.023

36. Liang WW, Cheng SC (2015) A novel mechanism for Prp5 function in prespliceosome formation and proofreading the branch site sequence. Genes Dev 29(1):81–93. https://doi.org/10.1101/gad.253708.114

37. Ivanov A, Memczak S, Wyler E, Torti F, Porath HT, Orejuela MR, Piechotta M, Levanon EY, Landthaler M, Dieterich C, Rajewsky N (2015) Analysis of intron sequences reveals hallmarks of circular RNA biogenesis in animals. Cell Rep 10(2):170–177. https://doi.org/10.1016/j.celrep.2014.12.019

38. Aktas T, Avsar Ilik I, Maticzka D, Bhardwaj V, Pessoa Rodrigues C, Mittler G, Manke T, Backofen R, Akhtar A (2017) DHX9 suppresses RNA processing defects originating from the Alu invasion of the human genome. Nature 544(7648):115–119. https://doi.org/10.1038/nature21715

39. Fei T, Chen Y, Xiao T, Li W, Cato L, Zhang P, Cotter MB, Bowden M, Lis RT, Zhao SG, Wu Q, Feng FY, Loda M, He HH, Liu XS, Brown M (2017) Genome-wide CRISPR screen identifies HNRNPL as a prostate cancer dependency regulating RNA splicing. Proc Natl Acad Sci U S A 114(26): E5207–E5215. https://doi.org/10.1073/pnas.1617467114

40. Stagsted LV, Nielsen KM, Daugaard I, Hansen TB (2019) Noncoding AUG circRNAs constitute an abundant and conserved subclass of circles. Life Sci Alliance 2(3): e201900398. https://doi.org/10.26508/lsa.201900398

41. Guo JU, Agarwal V, Guo H, Bartel DP (2014) Expanded identification and characterization of mammalian circular RNAs. Genome Biol 15(7):409. https://doi.org/10.1186/s13059-014-0409-z

42. Hansen TB, Jensen TI, Clausen BH, Bramsen JB, Finsen B, Damgaard CK, Kjems J (2013) Natural RNA circles function as efficient microRNA sponges. Nature 495 (7441):384–388. https://doi.org/10.1038/nature11993

43. Legnini I, Di Timoteo G, Rossi F, Morlando M, Briganti F, Sthandier O, Fatica A, Santini T, Andronache A, Wade M, Laneve P, Rajewsky N, Bozzoni I (2017) Circ-ZNF609 is a circular RNA that can be translated and functions in myogenesis. Mol Cell 66(1):22–37. e29. https://doi.org/10.1016/j.molcel.2017.02.017

44. Yang Y, Fan X, Mao M, Song X, Wu P, Zhang Y, Jin Y, Yang Y, Chen LL, Wang Y, Wong CC, Xiao X, Wang Z (2017) Extensive translation of circular RNAs driven by N(6)-methyladenosine. Cell Res 27(5):626–641. https://doi.org/10.1038/cr.2017.31

45. Yang Y, Gao X, Zhang M, Yan S, Sun C, Xiao F, Huang N, Yang X, Zhao K, Zhou H, Huang S, Xie B, Zhang N (2018) Novel role of FBXW7 circular RNA in repressing glioma tumorigenesis. J Natl Cancer Inst 110(3). https://doi.org/10.1093/jnci/djx166

46. You X, Vlatkovic I, Babic A, Will T, Epstein I, Tushev G, Akbalik G, Wang M, Glock C, Quedenau C, Wang X, Hou J, Liu H, Sun W, Sambandan S, Chen T, Schuman EM, Chen W (2015) Neural circular RNAs are derived from synaptic genes and regulated by development and plasticity. Nat Neurosci 18(4):603–610. https://doi.org/10.1038/nn.3975

47. Zheng Q, Bao C, Guo W, Li S, Chen J, Chen B, Luo Y, Lyu D, Li Y, Shi G, Liang L, Gu J, He X, Huang S (2016) Circular RNA profiling reveals an abundant circHIPK3 that regulates cell growth by sponging multiple miRNAs. Nat Commun 7:11215. https://doi.org/10.1038/ncomms11215

48. Bak RO, Mikkelsen JG (2014) miRNA sponges: soaking up miRNAs for regulation of gene expression. Wiley Interdiscip Rev RNA 5(3):317–333. https://doi.org/10.1002/wrna.1213

49. Zhu X, Shao P, Tang Y, Shu M, Hu WW, Zhang Y (2019) hsa_circRNA_100533 regulates GNAS by sponging hsa_miR_933 to prevent oral squamous cell carcinoma. J Cell Biochem 120(11):19159–19171. https://doi.org/10.1002/jcb.29245

50. Xu H, Sun Y, You B, Huang CP, Ye D, Chang C (2020) Androgen receptor reverses the oncometabolite R-2-hydroxyglutarate-induced prostate cancer cell invasion via suppressing the circRNA-51217/miRNA-646/TGFβ1/p-Smad2/3 signaling. Cancer Lett 472:151–164. https://doi.org/10.1016/j.canlet.2019.12.014

51. Xiang Q, Kang L, Wang J, Liao Z, Song Y, Zhao K, Wang K, Yang C, Zhang Y (2020) CircRNA-CIDN mitigated compression loading-induced damage in human nucleus pulposus cells via miR-34a-5p/SIRT1 axis. EBioMedicine 53:102679. https://doi.org/10.1016/j.ebiom.2020.102679

52. Lu J, Wang YH, Yoon C, Huang XY, Xu Y, Xie JW, Wang JB, Lin JX, Chen QY, Cao LL, Zheng CH, Li P, Huang CM (2020) Circular RNA circ-RanGAP1 regulates VEGFA expression by targeting miR-877-3p to facilitate gastric cancer invasion and metastasis. Cancer Lett 471:38–48. https://doi.org/10.1016/j.canlet.2019.11.038

53. Kong Z, Wan X, Lu Y, Zhang Y, Huang Y, Xu Y, Liu Y, Zhao P, Xiang X, Li L, Li Y (2020) Circular RNA circFOXO3 promotes prostate cancer progression through sponging miR-29a-3p. J Cell Mol Med 24(1):799–813. https://doi.org/10.1111/jcmm.14791

54. Ragan C, Goodall GJ, Shirokikh NE, Preiss T (2019) Insights into the biogenesis and potential functions of exonic circular RNA. Sci Rep 9(1):2048. https://doi.org/10.1038/s41598-018-37037-0

55. Kelly S, Greenman C, Cook PR, Papantonis A (2015) Exon Skipping Is Correlated with Exon Circularization. Journal of molecular biology 427(15):2414–2417. https://doi.org/10.1016/j.jmb.2015.02.018

56. Qu S, Yang X, Li X, Wang J, Gao Y, Shang R, Sun W, Dou K, Li H (2015) Circular RNA: a new star of noncoding RNAs. Cancer Lett 365(2):141–148. https://doi.org/10.1016/j.canlet.2015.06.003

57. Chao CW, Chan DC, Kuo A, Leder P (1998) The mouse formin (Fmn) gene: abundant circular RNA transcripts and gene-targeted deletion analysis. Mol Med 4(9):614–628

58. Moehle EA, Braberg H, Krogan NJ, Guthrie C (2014) Adventures in time and space: splicing efficiency and RNA polymerase II elongation rate. RNA Biol 11(4):313–319. https://doi.org/10.4161/rna.28646

59. Zhang Y, Xue W, Li X, Zhang J, Chen S, Zhang JL, Yang L, Chen LL (2016) The Biogenesis of Nascent Circular RNAs. Cell reports 15(3):611–624. https://doi.org/10.1016/j.celrep.2016.03.058

60. Huang A, Zheng H, Wu Z, Chen M, Huang Y (2020) Circular RNA-protein interactions: functions, mechanisms, and identification. Theranostics 10(8):3503–3517. https://doi.org/10.7150/thno.42174

61. Gualandi F, Trabanelli C, Rimessi P, Calzolari E, Toffolatti L, Patarnello T, Kunz G, Muntoni F, Ferlini A (2003) Multiple exon skipping and RNA circularisation contribute to the severe phenotypic expression of exon 5 dystrophin deletion. J Med Genet 40(8):e100. https://doi.org/10.1136/jmg.40.8.e100

62. Chen LL (2016) The biogenesis and emerging roles of circular RNAs. Nat Rev Mol Cell Biol 17(4):205–211. https://doi.org/10.1038/nrm.2015.32

63. Fan X, Weng X, Zhao Y, Chen W, Gan T, Xu D (2017) Circular RNAs in cardiovascular disease: an overview. Biomed Res Int 2017:5135781. https://doi.org/10.1155/2017/5135781

64. Ma N, Tie C, Yu B, Zhang W, Wan J (2020) Circular RNAs regulate its parental genes transcription in the AD mouse model using two methods of library construction. FASEB J 34(8):10342–10356. https://doi.org/10.1096/fj.201903157R

65. Chen N, Zhao G, Yan X, Lv Z, Yin H, Zhang S, Song W, Li X, Li L, Du Z, Jia L, Zhou L, Li W, Hoffman AR, Hu JF, Cui J (2018) A novel FLI1 exonic circular RNA promotes metastasis in breast cancer by coordinately regulating TET1 and DNMT1. Genome Biol 19(1):218. https://doi.org/10.1186/s13059-018-1594-y

66. Du WW, Zhang C, Yang W, Yong T, Awan FM, Yang BB (2017) Identifying and characterizing circRNA-protein interaction. Theranostics 7(17):4183–4191. https://doi.org/10.7150/thno.21299

67. Aufiero S, Reckman YJ, Pinto YM, Creemers EE (2019) Circular RNAs open a new chapter in cardiovascular biology. Nat Rev Cardiol 16 (8):503–514. https://doi.org/10.1038/s41569-019-0185-2

68. Du WW, Yang W, Chen Y, Wu ZK, Foster FS, Yang Z, Li X, Yang BB (2017) Foxo3 circular RNA promotes cardiac senescence by modulating multiple factors associated with stress and senescence responses. Eur Heart J 38 (18):1402–1412. https://doi.org/10.1093/eurheartj/ehw001

69. Hansen TB, Wiklund ED, Bramsen JB, Villadsen SB, Statham AL, Clark SJ, Kjems J (2011) miRNA-dependent gene silencing involving Ago2-mediated cleavage of a circular antisense RNA. EMBO J 30 (21):4414–4422. https://doi.org/10.1038/emboj.2011.359

70. Holdt LM, Stahringer A, Sass K, Pichler G, Kulak NA, Wilfert W, Kohlmaier A, Herbst A, Northoff BH, Nicolaou A, Gabel G, Beutner F, Scholz M, Thiery J, Musunuru K, Krohn K, Mann M, Teupser D (2016) Circular non-coding RNA ANRIL modulates ribosomal RNA maturation and atherosclerosis in humans. Nat Commun 7:12429. https://doi.org/10.1038/ncomms12429

71. Abdelmohsen K, Panda AC, Munk R, Grammatikakis I, Dudekula DB, De S, Kim J, Noh JH, Kim KM, Martindale JL, Gorospe M (2017) Identification of HuR target circular RNAs uncovers suppression of PABPN1 translation by CircPABPN1. RNA Biol 14(3):361–369. https://doi.org/10.1080/15476286.2017.1279788

72. Yu CY, Kuo HC (2019) The emerging roles and functions of circular RNAs and their generation. J Biomed Sci 26(1):29. https://doi.org/10.1186/s12929-019-0523-z

73. Zeng Y, Du WW, Wu Y, Yang Z, Awan FM, Li X, Yang W, Zhang C, Yang Q, Yee A, Chen Y, Yang F, Sun H, Huang R, Yee AJ, Li RK, Wu Z, Backx PH, Yang BB (2017) A circular RNA binds to and activates AKT phosphorylation and nuclear localization reducing apoptosis and enhancing cardiac repair. Theranostics 7(16):3842–3855. https://doi.org/10.7150/thno.19764

74. Yang ZG, Awan FM, Du WW, Zeng Y, Lyu J, Wu GS, Yang W, Yang BB (2017) The circular RNA interacts with STAT3, increasing its nuclear translocation and wound repair by modulating Dnmt3a and miR-17 function. Mol Ther 25(9):2062–2074. https://doi.org/10.1016/j.ymthe.2017.05.022

75. Du WW, Yang W, Li X, Awan FM, Yang Z, Fang L, Lyu J, Li F, Peng C, Krylov SN, Xie Y, Zhang Y, He C, Wu N, Zhang C, Sdiri M, Dong J, Ma J, Gao C, Hibberd S, Yang BB (2018) A circular RNA circ-DNMT1 enhances breast cancer progression by activating autophagy. Oncogene 37 (44):5829–5842. https://doi.org/10.1038/s41388-018-0369-y

76. Sun YM, Wang WT, Zeng ZC, Chen TQ, Han C, Pan Q, Huang W, Fang K, Sun LY, Zhou YF, Luo XQ, Luo C, Du X, Chen YQ (2019) circMYBL2, a circRNA from MYBL2, regulates FLT3 translation by recruiting PTBP1 to promote FLT3-ITD AML progression. Blood 134(18):1533–1546. https://doi.org/10.1182/blood.2019000802

77. Wang S, Zhang Y, Cai Q, Ma M, Jin LY, Weng M, Zhou D, Tang Z, Wang JD, Quan Z (2019) Circular RNA FOXP1 promotes tumor progression and Warburg effect in gallbladder cancer by regulating PKLR expression. Mol Cancer 18(1):145. https://doi.org/10.1186/s12943-019-1078-z

78. Garikipati VNS, Verma SK, Cheng Z, Liang D, Truongcao MM, Cimini M, Yue Y, Huang G, Wang C, Benedict C, Tang Y, Mallaredy V, Ibetti J, Grisanti L, Schumacher SM, Gao E, Rajan S, Wilusz JE, Goukassian D, Houser SR, Koch WJ, Kishore R (2019) Circular RNA CircFndc3b modulates cardiac repair after myocardial infarction via FUS/VEGF-A axis. Nat Commun 10 (1):4317. https://doi.org/10.1038/s41467-019-11777-7

79. Fang L, Du WW, Awan FM, Dong J, Yang BB (2019) The circular RNA circ-Ccnb1 dissociates Ccnb1/Cdk1 complex suppressing cell invasion and tumorigenesis. Cancer Lett

459:216–226. https://doi.org/10.1016/j.canlet.2019.05.036

80. Huang X, He M, Huang S, Lin R, Zhan M, Yang D, Shen H, Xu S, Cheng W, Yu J, Qiu Z, Wang J (2019) Circular RNA circERBB2 promotes gallbladder cancer progression by regulating PA2G4-dependent rDNA transcription. Mol Cancer 18(1):166. https://doi.org/10.1186/s12943-019-1098-8

81. Li H, Yang F, Hu A, Wang X, Fang E, Chen Y, Li D, Song H, Wang J, Guo Y, Liu Y, Li H, Huang K, Zheng L, Tong Q (2019) Therapeutic targeting of circ-CUX1/EWSR1/MAZ axis inhibits glycolysis and neuroblastoma progression. EMBO Mol Med 11(12): e10835. https://doi.org/10.15252/emmm.201910835

82. Hu X, Wu D, He X, Zhao H, He Z, Lin J, Wang K, Wang W, Pan Z, Lin H, Wang M (2019) circGSK3β promotes metastasis in esophageal squamous cell carcinoma by augmenting β-catenin signaling. Mol Cancer 18 (1):160. https://doi.org/10.1186/s12943-019-1095-y

83. Pandey PR, Yang JH, Tsitsipatis D, Panda AC, Noh JH, Kim KM, Munk R, Nicholson T, Hanniford D, Argibay D, Yang X, Martindale JL, Chang MW, Jones SW, Hernando E, Sen P, De S, Abdelmohsen K, Gorospe M (2020) circSamd4 represses myogenic transcriptional activity of PUR proteins. Nucleic Acids Res 48(7):3789–3805. https://doi.org/10.1093/nar/gkaa035

84. Wong CH, Lou UK, Li Y, Chan SL, Tong JH, To KF, Chen Y (2020) CircFOXK2 promotes growth and metastasis of pancreatic ductal adenocarcinoma by complexing with RNA-binding proteins and sponging MiR-942. Cancer Res 80(11):2138–2149. https://doi.org/10.1158/0008-5472.can-19-3268

85. Liu Z, Wang Q, Wang X, Xu Z, Wei X, Li J (2020) Circular RNA cIARS regulates ferroptosis in HCC cells through interacting with RNA binding protein ALKBH5. Cell Death Discov 6:72. https://doi.org/10.1038/s41420-020-00306-x

86. Gan X, Zhu H, Jiang X, Obiegbusi SC, Yong M, Long X, Hu J (2020) CircMUC16 promotes autophagy of epithelial ovarian cancer via interaction with ATG13 and miR-199a. Mol Cancer 19(1):45. https://doi.org/10.1186/s12943-020-01163-z

87. Lou J, Hao Y, Lin K, Lyu Y, Chen M, Wang H, Zou D, Jiang X, Wang R, Jin D, Lam EW, Shao S, Liu Q, Yan J, Wang X, Chen P, Zhang B, Jin B (2020) Circular RNA CDR1as disrupts the p53/MDM2 complex to inhibit Gliomagenesis. Mol Cancer 19(1):138. https://doi.org/10.1186/s12943-020-01253-y

88. Chen CY, Sarnow P (1995) Initiation of protein synthesis by the eukaryotic translational apparatus on circular RNAs. Science 268 (5209):415–417

89. Pamudurti NR, Bartok O, Jens M, Ashwal-Fluss R, Stottmeister C, Ruhe L, Hanan M, Wyler E, Perez-Hernandez D, Ramberger E, Shenzis S, Samson M, Dittmar G, Landthaler M, Chekulaeva M, Rajewsky N, Kadener S (2017) Translation of CircRNAs. Mol Cell 66(1):9–21.e7. https://doi.org/10.1016/j.molcel.2017.02.021

90. Begum S, Yiu A, Stebbing J, Castellano L (2018) Novel tumour suppressive protein encoded by circular RNA, circ-SHPRH, in glioblastomas. Oncogene 37 (30):4055–4057. https://doi.org/10.1038/s41388-018-0230-3

91. Lei M, Zheng G, Ning Q, Zheng J, Dong D (2020) Translation and functional roles of circular RNAs in human cancer. Mol Cancer 19(1):30. https://doi.org/10.1186/s12943-020-1135-7

92. Di Timoteo G, Dattilo D, Centrón-Broco A, Colantoni A, Guarnacci M, Rossi F, Incarnato D, Oliviero S, Fatica A, Morlando M, Bozzoni I (2020) Modulation of circRNA Metabolism by m(6)A modification. Cell Rep 31(6):107641. https://doi.org/10.1016/j.celrep.2020.107641

93. Kristensen LS, Andersen MS, Stagsted LVW, Ebbesen KK, Hansen TB, Kjems J (2019) The biogenesis, biology and characterization of circular RNAs. Nat Rev Genet 20 (11):675–691. https://doi.org/10.1038/s41576-019-0158-7

94. Zhang M, Zhao K, Xu X, Yang Y, Yan S, Wei P, Liu H, Xu J, Xiao F, Zhou H, Yang X, Huang N, Liu J, He K, Xie K, Zhang G, Huang S, Zhang N (2018) A peptide encoded by circular form of LINC-PINT suppresses oncogenic transcriptional elongation in glioblastoma. Nat Commun 9 (1):4475. https://doi.org/10.1038/s41467-018-06862-2

95. Zhang M, Huang N, Yang X, Luo J, Yan S, Xiao F, Chen W, Gao X, Zhao K, Zhou H,

Li Z, Ming L, Xie B, Zhang N (2018) A novel protein encoded by the circular form of the SHPRH gene suppresses glioma tumorigenesis. Oncogene 37(13):1805–1814. https://doi.org/10.1038/s41388-017-0019-9

96. Liang WC, Wong CW, Liang PP, Shi M, Cao Y, Rao ST, Tsui SK, Waye MM, Zhang Q, Fu WM, Zhang JF (2019) Translation of the circular RNA circβ-catenin promotes liver cancer cell growth through activation of the Wnt pathway. Genome Biol 20(1):84. https://doi.org/10.1186/s13059-019-1685-4

97. Zheng X, Chen L, Zhou Y, Wang Q, Zheng Z, Xu B, Wu C, Zhou Q, Hu W, Wu C, Jiang J (2019) A novel protein encoded by a circular RNA circPPP1R12A promotes tumor pathogenesis and metastasis of colon cancer via Hippo-YAP signaling. Mol Cancer 18(1):47. https://doi.org/10.1186/s12943-019-1010-6

98. Pan Z, Cai J, Lin J, Zhou H, Peng J, Liang J, Xia L, Yin Q, Zou B, Zheng J, Qiao L, Zhang L (2020) A novel protein encoded by circFNDC3B inhibits tumor progression and EMT through regulating Snail in colon cancer. Mol Cancer 19(1):71. https://doi.org/10.1186/s12943-020-01179-5

99. Cocquerelle C, Mascrez B, Hetuin D, Bailleul B (1993) Mis-splicing yields circular RNA molecules. FASEB J 7(1):155–160

100. Memczak S, Papavasileiou P, Peters O, Rajewsky N (2015) Identification and characterization of circular RNAs as a new class of putative biomarkers in human blood. PLoS One 10(10):e0141214. https://doi.org/10.1371/journal.pone.0141214

101. Li Y, Zheng Q, Bao C, Li S, Guo W, Zhao J, Chen D, Gu J, He X, Huang S (2015) Circular RNA is enriched and stable in exosomes: a promising biomarker for cancer diagnosis. Cell Res 25(8):981–984. https://doi.org/10.1038/cr.2015.82

102. Zhang X, Xu Y, Qian Z, Zheng W, Wu Q, Chen Y, Zhu G, Liu Y, Bian Z, Xu W, Zhang Y, Sun F, Pan Q, Wang J, Du L, Yu Y (2018) circRNA_104075 stimulates YAP-dependent tumorigenesis through the regulation of HNF4a and may serve as a diagnostic marker in hepatocellular carcinoma. Cell Death Dis 9(11):1091. https://doi.org/10.1038/s41419-018-1132-6

103. Chen X, Chen RX, Wei WS, Li YH, Feng ZH, Tan L, Chen JW, Yuan GJ, Chen SL, Guo SJ, Xiao KH, Liu ZW, Luo JH, Zhou FJ, Xie D (2018) PRMT5 circular RNA promotes metastasis of urothelial carcinoma of the bladder through sponging miR-30c to induce epithelial-mesenchymal transition. Clin Cancer Res 24(24):6319–6330. https://doi.org/10.1158/1078-0432.ccr-18-1270

104. Luo YH, Yang YP, Chien CS, Yarmishyn AA, Ishola AA, Chien Y, Chen YM, Huang TW, Lee KY, Huang WC, Tsai PH, Lin TW, Chiou SH, Liu CY, Chang CC, Chen MT, Wang ML (2020) Plasma level of circular RNA hsa_circ_0000190 correlates with tumor progression and poor treatment response in advanced lung cancers. Cancers 12(7):1740. https://doi.org/10.3390/cancers12071740

105. Rong D, Lu C, Zhang B, Fu K, Zhao S, Tang W, Cao H (2019) CircPSMC3 suppresses the proliferation and metastasis of gastric cancer by acting as a competitive endogenous RNA through sponging miR-296-5p. Mol Cancer 18(1):25. https://doi.org/10.1186/s12943-019-0958-6

106. Pan B, Qin J, Liu X, He B, Wang X, Pan Y, Sun H, Xu T, Xu M, Chen X, Xu X, Zeng K, Sun L, Wang S (2019) Identification of serum exosomal hsa-circ-0004771 as a novel diagnostic biomarker of colorectal cancer. Front Genet 10:1096. https://doi.org/10.3389/fgene.2019.01096

107. Han D, Li J, Wang H, Su X, Hou J, Gu Y, Qian C, Lin Y, Liu X, Huang M, Li N, Zhou W, Yu Y, Cao X (2017) Circular RNA circMTO1 acts as the sponge of microRNA-9 to suppress hepatocellular carcinoma progression. Hepatology 66(4):1151–1164. https://doi.org/10.1002/hep.29270

108. Liang G, Liu Z, Tan L, Su AN, Jiang WG, Gong C (2017) HIF1alpha-associated circDENND4C promotes proliferation of breast cancer cells in hypoxic environment. Anticancer Res 37(8):4337–4343. https://doi.org/10.21873/anticanres.11827

109. Yao Z, Luo J, Hu K, Lin J, Huang H, Wang Q, Zhang P, Xiong Z, He C, Huang Z, Liu B, Yang Y (2017) ZKSCAN1 gene and its related circular RNA (circZKSCAN1) both inhibit hepatocellular carcinoma cell growth, migration, and invasion but through different signaling pathways. Mol Oncol 11(4):422–437. https://doi.org/10.1002/1878-0261.12045

110. Liang HF, Zhang XZ, Liu BG, Jia GT, Li WL (2017) Circular RNA circ-ABCB10 promotes breast cancer proliferation and progression through sponging miR-1271. Am J Cancer Res 7(7):1566–1576

111. Huang XY, Huang ZL, Xu YH, Zheng Q, Chen Z, Song W, Zhou J, Tang ZY, Huang XY (2017) Comprehensive circular RNA profiling reveals the regulatory role of the circRNA-100338/miR-141-3p pathway in hepatitis B-related hepatocellular carcinoma. Sci Rep 7(1):5428. https://doi.org/10.1038/s41598-017-05432-8

112. Liu W, Zhang J, Zou C, Xie X, Wang Y, Wang B, Zhao Z, Tu J, Wang X, Li H, Shen J, Yin J (2017) Microarray expression profile and functional analysis of circular RNAs in osteosarcoma. Cell Physiol Biochem 43(3):969–985. https://doi.org/10.1159/000481650

113. Huang G, Zhu H, Shi Y, Wu W, Cai H, Chen X (2015) cir-ITCH plays an inhibitory role in colorectal cancer by regulating the Wnt/beta-catenin pathway. PLoS One 10(6):e0131225. https://doi.org/10.1371/journal.pone.0131225

114. Wan L, Zhang L, Fan K, Cheng ZX, Sun QC, Wang JJ (2016) Circular RNA-ITCH suppresses lung cancer proliferation via inhibiting the Wnt/beta-catenin pathway. Biomed Res Int 2016:1579490. https://doi.org/10.1155/2016/1579490

115. Pan H, Li T, Jiang Y, Pan C, Ding Y, Huang Z, Yu H, Kong D (2018) Overexpression of circular RNA ciRS-7 abrogates the tumor suppressive effect of miR-7 on gastric cancer via PTEN/PI3K/AKT signaling pathway. J Cell Biochem 119(1):440–446. https://doi.org/10.1002/jcb.26201

116. Zhong Z, Lv M, Chen J (2016) Screening differential circular RNA expression profiles reveals the regulatory role of circTCF25-miR-103a-3p/miR-107-CDK6 pathway in bladder carcinoma. Sci Rep 6:30919. https://doi.org/10.1038/srep30919

117. Barrett SP, Parker KR, Horn C, Mata M, Salzman J (2017) ciRS-7 exonic sequence is embedded in a long non-coding RNA locus. PLoS Genet 13(12):e1007114. https://doi.org/10.1371/journal.pgen.1007114

118. Hanniford D, Ulloa-Morales A, Karz A, Berzoti-Coelho MG, Moubarak RS, Sánchez-Sendra B, Kloetgen A, Davalos V, Imig J, Wu P, Vasudevaraja V, Argibay D, Lilja K, Tabaglio T, Monteagudo C, Guccione E, Tsirigos A, Osman I, Aifantis I, Hernando E (2020) Epigenetic silencing of CDR1as drives IGF2BP3-mediated melanoma invasion and metastasis. Cancer Cell 37(1):55–70.e15. https://doi.org/10.1016/j.ccell.2019.12.007

119. Uhr K, Sieuwerts AM, de Weerd V, Smid M, Hammerl D, Foekens JA, Martens JWM (2018) Association of microRNA-7 and its binding partner CDR1-AS with the prognosis and prediction of 1(st)-line tamoxifen therapy in breast cancer. Sci Rep 8(1):9657. https://doi.org/10.1038/s41598-018-27987-w

120. Yang W, Yang X, Wang X, Gu J, Zhou D, Wang Y, Yin B, Guo J, Zhou M (2019) Silencing CDR1as enhances the sensitivity of breast cancer cells to drug resistance by acting as a miR-7 sponge to down-regulate REGgamma. J Cell Mol Med 23(8):4921–4932. https://doi.org/10.1111/jcmm.14305

121. Zhang X, Yang D, Wei Y (2018) Overexpressed CDR1as functions as an oncogene to promote the tumor progression via miR-7 in non-small-cell lung cancer. Onco Targets Ther 11:3979–3987. https://doi.org/10.2147/ott.s158316

122. Weng W, Wei Q, Toden S, Yoshida K, Nagasaka T, Fujiwara T, Cai S, Qin H, Ma Y, Goel A (2017) Circular RNA ciRS-7- A promising prognostic biomarker and a potential therapeutic target in colorectal cancer. Clin Cancer Res 23(14):3918–3928. https://doi.org/10.1158/1078-0432.ccr-16-2541

123. Yu L, Gong X, Sun L, Zhou Q, Lu B, Zhu L (2016) The circular RNA Cdr1as act as an oncogene in hepatocellular carcinoma through targeting miR-7 expression. PLoS One 11(7):e0158347. https://doi.org/10.1371/journal.pone.0158347

124. Yang X, Xiong Q, Wu Y, Li S, Ge F (2017) Quantitative proteomics reveals the regulatory networks of circular RNA CDR1as in hepatocellular carcinoma cells. J Proteome Res 16(10):3891–3902. https://doi.org/10.1021/acs.jproteome.7b00519

125. Zhong Q, Huang J, Wei J, Wu R (2019) Circular RNA CDR1as sponges miR-7-5p to enhance E2F3 stability and promote the growth of nasopharyngeal carcinoma. Cancer Cell Int 19:252. https://doi.org/10.1186/s12935-019-0959-y

126. Yang X, Li S, Wu Y, Ge F, Chen Y, Xiong Q (2020) The circular RNA CDR1as regulate cell proliferation via TMED2 and TMED10. BMC Cancer 20(1):312. https://doi.org/10.1186/s12885-020-06794-5

127. Han JY, Guo S, Wei N, Xue R, Li W, Dong G, Li J, Tian X, Chen C, Qiu S, Wang T, Xiao Q, Liu C, Xu J, Chen KS (2020) ciRS-7 promotes the proliferation and migration of papillary thyroid cancer by negatively regulating the miR-7/epidermal growth factor receptor axis. Biomed Res Int 2020:9875636. https://doi.org/10.1155/2020/9875636

128. Huang H, Wei L, Qin T, Yang N, Li Z, Xu Z (2019) Circular RNA ciRS-7 triggers the migration and invasion of esophageal squamous cell carcinoma via miR-7/KLF4 and NF-κB signals. Cancer Biol Ther 20 (1):73–80. https://doi.org/10.1080/15384047.2018.1507254

129. Li C, Li M, Xue Y (2019) Downregulation of CircRNA CDR1as specifically triggered low-dose Diosbulbin-B induced gastric cancer cell death by regulating miR-7-5p/REGγ axis. Biomed Pharmacother 120:109462. https://doi.org/10.1016/j.biopha.2019.109462

130. Yang W, Gu J, Wang X, Wang Y, Feng M, Zhou D, Guo J, Zhou M (2019) Inhibition of circular RNA CDR1as increases chemosensitivity of 5-FU-resistant BC cells through up-regulating miR-7. J Cell Mol Med 23 (5):3166–3177. https://doi.org/10.1111/jcmm.14171

131. Zou Y, Zheng S, Deng X, Yang A, Kong Y, Kohansal M, Hu X, Xie X (2020) Diagnostic and prognostic value of circular RNA CDR1as/ciRS-7 for solid tumours: a systematic review and meta-analysis. J Cell Mol Med 24(17):9507–9517. https://doi.org/10.1111/jcmm.15619

132. Tian G, Li G, Guan L, Wang Z, Li N (2020) Prognostic value of circular RNA ciRS-7 in various cancers: a PRISMA-compliant meta-analysis. Biomed Res Int 2020:1487609. https://doi.org/10.1155/2020/1487609

133. Su C, Han Y, Zhang H, Li Y, Yi L, Wang X, Zhou S, Yu D, Song X, Xiao N, Cao X, Liu Z (2018) CiRS-7 targeting miR-7 modulates the progression of non-small cell lung cancer in a manner dependent on NF-κB signalling. J Cell Mol Med 22(6):3097–3107. https://doi.org/10.1111/jcmm.13587

134. Tang W, Ji M, He G, Yang L, Niu Z, Jian M, Wei Y, Ren L, Xu J (2017) Silencing CDR1as inhibits colorectal cancer progression through regulating microRNA-7. Onco Targets Ther 10:2045–2056. https://doi.org/10.2147/ott.s131597

135. Zhao Z, Ji M, Wang Q, He N, Li Y (2019) Circular RNA Cdr1as upregulates SCAI to suppress cisplatin resistance in ovarian cancer via miR-1270 suppression. Mol Ther Nucleic Acids 18:24–33. https://doi.org/10.1016/j.omtn.2019.07.012

136. Wenzhe G, Jiahao X, Cheng P, Hongwei Z, Xiao Y (2020) Circular RNA HIPK3 is a prognostic and clinicopathological predictor in malignant tumor patients. J Cancer 11 (14):4230–4239. https://doi.org/10.7150/jca.40001

137. Jin P, Huang Y, Zhu P, Zou Y, Shao T, Wang O (2018) CircRNA circHIPK3 serves as a prognostic marker to promote glioma progression by regulating miR-654/IGF2BP3 signaling. Biochem Biophys Res Commun 503(3):1570–1574. https://doi.org/10.1016/j.bbrc.2018.07.081

138. Wei J, Xu H, Wei W, Wang Z, Zhang Q, De W, Shu Y (2020) circHIPK3 promotes cell proliferation and migration of gastric cancer by sponging miR-107 and regulating BDNF expression. Onco Targets Ther 13:1613–1624. https://doi.org/10.2147/ott.s226300

139. Cheng J, Zhuo H, Xu M, Wang L, Xu H, Peng J, Hou J, Lin L, Cai J (2018) Regulatory network of circRNA-miRNA-mRNA contributes to the histological classification and disease progression in gastric cancer. J Transl Med 16(1):216. https://doi.org/10.1186/s12967-018-1582-8

140. Liu Y, Xia L, Dong L, Wang J, Xiao Q, Yu X, Zhu H (2020) CircHIPK3 promotes gemcitabine (GEM) resistance in pancreatic cancer cells by sponging miR-330-5p and targets RASSF1. Cancer Manag Res 12:921–929. https://doi.org/10.2147/cmar.s239326

141. Liu N, Zhang J, Zhang LY, Wang L (2018) CircHIPK3 is upregulated and predicts a poor prognosis in epithelial ovarian cancer. Eur Rev Med Pharmacol Sci 22(12):3713–3718. https://doi.org/10.26355/eurrev_201806_15250

142. Zeng K, Chen X, Xu M, Liu X, Hu X, Xu T, Sun H, Pan Y, He B, Wang S (2018) CircHIPK3 promotes colorectal cancer growth and metastasis by sponging miR-7. Cell Death Dis 9(4):417. https://doi.org/10.1038/s41419-018-0454-8

143. Zhang Y, Li C, Liu X, Wang Y, Zhao R, Yang Y, Zheng X, Zhang Y, Zhang X (2019) circHIPK3 promotes oxaliplatin-resistance in colorectal cancer through autophagy by sponging miR-637. EBioMedicine 48:277–288. https://doi.org/10.1016/j.ebiom.2019.09.051

144. Chen D, Lu X, Yang F, Xing N (2019) Circular RNA circHIPK3 promotes cell proliferation and invasion of prostate cancer by sponging miR-193a-3p and regulating MCL1 expression. Cancer Manag Res 11:1415–1423. https://doi.org/10.2147/cmar.s190669

145. Li Y, Zheng F, Xiao X, Xie F, Tao D, Huang C, Liu D, Wang M, Wang L, Zeng F, Jiang G (2017) CircHIPK3 sponges miR-558 to suppress heparanase expression in bladder cancer cells. EMBO Rep 18(9):1646–1659.

https://doi.org/10.15252/embr.
201643581

146. Xie F, Zhao N, Zhang H, Xie D (2020) Circular RNA CircHIPK3 promotes gemcitabine sensitivity in bladder cancer. J Cancer 11 (7):1907–1912. https://doi.org/10.7150/jca.39722

147. Xiao-Long M, Kun-Peng Z, Chun-Lin Z (2018) Circular RNA circ_HIPK3 is downregulated and suppresses cell proliferation, migration and invasion in osteosarcoma. J Cancer 9(10):1856–1862. https://doi.org/10.7150/jca.24619

148. Hu J, Wang L, Chen J, Gao H, Zhao W, Huang Y, Jiang T, Zhou J, Chen Y (2018) The circular RNA circ-ITCH suppresses ovarian carcinoma progression through targeting miR-145/RASA1 signaling. Biochem Biophys Res Commun 505(1):222–228. https://doi.org/10.1016/j.bbrc.2018.09.060

149. Lin C, Xu X, Yang Q, Liang L, Qiao S (2020) Circular RNA ITCH suppresses proliferation, invasion, and glycolysis of ovarian cancer cells by up-regulating CDH1 via sponging miR-106a. Cancer Cell Int 20:336. https://doi.org/10.1186/s12935-020-01420-7

150. Yang C, Yuan W, Yang X, Li P, Wang J, Han J, Tao J, Li P, Yang H, Lv Q, Zhang W (2018) Circular RNA circ-ITCH inhibits bladder cancer progression by sponging miR-17/miR-224 and regulating p21, PTEN expression. Mol Cancer 17(1):19. https://doi.org/10.1186/s12943-018-0771-7

151. Li F, Ma K, Sun M, Shi S (2018) Identification of the tumor-suppressive function of circular RNA ITCH in glioma cells through sponging miR-214 and promoting linear ITCH expression. Am J Transl Res 10 (5):1373–1386

152. Hao C, Wangzhou K, Liang Z, Liu C, Wang L, Gong L, Tan Y, Li C, Lai Z, Hu G (2020) Circular RNA ITCH suppresses cell proliferation but induces apoptosis in oral squamous cell carcinoma by regulating miR-421/PDCD4 Axis. Cancer Manag Res 12:5651–5658. https://doi.org/10.2147/cmar.s258887

153. Wang X, Wang R, Wu Z, Bai P (2019) Circular RNA ITCH suppressed prostate cancer progression by increasing HOXB13 expression via spongy miR-17-5p. Cancer Cell Int 19:328. https://doi.org/10.1186/s12935-019-0994-8

154. Wang M, Chen B, Ru Z, Cong L (2018) CircRNA circ-ITCH suppresses papillary thyroid cancer progression through miR-22-3p/CBL/beta-catenin pathway. Biochem

Biophys Res Commun 504(1):283–288. https://doi.org/10.1016/j.bbrc.2018.08.175

155. Zeng W, Liu Y, Li WT, Li Y, Zhu JF (2020) CircFNDC3B sequestrates miR-937-5p to derepress TIMP3 and inhibit colorectal cancer progression. Mol Oncol 14 (11):2960–2984. https://doi.org/10.1002/1878-0261.12796

156. Liu H, Bi J, Dong W, Yang M, Shi J, Jiang N, Lin T, Huang J (2018) Invasion-related circular RNA circFNDC3B inhibits bladder cancer progression through the miR-1178-3p/G3BP2/SRC/FAK axis. Mol Cancer 17 (1):161. https://doi.org/10.1186/s12943-018-0908-8

157. Chen T, Yu Q, Shao S, Guo L (2020) Circular RNA circFNDC3B protects renal carcinoma by miR-99a downregulation. J Cell Physiol 235(5):4399–4406. https://doi.org/10.1002/jcp.29316

158. Hong Y, Qin H, Li Y, Zhang Y, Zhuang X, Liu L, Lu K, Li L, Deng X, Liu F, Shi S, Liu G (2019) FNDC3B circular RNA promotes the migration and invasion of gastric cancer cells via the regulation of E-cadherin and CD44 expression. J Cell Physiol 234 (11):19895–19910. https://doi.org/10.1002/jcp.28588

159. Wu G, Zhou W, Pan X, Sun Z, Sun Y, Xu H, Shi P, Li J, Gao L, Tian X (2020) Circular RNA profiling reveals exosomal circ_0006156 as a novel biomarker in papillary thyroid cancer. Mol Ther Nucleic Acids 19:1134–1144. https://doi.org/10.1016/j.omtn.2019.12.025

160. He YX, Ju H, Li N, Jiang YF, Zhao WJ, Song TT, Ren WH (2020) Association between hsa_circ_0006156 expression and incidence of gastric cancer. Eur Rev Med Pharmacol Sci 24(6):3030–3036. https://doi.org/10.26355/eurrev_202003_20667

161. Liu T, Song Z, Gai Y (2018) Circular RNA circ_0001649 acts as a prognostic biomarker and inhibits NSCLC progression via sponging miR-331-3p and miR-338-5p. Biochem Biophys Res Commun 503(3):1503–1509. https://doi.org/10.1016/j.bbrc.2018.07.070

162. Xing L, Zhang L, Feng Y, Cui Z, Ding L (2018) Downregulation of circular RNA hsa_circ_0001649 indicates poor prognosis for retinoblastoma and regulates cell proliferation and apoptosis via AKT/mTOR signaling pathway. Biomed Pharmacother 105:326–333. https://doi.org/10.1016/j.biopha.2018.05.141

163. Su Y, Xu C, Liu Y, Hu Y, Wu H (2019) Circular RNA hsa_circ_0001649 inhibits hepatocellular carcinoma progression via multiple miRNAs sponge. Aging 11 (10):3362–3375. https://doi.org/10.18632/aging.101988

164. Qin M, Liu G, Huo X, Tao X, Sun X, Ge Z, Yang J, Fan J, Liu L, Qin W (2016) Hsa_circ_0001649: A circular RNA and potential novel biomarker for hepatocellular carcinoma. Cancer Biomarkers 16(1):161–169. https://doi.org/10.3233/cbm-150552

165. Xu Y, Yao Y, Zhong X, Leng K, Qin W, Qu L, Cui Y, Jiang X (2018) Downregulated circular RNA hsa_circ_0001649 regulates proliferation, migration and invasion in cholangiocarcinoma cells. Biochem Biophys Res Commun 496(2):455–461. https://doi.org/10.1016/j.bbrc.2018.01.077

166. Hao L, Rong W, Bai L, Cui H, Zhang S, Li Y, Chen D, Meng X (2019) Upregulated circular RNA circ_0007534 indicates an unfavorable prognosis in pancreatic ductal adenocarcinoma and regulates cell proliferation, apoptosis, and invasion by sponging miR-625 and miR-892b. J Cell Biochem 120(3):3780–3789. https://doi.org/10.1002/jcb.27658

167. Li GF, Li L, Yao ZQ, Zhuang SJ (2018) Hsa_circ_0007534/miR-761/ZIC5 regulatory loop modulates the proliferation and migration of glioma cells. Biochem Biophys Res Commun 499(4):765–771. https://doi.org/10.1016/j.bbrc.2018.03.219

168. Li B, Li X (2018) Overexpression of hsa_circ_0007534 predicts unfavorable prognosis for osteosarcoma and regulates cell growth and apoptosis by affecting AKT/GSK-3beta signaling pathway. Biomed Pharmacother 107:860–866. https://doi.org/10.1016/j.biopha.2018.08.086

169. Ding DY, Wang D, Shu ZB (2020) Hsa_circ_0007534 knockdown represses the development of colorectal cancer cells through regulating miR-613/SLC25A22 axis. Eur Rev Med Pharmacol Sci 24 (6):3004–3022. https://doi.org/10.26355/eurrev_202003_20665

170. Westholm JO, Miura P, Olson S, Shenker S, Joseph B, Sanfilippo P, Celniker SE, Graveley BR, Lai EC (2014) Genome-wide analysis of drosophila circular RNAs reveals their structural and sequence properties and age-dependent neural accumulation. Cell Rep 9(5):1966–1980. https://doi.org/10.1016/j.celrep.2014.10.062

171. Xiao MS, Wilusz JE (2019) An improved method for circular RNA purification using RNase R that efficiently removes linear RNAs containing G-quadruplexes or structured 3′ ends. Nucleic Acids Res 47 (16):8755–8769. https://doi.org/10.1093/nar/gkz576

172. Szabo L, Salzman J (2016) Detecting circular RNAs: bioinformatic and experimental challenges. Nat Rev Genet 17(11):679–692. https://doi.org/10.1038/nrg.2016.114

173. Panda AC, De S, Grammatikakis I, Munk R, Yang X, Piao Y, Dudekula DB, Abdelmohsen K, Gorospe M (2017) High-purity circular RNA isolation method (RPAD) reveals vast collection of intronic circRNAs. Nucleic Acids Res 45(12):e116. https://doi.org/10.1093/nar/gkx297

174. Pandey PR, Rout PK, Das A, Gorospe M, Panda AC (2019) RPAD (RNase R treatment, polyadenylation, and poly(A)+ RNA depletion) method to isolate highly pure circular RNA. Methods (San Diego, Calif) 155:41–48. https://doi.org/10.1016/j.ymeth.2018.10.022

175. Gao Y, Wang J, Zhao F (2015) CIRI: an efficient and unbiased algorithm for de novo circular RNA identification. Genome Biol 16 (1):4. https://doi.org/10.1186/s13059-014-0571-3

176. Chuang TJ, Wu CS, Chen CY, Hung LY, Chiang TW, Yang MY (2016) NCLscan: accurate identification of non-co-linear transcripts (fusion, trans-splicing and circular RNA) with a good balance between sensitivity and precision. Nucleic Acids Res 44(3):e29. https://doi.org/10.1093/nar/gkv1013

177. Szabo L, Morey R, Palpant NJ, Wang PL, Afari N, Jiang C, Parast MM, Murry CE, Laurent LC, Salzman J (2015) Statistically based splicing detection reveals neural enrichment and tissue-specific induction of circular RNA during human fetal development. Genome Biol 16(1):126. https://doi.org/10.1186/s13059-015-0690-5

178. Song X, Zhang N, Han P, Moon BS, Lai RK, Wang K, Lu W (2016) Circular RNA profile in gliomas revealed by identification tool UROBORUS. Nucleic Acids Res 44(9):e87. https://doi.org/10.1093/nar/gkw075

179. Carrara M, Fuschi P, Ivan C, Martelli F (2018) Circular RNAs: methodological challenges and perspectives in cardiovascular diseases. J Cell Mol Med 22(11):5176–5187. https://doi.org/10.1111/jcmm.13789

180. Gao Y, Zhang J, Zhao F (2018) Circular RNA identification based on multiple seed matching. Brief Bioinform 19(5):803–810. https://doi.org/10.1093/bib/bbx014

181. Zeng X, Lin W, Guo M, Zou Q (2017) A comprehensive overview and evaluation of circular RNA detection tools. PLoS Comput Biol 13(6):e1005420. https://doi.org/10.1371/journal.pcbi.1005420

182. Hansen TB, Veno MT, Damgaard CK, Kjems J (2016) Comparison of circular RNA prediction tools. Nucleic Acids Res 44(6):e58. https://doi.org/10.1093/nar/gkv1458

183. Gao Y, Zhao F (2018) Computational strategies for exploring circular RNAs. Trends Genet 34(5):389–400. https://doi.org/10.1016/j.tig.2017.12.016

184. Chen B, Wei W, Huang X, Xie X, Kong Y, Dai D, Yang L, Wang J, Tang H, Xie X (2018) circEPSTI1 as a prognostic marker and mediator of triple-negative breast cancer progression. Theranostics 8(14):4003–4015. https://doi.org/10.7150/thno.24106

185. Chen L, Zhang S, Wu J, Cui J, Zhong L, Zeng L, Ge S (2017) circRNA_100290 plays a role in oral cancer by functioning as a sponge of the miR-29 family. Oncogene 36(32):4551–4561. https://doi.org/10.1038/onc.2017.89

186. Dou C, Cao Z, Yang B, Ding N, Hou T, Luo F, Kang F, Li J, Yang X, Jiang H, Xiang J, Quan H, Xu J, Dong S (2016) Changing expression profiles of lncRNAs, mRNAs, circRNAs and miRNAs during osteoclastogenesis. Sci Rep 6:21499. https://doi.org/10.1038/srep21499

187. Cortes-Lopez M, Miura P (2016) Emerging functions of circular RNAs. Yale J Biol Med 89(4):527–537

188. Lin J, Liao S, Li E, Liu Z, Zheng R, Wu X, Zeng W (2020) circCYFIP2 acts as a sponge of miR-1205 and affects the expression of its target gene E2F1 to regulate gastric cancer metastasis. Mol Ther Nucleic Acids 21:121–132. https://doi.org/10.1016/j.omtn.2020.05.007

189. Li G, Xue M, Yang F, Jin Y, Fan Y, Li W (2019) CircRBMS3 promotes gastric cancer tumorigenesis by regulating miR-153-SNAI1 axis. J Cell Physiol 234(3):3020–3028. https://doi.org/10.1002/jcp.27122

190. Wei S, Zheng Y, Jiang Y, Li X, Geng J, Shen Y, Li Q, Wang X, Zhao C, Chen Y, Qian Z, Zhou J, Li W (2019) The circRNA circPTPRA suppresses epithelial-mesenchymal transitioning and metastasis of NSCLC cells by sponging miR-96-5p. EBioMedicine 44:182–193. https://doi.org/10.1016/j.ebiom.2019.05.032

191. Li L, Wei H, Zhang H, Xu F, Che G (2020) Circ_100565 promotes proliferation, migration and invasion in non-small cell lung cancer through upregulating HMGA2 via sponging miR-506-3p. Cancer Cell Int 20:160. https://doi.org/10.1186/s12935-020-01241-8

192. Liu YT, Han XH, Xing PY, Hu XS, Hao XZ, Wang Y, Li JL, Zhang ZS, Yang ZH, Shi YK (2019) Circular RNA profiling identified as a biomarker for predicting the efficacy of Gefitinib therapy for non-small cell lung cancer. J Thoracic Dis 11(5):1779–1787. https://doi.org/10.21037/jtd.2019.05.22

193. Dai X, Liu J, Guo X, Cheng A, Deng X, Guo L, Wang Z (2020) Circular RNA circFGD4 suppresses gastric cancer progression via modulating miR-532-3p/APC/β-catenin signalling pathway. Clin Sci (London, England: 1979) 134(13):1821–1839. https://doi.org/10.1042/cs20191043

194. Dudekula DB, Panda AC, Grammatikakis I, De S, Abdelmohsen K, Gorospe M (2016) CircInteractome: a web tool for exploring circular RNAs and their interacting proteins and microRNAs. RNA Biol 13(1):34–42. https://doi.org/10.1080/15476286.2015.1128065

195. Zhong S, Wang J, Zhang Q, Xu H, Feng J (2018) CircPrimer: a software for annotating circRNAs and determining the specificity of circRNA primers. BMC Bioinformatics 19(1):292. https://doi.org/10.1186/s12859-018-2304-1

196. Chuang TJ, Chen YJ, Chen CY, Mai TL, Wang YD, Yeh CS, Yang MY, Hsiao YT, Chang TH, Kuo TC, Cho HH, Shen CN, Kuo HC, Lu MY, Chen YH, Hsieh SC, Chiang TW (2018) Integrative transcriptome sequencing reveals extensive alternative transsplicing and cis-backsplicing in human cells. Nucleic Acids Res 46(7):3671–3691. https://doi.org/10.1093/nar/gky032

197. Huang R, Zhang Y, Han B, Bai Y, Zhou R, Gan G, Chao J, Hu G, Yao H (2017) Circular RNA HIPK2 regulates astrocyte activation via cooperation of autophagy and ER stress by targeting MIR124-2HG. Autophagy 13(10):1722–1741. https://doi.org/10.1080/15548627.2017.1356975

198. Panda AC, Abdelmohsen K, Gorospe M (2017) RT-qPCR Detection of Senescence-Associated Circular RNAs. Methods Mol Biol (Clifton, NJ) 1534:79–87. https://doi.org/10.1007/978-1-4939-6670-7_7

199. Panda AC, Gorospe M (2018) Detection and Analysis of Circular RNAs by RT-PCR. Bio Protoc 8(6):e2775. https://doi.org/10.21769/BioProtoc.2775

200. Bachmayr-Heyda A, Reiner AT, Auer K, Sukhbaatar N, Aust S, Bachleitner-Hofmann-T, Mesteri I, Grunt TW, Zeillinger R, Pils D (2015) Correlation of circular RNA abundance with proliferation--exemplified with colorectal and ovarian cancer, idiopathic lung fibrosis, and normal human tissues. Sci Rep 5:8057. https://doi.org/10.1038/srep08057

201. Ma HB, Yao YN, Yu JJ, Chen XX, Li HF (2018) Extensive profiling of circular RNAs and the potential regulatory role of circRNA-000284 in cell proliferation and invasion of cervical cancer via sponging miR-506. Am J Transl Res 10(2):592–604

202. Rochow H, Franz A, Jung M, Weickmann S, Ralla B, Kilic E, Stephan C, Fendler A, Jung K (2020) Instability of circular RNAs in clinical tissue samples impairs their reliable expression analysis using RT-qPCR: from the myth of their advantage as biomarkers to reality. Theranostics 10(20):9268–9279. https://doi.org/10.7150/thno.46341

203. Zhong S, Zhou S, Yang S, Yu X, Xu H, Wang J, Zhang Q, Lv M, Feng J (2019) Identification of internal control genes for circular RNAs. Biotechnol Lett 41(10):1111–1119. https://doi.org/10.1007/s10529-019-02723-0

204. Panda AC, Grammatikakis I, Kim KM, De S, Martindale JL, Munk R, Yang X, Abdelmohsen K, Gorospe M (2017) Identification of senescence-associated circular RNAs (SAC-RNAs) reveals senescence suppressor CircPVT1. Nucleic Acids Res 45(7):4021–4035. https://doi.org/10.1093/nar/gkw1201

205. Wang PL, Bao Y, Yee MC, Barrett SP, Hogan GJ, Olsen MN, Dinneny JR, Brown PO, Salzman J (2014) Circular RNA is expressed across the eukaryotic tree of life. PLoS One 9(6):e90859. https://doi.org/10.1371/journal.pone.0090859

206. Roy CK, Olson S, Graveley BR, Zamore PD, Moore MJ (2015) Assessing long-distance RNA sequence connectivity via RNA-templated DNA-DNA ligation. eLife 4:e03700. https://doi.org/10.7554/eLife.03700

207. Cocquet J, Chong A, Zhang G, Veitia RA (2006) Reverse transcriptase template switching and false alternative transcripts. Genomics 88(1):127–131. https://doi.org/10.1016/j.ygeno.2005.12.013

208. Abe N, Matsumoto K, Nishihara M, Nakano Y, Shibata A, Maruyama H, Shuto S, Matsuda A, Yoshida M, Ito Y, Abe H (2015) Rolling circle translation of circular RNA in living human cells. Sci Rep 5:16435. https://doi.org/10.1038/srep16435

209. Quail MA, Kozarewa I, Smith F, Scally A, Stephens PJ, Durbin R, Swerdlow H, Turner DJ (2008) A large genome center's improvements to the Illumina sequencing system. Nat Methods 5(12):1005–1010. https://doi.org/10.1038/nmeth.1270

210. Hindson BJ, Ness KD, Masquelier DA, Belgrader P, Heredia NJ, Makarewicz AJ, Bright IJ, Lucero MY, Hiddessen AL, Legler TC, Kitano TK, Hodel MR, Petersen JF, Wyatt PW, Steenblock ER, Shah PH, Bousse LJ, Troup CB, Mellen JC, Wittmann DK, Erndt NG, Cauley TH, Koehler RT, So AP, Dube S, Rose KA, Montesclaros L, Wang S, Stumbo DP, Hodges SP, Romine S, Milanovich FP, White HE, Regan JF, Karlin-Neumann GA, Hindson CM, Saxonov S, Colston BW (2011) High-throughput droplet digital PCR system for absolute quantitation of DNA copy number. Anal Chem 83(22):8604–8610. https://doi.org/10.1021/ac202028g

211. Quan PL, Sauzade M, Brouzes E (2018) dPCR: A Technology Review. Sensors (Basel) 18(4):1271. https://doi.org/10.3390/s18041271

212. Li T, Shao Y, Fu L, Xie Y, Zhu L, Sun W, Yu R, Xiao B, Guo J (2018) Plasma circular RNA profiling of patients with gastric cancer and their droplet digital RT-PCR detection. J Mol Med (Berl) 96(1):85–96. https://doi.org/10.1007/s00109-017-1600-y

213. Trayhurn P (1996) Northern blotting. Proc Nutr Soc 55(1B):583–589. https://doi.org/10.1079/pns19960051

214. Schneider T, Schreiner S, Preußer C, Bindereif A, Rossbach O (2018) Northern blot analysis of circular RNAs. Methods Mol Biol 1724:119–133. https://doi.org/10.1007/978-1-4939-7562-4_10

215. Wang X, Shan G (2018) Nonradioactive Northern Blot of circRNAs. Methods Mol Biol 1724:135–141. https://doi.org/10.1007/978-1-4939-7562-4_11

216. Tabak HF, Van der Horst G, Smit J, Winter AJ, Mul Y, Groot Koerkamp MJ (1988) Discrimination between RNA circles, interlocked RNA circles and lariats using two-dimensional polyacrylamide gel electrophoresis. Nucleic Acids Res 16(14A):6597–6605. https://doi.org/10.1093/nar/16.14.6597

217. Zirkel A, Papantonis A (2018) Detecting circular RNAs by RNA fluorescence in situ hybridization. Methods Mol Biol 1724:69–75. https://doi.org/10.1007/978-1-4939-7562-4_6

218. Zhang J, Liu H, Hou L, Wang G, Zhang R, Huang Y, Chen X, Zhu J (2017) Circular RNA_LARP4 inhibits cell proliferation and invasion of gastric cancer by sponging miR-424-5p and regulating LATS1 expression. Mol Cancer 16(1):151. https://doi.org/10.1186/s12943-017-0719-3

219. Liu H, Liu Y, Bian Z, Zhang J, Zhang R, Chen X, Huang Y, Wang Y, Zhu J (2018) Circular RNA YAP1 inhibits the proliferation and invasion of gastric cancer cells by regulating the miR-367-5p/p27 (Kip1) axis. Mol Cancer 17(1):151. https://doi.org/10.1186/s12943-018-0902-1

220. Zhang J, Hou L, Liang R, Chen X, Zhang R, Chen W, Zhu J (2019) CircDLST promotes the tumorigenesis and metastasis of gastric cancer by sponging miR-502-5p and activating the NRAS/MEK1/ERK1/2 signaling. Mol Cancer 18(1):80. https://doi.org/10.1186/s12943-019-1015-1

221. Liu Z, Zhou Y, Liang G, Ling Y, Tan W, Tan L, Andrews R, Zhong W, Zhang X, Song E, Gong C (2019) Circular RNA hsa_circ_001783 regulates breast cancer progression via sponging miR-200c-3p. Cell Death Dis 10(2):55. https://doi.org/10.1038/s41419-018-1287-1

222. Kocks C, Boltengagen A, Piwecka M, Rybak-Wolf A, Rajewsky N (2018) Single-Molecule Fluorescence In Situ Hybridization (FISH) of Circular RNA CDR1as. Methods Mol Biol 1724:77–96. https://doi.org/10.1007/978-1-4939-7562-4_7

223. Wang L, Long H, Zheng Q, Bo X, Xiao X, Li B (2019) Circular RNA circRHOT1 promotes hepatocellular carcinoma progression by initiation of NR2F6 expression. Mol Cancer 18(1):119. https://doi.org/10.1186/s12943-019-1046-7

224. Florkowski CM (2008) Sensitivity, specificity, receiver-operating characteristic (ROC) curves and likelihood ratios: communicating the performance of diagnostic tests. Clin Biochem Rev 29 Suppl 1(Suppl 1):S83–S87

225. Shiu SY, Gatsonis C (2008) The predictive receiver operating characteristic curve for the joint assessment of the positive and negative predictive values. Phil Trans A Math Phys Eng Sci 366(1874):2313–2333. https://doi.org/10.1098/rsta.2008.0043

226. Goel MK, Khanna P, Kishore J (2010) Understanding survival analysis: Kaplan-Meier estimate. Int J Ayurveda Res 1(4):274–278. https://doi.org/10.4103/0974-7788.76794

227. Bland JM, Altman DG (2004) The logrank test. BMJ 328(7447):1073. https://doi.org/10.1136/bmj.328.7447.1073

228. Savas S, Liu G, Xu W (2013) Special considerations in prognostic research in cancer involving genetic polymorphisms. BMC Med 11:149. https://doi.org/10.1186/1741-7015-11-149

229. Costa MC, Enguita FJ (2020) Towards a universal nomenclature standardization for circular RNAs. Non-coding RNA Investig 4

230. Jiang XM, Li ZL, Li JL, Xu Y, Leng KM, Cui YF, Sun DJ (2018) A novel prognostic biomarker for cholangiocarcinoma: circRNA Cdr1as. Eur Rev Med Pharmacol Sci 22(2):365–371. https://doi.org/10.26355/eurrev_201801_14182

231. Sang M, Meng L, Liu S, Ding P, Chang S, Ju Y, Liu F, Gu L, Lian Y, Geng C (2018) Circular RNA ciRS-7 maintains metastatic phenotypes as a ceRNA of miR-1299 to target MMPs. Mol Cancer Res 16(11):1665–1675. https://doi.org/10.1158/1541-7786.mcr-18-0284

232. Xu L, Zhang M, Zheng X, Yi P, Lan C, Xu M (2017) The circular RNA ciRS-7 (Cdr1as) acts as a risk factor of hepatic microvascular invasion in hepatocellular carcinoma. J Cancer Res Clin Oncol 143(1):17–27. https://doi.org/10.1007/s00432-016-2256-7

233. Zhang J, Hu H, Zhao Y, Zhao Y (2018) CDR1as is overexpressed in laryngeal squamous cell carcinoma to promote the tumour's progression via miR-7 signals. Cell proliferation 51(6):e12521. https://doi.org/10.1111/cpr.12521

234. Xu B, Yang T, Wang Z, Zhang Y, Liu S, Shen M (2018) CircRNA CDR1as/miR-7 signals promote tumor growth of osteosarcoma with a potential therapeutic and diagnostic value. Cancer Manag Res 10:4871–4880. https://doi.org/10.2147/cmar.s178213

235. Li J, Guo R, Liu Q, Sun J, Wang H (2020) Circular RNA Circ-ITCH inhibits the malignant behaviors of cervical cancer by microRNA-93-5p/FOXK2 axis. Reprod Sci 27(3):860–868. https://doi.org/10.1007/s43032-020-00140-7

236. Ren C, Liu J, Zheng B, Yan P, Sun Y, Yue B (2019) The circular RNA circ-ITCH acts as a tumour suppressor in osteosarcoma via regulating miR-22. Artif Cells Nanomed Biotechnol 47(1):3359–3367. https://doi.org/10.1080/21691401.2019.1649273

237. Zhang R, Xu J, Zhao J, Wang X (2018) Silencing of hsa_circ_0007534 suppresses proliferation and induces apoptosis in

colorectal cancer cells. Eur Rev Med Pharmacol Sci 22(1):118–126. https://doi.org/10.26355/eurrev_201801_14108

238. Rong X, Gao W, Yang X, Guo J (2019) Downregulation of hsa_circ_0007534 restricts the proliferation and invasion of cervical cancer through regulating miR-498/BMI-1 signaling. Life Sci 235:116785. https://doi.org/10.1016/j.lfs.2019.116785

239. Song L, Xiao Y (2018) Downregulation of hsa_circ_0007534 suppresses breast cancer cell proliferation and invasion by targeting miR-593/MUC19 signal pathway. Biochem Biophys Res Commun 503(4):2603–2610. https://doi.org/10.1016/j.bbrc.2018.08.007

# Chapter 22

## Bioinformatic Analysis of Circular RNA Expression

### Enrico Gaffo, Alessia Buratin, Anna Dal Molin, and Stefania Bortoluzzi

### Abstract

Circular RNAs (circRNAs) are stable RNA molecules generated by backsplicing that play regulatory functions through interaction with other RNA and proteins, as well as by encoding peptides. Dysregulation of circRNA expression can drive cancer development and progression with different mechanisms. CircRNAs are currently regarded as extremely attractive molecules in cancer research for the identification of new and possibly targetable disease regulatory networks and for the development of biomarkers for cancer diagnosis, prognosis definition, and monitoring. Using specific experimental and computational protocols, circRNAs can be identified through RNA-seq by spotting the reads spanning backsplice junctions, which are specific to circular molecules. In this chapter, we report a state-of-the-art computational protocol for a genome-wide analysis of circRNAs from RNA-seq data, which considers circRNA detection, quantification, and differential expression testing. Finally, we indicate how to determine circular transcript sequences and the resources for an in silico functional characterization of circRNAs.

**Key words** Circular RNA, RNA-seq, Bioinformatics, Computational pipeline

## 1  Introduction

Circular RNAs (circRNAs) are transcripts in which a downstream splice donor site is covalently bound to an upstream acceptor site by a process called backsplicing (Fig. 1). Pervasive circRNAs expression has been recently described in Eukaryotes with expression variations among tissues and throughout differentiation stages [1, 2]. CircRNAs are particularly stable molecules that can play regulatory functions by interacting with microRNAs [3] and proteins [4] and by encoding biologically active specific peptides [5–8].

In the last years, we witnessed a rising interest of the scientific community on circRNAs, mainly with the aim of identifying new and possibly targetable disease mechanisms [9]. Robust evidence about circRNAs dysregulation and function in solid [10–13] and hematologic cancer [9, 14–17], as well as other diseases, is quickly accumulating. Moreover, the stability and detectability in body fluids of circRNAs make them ideal biomarkers [18].

Alfons Navarro (ed.), *Long Non-Coding RNAs in Cancer*, Methods in Molecular Biology, vol. 2348,
https://doi.org/10.1007/978-1-0716-1581-2_22, © Springer Science+Business Media, LLC, part of Springer Nature 2021

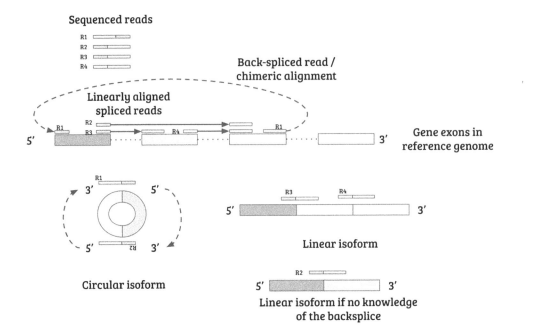

**Fig. 1** Backsplice reads identify circRNAs. CircRNAs can be identified through RNA-seq reads spanning the backsplice junctions (green-pink read R1), which are specific to circular transcripts. It is not possible to determine which is the origin of reads from exons common to linear and circular transcripts (pink-green read R2)

Genome-wide investigation of circRNA expression can be performed by means of RNA-seq of total RNA libraries. Lacking a polyadenylated tail, circRNAs are depleted by traditional mRNA enrichment library protocols (poly(A) + sequencing). The resistance of circRNAs to RNase R activity allows enriching the circular RNA fraction by RNase R treatment [19]. However, circRNAs sensitive to the enzyme [20] would be lost. A wider picture of global expression can be achieved by the use of ribosomal RNA depleted (rRNA-) and/or poly(A)- sequencing protocols, which allow the study of both circular and linear RNAs within the same experiment. However, sequence overlap between circRNAs and their parent-gene linear transcripts (Fig. 1) makes it hard to disentangle circular and linear expression [21, 22].

In this chapter, we describe a computational protocol for circRNA detection and quantification from RNA-seq data. Next, we show how to test for circRNA differential expression and study the relationship between linear and circular transcript expression. Finally, we indicate how to reconstruct the sequence of circRNAs and provide some hints on in silico circRNA functional characterization.

# 2   Materials

## 2.1   Hardware Requirements

To perform all the bioinformatics analyses, you will need a workstation with this minimal hardware.

1. $\geq 2$ CPU cores (*see* **Note 1**).
2. $\geq 8$ GBytes of RAM (*see* **Note 2**).
3. $\geq 200$ GBytes of free disk space (*see* **Note 3**).
4. Internet connection for software installation and data retrieval.

## 2.2   CircRNA Detection

### 2.2.1   Software Requirements and Installation

Most software run on the Linux operating system (OS) (*see* **Note 4**). The next commands were tested on an Ubuntu 16.04 and 20.04 Linux OS (*see* **Note 5**) and will install the software composing a circRNA analysis pipeline.

1. Most circRNA detection tools execute from a command line interface, so if working from a graphical user interface (GUI) environment (such as a Ubuntu desktop), you will need to open a terminal emulator window, such as the gnome-terminal. In Ubuntu 16.04, you can use the keyboard shortcut combination CTRL+ALT+T or search "terminal" in the search dashboard. All the following commands will be input to the command line prompt (*see* **Notes 6–10**).

2. Create a directory where to install the software; then, enter the directory.

```
user@mypc:~$ mkdir tools
user@mypc:~$ cd tools
```

3. Download CIRI2 [23], extract the package, and (optionally) make a link to the main script into the tools directory (*see* **Notes 11** and **12**).

```
user@mypc:tools$ wget http://downloads.sourceforge.net/pro-
ject/ciri/CIRI2/CIRI_v2.0.6.zip
user@mypc:tools$ unzip CIRI_v2.0.6.zip
user@mypc:tools$ ln -s CIRI_v2.0.6/CIRI2.pl
```

4. Download BWA [24] (*see* **Notes 13** and **14**), extract the package, and (optionally) make a link to the main script into the tools directory (*see* **Note 12**).

```
user@mypc:tools$ wget https://sourceforge.net/projects/bio-
bwa/files/bwakit/bwakit-0.7.15_x64-linux.tar.bz2
user@mypc:tools$ tar -xf bwakit-0.7.15_x64-linux.tar.bz2
user@mypc:tools$ ln -s bwa.kit/bwa
```

5. Download BEDTools [25], extract the package, compile the source code, and (optionally) make a link to the main script into the tools directory (*see* **Notes 15** and **16**).

```
user@mypc:tools$ wget https://github.com/arq5x/bedtools2/re-
leases/download/v2.29.2/bedtools-2.29.2.tar.gz
user@mypc:tools$ tar -xf bedtools-2.29.2.tar.gz
user@mypc:tools$ cd bedtools2
user@mypc:bedtools2$ make
user@mypc:bedtools2$ cd ..
user@mypc:tools$ ln -s bedtools2/bin/bedtools
```

6. Download Samtools [26], extract the package, and generate the executable files by compiling the code (*see* **Notes 17–19**). Optionally, make a link to the main script into the tools directory.

```
user@mypc:tools$ wget https://github.com/samtools/samtools/
releases/download/1.10/samtools-1.10.tar.bz2
user@mypc:tools$ tar -xf samtools-1.10.tar.bz2
user@mypc:tools$ cd samtools-1.10
user@mypc:samtools-1.10$ make prefix=$PWD install
user@mypc:samtools-1.10$ cd ..
user@mypc:tools$ ln -s samtools-1.10/samtools
```

7. Download HISAT2 [27] (*see* **Note 20**), extract the package and (optionally) make a link to the main scripts into the tools directory (*see* **Note 21**).

```
user@mypc:tools$ wget https://cloud.biohpc.swmed.edu/index.
php/s/hisat2-210-Linux_x86_64/download -O hisat2-2.1.0-Li-
nux_x86_64.zip
user@mypc:tools$ unzip hisat2-2.1.0-Linux_x86_64.zip
user@mypc:tools$ ln -s hisat2-2.1.0/hisat2
user@mypc:tools$ ln -s hisat2-2.1.0/hisat2-build
```

8. Download FASTQC [28], extract the package and (optionally) make a link to the main script into the tools directory (*see* **Notes 22** and **23**).

```
user@mypc:tools$ wget http://www.bioinformatics.babraham.ac.
uk/projects/fastqc/fastqc_v0.11.9.zip
user@mypc:tools$ unzip fastqc_v0.11.9.zip
user@mypc:tools$ chmod +x FastQC/fastqc
user@mypc:tools$ ln -s FastQC/fastqc
```

9. Download SRAToolkit [29], extract the package, and configure the installation (*see* **Notes 24** and **25**).

```
user@mypc:tools$ wget https://ftp-trace.ncbi.nlm.nih.gov/sra/
sdk/2.10.8/sratoolkit.2.10.8-ubuntu64.tar.gz
```

```
user@mypc:tools$ tar -xf sratoolkit.2.10.8-ubuntu64.tar.gz
user@mypc:tools$ cd sratoolkit.2.10.8-ubuntu64/
user@mypc:sratoolkit.2.10.8-ubuntu64$ ./bin/vdb-config -i
```

Then follow the instructions on the screen to complete the configuration.

10. Download Trimmomatic [30] and extract the package.

```
user@mypc:tools$ wget http://www.usadellab.org/cms/uploads/
supplementary/Trimmomatic/Trimmomatic-0.39.zip
user@mypc:tools$ unzip Trimmomatic-0.39.zip
```

11. Add the tools directory to the environment path so that you can avoid writing the whole path of the tool (*see* **Notes 26** and **27**).

```
user@mypc:tools$ export PATH='pwd':$PATH
```

2.2.2  *Input Data*

1. Open a terminal as in **item 1** of Subheading 2.2.1 (Software requirements and installation).

2. To keep files in order, create a directory where to store the data and processing files, and enter it.

```
user@mypc:~$ mkdir data
user@mypc:~$ cd data
```

3. Download and decompress the reference genome (*see* **Note 28**).

```
user@mypc:data$ wget ftp://ftp.ensembl.org/pub/release-
100/fasta/homo_sapiens/dna/Homo_sapiens.GRCh38.dna.pri-
mary_assembly.fa.gz
user@mypc:data$ gunzip Homo_sapiens.GRCh38.dna.primary_assem-
bly.fa.gz
```

4. Download and decompress the gene annotation in GTF format (*see* **Note 29**).

```
user@mypc:data$ wget ftp://ftp.ensembl.org/pub/release-
100/gtf/homo_sapiens/Homo_sapiens.GRCh38.100.gtf.gz
user@mypc:data$ gunzip Homo_sapiens.GRCh38.100.gtf.gz
```

5. Get the RNA-seq data from SRA and convert into compressed FASTQ files (*see* **Notes 30–32**).

```
user@mypc:data$ fastq-dump --split-files --gzip SRR6674620
user@mypc:data$ cd ..
```

### 2.3  CircRNA Expression Analysis

1. First install R. Open a terminal and run the following in the command line to install base R.

*2.3.1  Software Requirements and Installation*

```
user@mypc:~$ sudo apt -y install r-base
```

2. Open an R session.

```
user@mypc$ R
```

3. Install the following CRAN packages: BiocManager, data.table, dplyr, plyr, tidyverse. From the R command line, install the packages from CRAN by typing in the console or using the graphical interface, you can use the following function to install them one by one (*see* **Note 33**).

```
install.packages("BiocManager")
install.packages("data.table")
install.packages("dplyr")
install.packages("plyr")
install.packages("tidyverse")
```

4. Install the DESeq2 package from Bioconductor, using Bioc-Manager::install() function for each package (*see* **Note 33**).

```
install.packages("BiocManager")
BiocManager::install("DESeq2")
```

5. From the R command line, Install CircTest package. You will need also the devtool package to be installed and loaded, as the CircTest code is available from GitHub (*see* **Note 34**).

```
install.packages("devtools")
require(devtools)
install_github('dieterich-lab/CircTest')
```

*2.3.2  Input  Data*

1. Open a terminal.

2. Enter the created data directory:

```
user@mypc:~$ cd data
```

3. Repeat **item 5** of Subheading 2.2.2 (CircRNA detection: input data). to get the RNA-seq data from SRA for each sample.

4. Repeat **items 1–11** of Subheading 2.2.1 to quantify circRNA expression for each sample.

**2.4  CircRNA Characterization**

*2.4.1  Software Requirements and Installation*

1. Open a terminal as in **item 1** of Subheading 2.2.1(Software requirements and installation).
2. Install Perl (*see* **Note 73**).

```
user@mypc:~$ sudo apt-get install perl
```

3. Enter the directory where the software is installed.

```
user@mypc:~$ cd tools
```

4. Download CIRI-AS [23, 31] from https://sourceforge.net/ projects/ciri/files/CIRI-AS/, extract the package and (optionally) make a link to the main script into the tools directory (*see* **Note 12**).

```
user@mypc:tools$ jar xf rt.jar CIRI-vis_v1.4.jar
user@mypc:tools$ ln -s CIRI-vis_v1.4/CIRI_AS_1.2.pl
```

5. Download BEDTools as in **item 5** of Subheading 2.2.1.

*2.4.2  Input Data*

1. Open a terminal as in **item 1** of Subheading 2.2.1(Software requirements and installation).
2. Enter the directory where data are stored.

```
user@mypc:~$ cd data
```

3. Make sure to have these four files in the directory.

```
user@mypc:data$ ls
```

- "SRR6674620_bwa.sam" (the SAM file of chimeric alignment records generated by BWA-MEM).
- "SRR6674620_ciri.out" (the circRNA list generated by CIRI2 by processing the alignment file).
- "Homo_sapiens.GRCh38.dna.primary_assembly. fa" (the reference genome in FASTA format).
- "Homo_sapiens.GRCh38.100.gtf" (the genome annotation in GTF format).

# 3  Methods

To identify putative backsplicing events, many computational methods have been developed since the first genome-wide characterization of a circular transcriptome [32]. Almost all methods rely on the identification of chimeric alignments in which the read segments are aligned in chiastic order (Fig. 1).

CircRNA characterization adds up to a traditional RNA-seq analysis (Fig. 2). CircRNA detection methods usually consider a prefiltering of the reads that align collinearly to the genome, for later processing the unmapped reads, which likely bear backsplice junctions. The amount of backsplicing reads serve to determine circular transcripts' expression level, as well as their correlation with the parent gene linear transcripts; while the backsplice genome coordinates allow downstream characterization of the circRNA.

In the following sections, we will consider one of the most popular tools for circRNA detection. Nevertheless, the procedure is similar to other methods.

**3.1 Input Preprocessing and circRNA Detection**

**Steps 1**–**7** indicate how to clean raw reads and filter out reads belonging to linear transcripts or reads that cannot be uniquely assigned to either linear or circular transcripts. Start from **step 8** if you were provided with an alignment file. Start from **step 9** if you already have clean reads purged from linear transcript reads (*see* **Note 35**).

1. Open a terminal session. All commands are assumed to be run in the same directory where the data is stored.

2. Assess the quality of the sequencing by inspecting FASTQC reports (*see* **Notes 36** and **37**).

```
user@mypc:data$ mkdir read_stats
user@mypc:data$ cd read_stats
user@mypc:read_stats$ fastqc ../data/SRR6674620_1.fastq.gz -o
fastqc_stats --extract > SRR6674620_1.fastq_fastqc.log 2>
SRR6674620_1.fastq_fastqc.err
user@mypc:read_stats$ fastqc ../data/SRR6674620_2.fastq.gz -o
fastqc_stats --extract > SRR6674620_2.fastq_fastqc.log 2>
SRR6674620_2.fastq_fastqc.err
user@mypc:read_stats$ cd ..
```

3. Remove low quality reads, residual adapter sequences and trim low quality read segments (*see* **Notes 38** and **39**) (optional).

```
user@mypc:data$ mkdir trimmomatic
user@mypc:data$ java -jar ../tools/Trimmomatic-0.39/trimmo-
matic-0.39.jar PE -threads 4
  SRR6674620_1.fastq.gz SRR6674620_2.fastq.gz trimmomatic/
SRR6674620_1.fq.P.qtrim.gz
trimmomatic/SRR6674620_1.fq.U.qtrim.gz trimmomatic/
SRR6674620_2.fq.P.qtrim.gz
trimmomatic/SRR6674620_2.fq.U.qtrim.gz ILLUMINACLIP:../tools/
Trimmomatic-0.39/adapters/TruSeq3-
PE-2.fa:2:30:10 MAXINFO:40:0.5 LEADING:20 TRAILING:20 SLIDING
WINDOW:4:30 MINLEN:35 AVGQUAL:30 2> trimmomatic.log
```

4. Check the clean read quality to evaluate the effect of the cleaning procedure.

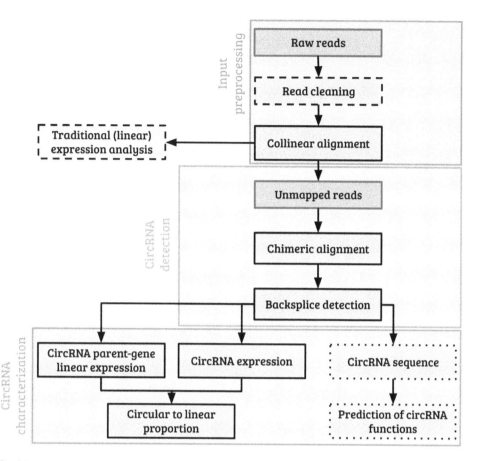

**Fig. 2** CircRNA analysis bioinformatics pipeline

```
user@mypc:data$ fastqc trimmomatic/SRR6674620_1.fq.P.qtrim.gz
-o fastqc_stats --extract > fastqc_stats/SRR6674620_1.fq.P.
qtrim_fastqc.log 2> fastqc_stats/SRR6674620_1.fq.P.qtrim_-
fastqc.err
user@mypc:data$ fastqc trimmomatic/SRR6674620_2.fq.P.qtrim.gz
-o fastqc_stats --extract > fastqc_stats/SRR6674620_2.fq.P.
qtrim_fastqc.log 2> fastqc_stats/SRR6674620_2.fq.P.qtrim_-
fastqc.err
```

5. Generate genome index for HISAT2 (*see* **Notes 40–43**).

```
user@mypc:data$ mkdir -p indexes/hisat2
user@mypc:data$ hisat2-build -f --seed 123 -p 4 Homo_sapiens.
GRCh38.dna.primary_
assembly.fa
indexes/hisat2/Homo_sapiens.GRCh38.dna.primary_assembly
```

6. Generate genome index for BWA (*see* **Note 44**).

```
user@mypc:data$ mkdir -p indexes/bwa
```

```
user@mypc:data$ bwa index -a bwtsw -p indexes/bwa/Homo_sa-
piens.GRCh38.dna.
primary_assembly
Homo_sapiens.GRCh38.dna.primary_assembly.fa
```

7. Align reads to filter out collinearly aligned reads (*see* **Notes 45–48**). If you preprocessed the reads with Trimmomatic, use as input the SRR6674620_1.fq.P.qtrim.gz and the SRR6674620_1.fq.P.qtrim.gz files in place of the SRR6674620_2.fastq.gz and the SRR6674620_2.fastq.gz files.

```
user@mypc:data$ mkdir hisat2_out
user@mypc:data$ cd hisat2_out
user@mypc:hisat2_out$ ../../tools/hisat2 -x ../grch38/genome
-p 6 --no-discordant --no-mixed -1 ../SRR6674620_1.fastq.gz -2
../SRR6674620_2.fastq.gz --un-conc-gz unmapped_%.fq.gz >
SRR6674620_hisat2.sam 2> SRR6674620_hisat2.log
```

    (a) Convert the alignment file into a sorted BAM (*see* **Notes 49–51**). You will need a BAM formatted file later in this sample analysis.

```
user@mypc:hisat2_out$ samtools sort -m 768M -O 'bam' -@ 4 -T
hisat2_SRR6674620 SRR6674620_hisat2.sam > SRR6674620_hisat2.
bam
user@mypc:hisat2_out$ cd ..
```

    (b) Generate an index of the alignment file for a fast parsing by downstream methods.

```
user@mypc:data$ samtools index hisat2_out/SRR6674620_hisat2.
bam
hisat2_out/SRR6674620_hisat2.bam.bai
```

8. If you were provided already with an alignment file in SAM/-BAM format you can extract the collinearly unmapped reads from it by using Samtools.

    (a) Filter out collinearly aligned reads, extract unmapped reads and convert them in FASTQ format (*see* **Notes 52 and 53**):

```
user@mypc:data$ samtools fastq -f 12 -F 3328 -n -s singleton.
fastq -1 unmapped_1.fastq -2
 unmapped_2.fastq hisat2_out/SRR6674620_hisat2.bam
```

    (b) Compress the unmapped read files to save disk space (optional).

```
user@mypc:data$ gzip unmapped_1.fastq
user@mypc:data$ gzip unmapped_2.fastq
user@mypc:data$ gzip singleton.fastq
```

9. Align collinearly unmapped reads allowing chimeric alignments (*see* **Note 54**).

```
user@mypc:data$ mkdir bwa_out
user@mypc:data$ ../tools/bwa mem -t 4 -T 19 indexes/bwa/Homo_-
sapiens.GRCh38.dna.primary_assembly hisat2_out/unmapped_1.fq.
gz hisat2_out/unmapped_2.fq.gz > bwa_out/SRR6674620_bwa.sam
```

10. CircRNA detection: detect backsplices (*see* **Notes 55** and **56**).

```
user@mypc:data$ mkdir ciri_out
user@mypc:data$ cd ciri_out
user@mypc:ciri_out$ perl ../tools/CIRI2.pl -T 1 -I
SRR6674620_bwa.sam -O SRR6674620_ciri.out -F data/Homo_sa-
piens.GRCh38.dna.primary_assembly.fa -A data/Homo_sapiens.
GRCh38.100.gtf
user@mypc:ciri_out$ cd ..
```

CircRNA identifiers will be stored in the SRR6674620_ciri.out file. Each circRNA is identified by the backsplicing junction genomic coordinates reported as chromosome, start position (the end base of the backsplice), end position (actually where the backsplice begins), and strand.

Postdetection filters might be applied, such as the following.

(a) Maximum and minimum backsplice/circRNA length (a transcript does not usually span more than 100/200 kbp, while the minimal length should be set according to the size of the sequenced fragments, which consider read length and insert size, usually 200 bp in current sequencing experiments).

(b) Minimum expression (at least 2 reads spanning the backsplice).

(c) Discard circRNAs from circular chromosomes, such as the mitochondrial genome.

11. Collinear read counts on backsplice junctions (for later computing of CLP) (*see* **Note 57**)

(a) Generate a .genome file, which is required by some BED-Tools functions.

```
user@mypc:data$ grep "^@SQ" bwa_out/SRR6674620_bwa.sam | sed
-r 's/.*SN:([^\t]+)\tLN:([^ ]+)/\1\t\2/' &gt; chr_len.genome
```

(b) Convert CIRI2 output into BED intervals.

```
user@mypc:data$ grep -v '^circRNA_ID' ciri_out/
SRR6674620_ciri.out | awk 'OFS="\t" {print $2,$3-=1,$4,$1,$5,
```

```
$11}' | sort -k1,1 -k2,2n | uniq > ciri_out/SRR6674620_ciri.
bed
```

    (c)  Generate single nucleotide intervals to identify the bases flanking the backsplice junctions (i.e., last intron base of the start coordinate and first intron base for the end coordinate).

```
user@mypc:data$ bedtools flank -i ciri_out/SRR6674620_ciri.bed
-g chr_len.genome -s -b 1 | bedtools sort -faidx chr_len.genome
-i stdin > sorted_sn_circ.bed
```

    (d)  Count reads spanning the nucleotides flanking the backsplice junctions. Using the collinear alignment file we will count reads from linear transcripts (*see* **Notes 58** and **59**).

```
user@mypc:data$ bedtools coverage -counts -sorted -g chr_len.
genome -a sorted_sn_circ.bed -b hisat2_out/SRR6674620_hisat2.
bam > SRR6674620_bks_linear_counts.tab
```

## 3.2 CircRNA Expression Analysis

After circRNA detection and quantification, a common task is the definition of circRNAs differentially expressed among conditions.

Several Bioconductor packages for DE analysis of RNA-Seq data (DESeq2 [33], edgeR [34], limma [35], and baySeq [36]) implement whole RNA-Seq data analysis pipelines which can be used to identify DE circRNAs from the count of reads spanning the backsplices. DESeq2 is used in the following example code.

1. Open a terminal. All commands are assumed to be run in the same directory where the data is stored.

2. Create a new directory for the analyses.

```
user@mypc:~$ cd data
user@mypc:data~$ mkdir analyses
user@mypc:data~$ cd analyses
```

3. Open an R session.

```
user@mypc:data/analyses~$ R
```

4. Load required Packages.

```
library("BiocManager")
library("dplyr")
library("tidyverse")
library("plyr")
library("data.table")
library("DESEq2")
```

5. Merge the backsplicing spanning read counts into one matrix having one row for each circRNA and one column for each

sample. At first, you have to search within the sample folders the files of circRNA predictions.

```
Samples <- c("SRR6674618","SRR6674619","SRR6674620",
 "SRR6674622","SRR6674623","SRR6674624")
```

6. Create an input list of CIRI outputs.

```
inputs <- list()
for(i in 1:length(Samples)){
inputs[[i]] <- paste0("../data/", Samples[i],"ciri.out/",Sam-
ples[i],"_ciri.out")
}
names(input) <- Samples
```

7. Then, a joined backspliced count table can be created from different samples (*see* **Note 60**).

```
combined.df <- ldply(input, function(x){
 a <- read.table(file=x, sep="\t", header=T, comment.char="",
stringsAsFactors=F)[,c(1:11)]; a})
colnames(combined.df)[1] <- "sampleID"
```

8. DESeq2 requires an object of class DESeqDataSet to perform the analysis. We will use the DESeqDataSetFromMatrix function to build such an object, as we already have a matrix of read counts. Also, we need to specify the sample information table, which we name coldata (*see* **Note 61**).

```
counts <- as.matrix(combined.df)
coldata <- data.frame(sample_id=Samples,
 condition=c("B","B","B","M","M","M"))
rownames(coldata) <- coldata$sample_id
coldata <- coldata[,c("condition")]
coldata$condition <- factor(coldata$condition)
```

9. Build up a DESeqDataSet object.

```
dds <- DESeqDataSetFromMatrix(countData = counts,
 colData = coldata,
 design = ~ condition)
```

10. Perform a basic filtering to discard circRNAs with few BS-supporting reads, for instance, at least 5 reads in total (*see* **Note 62**).

```
keep <- rowSums(counts(dds)) >= 5
dds <- dds[keep,]
```

11. The standard differential expression analysis steps are wrapped into a single function, *DESeq*. (*see* **Note 63**).

```
dds <- DESeq(dds)
```

12. The *results* function returns a table with log2 fold change, p-values, and adjusted p-values of the test, for each circRNA (*see* **Notes 64** and **65**).

```
res <- results(dds)
```

### 3.3 Circular to Linear Transcript Differential Proportion Analysis

Recent study suggests that the circRNA–linear mRNA balance control contributes to the post-transcriptional gene regulation [37]. The information of parental genes could potentially provide biological insights of circRNA–linear mRNA interplay. To discern which circular and linear RNA isoform expressions diverge, counts of the reads that are linearly spliced on the backsplice junctions are used as an estimate of the parental gene expression.

Let $x_{ij}$ be the observed circular read counts and $n_{ij}$ the total read counts (circRNA plus mRNA) of $i$th circRNA in $j$th condition. Then, the circular to linear expression proportion (CLP) is calculated as $\mathrm{CLP}_{ij} = x_{ij}/n_{ij}$ (Fig. 3).

A CLP > 0.5 will indicate circRNAs that are more expressed than the linear counterpart. To test whether the proportion is significantly varied across experimental conditions, a likelihood ratio test (ANOVA) can be used (*see* **Note 66**), as the one implemented in the CircTest R package [38]. To run the *Circ.test* function you need the table with the backspliced read counts and the corresponding host-gene linearly spliced read counts. For both matrices a column named "circ_id" that contains the circRNA identifiers has to be added as a non–read count column. Both matrices must have the same order of rows (*see* **Note 67**).

1. Load the package and the required matrices.

```
library(CircTest)
Circ <- as.matrix(combined.df)
Circ <- Circ[order(Circ$circ_id), ]
circ.lin.xpr <- data.table(ciri_bks_linexp)
```

2. A joined host-gene read count table will be created from different samples using the "*_bks_linear_counts.tab" generated for each sample in **step 11**. of Input preprocessing and circRNA detection.

```
input <- list()
```

```
for(i in 1:length(Samples)){
 input[[i]] <- paste0("../data/",
 Samples[i],"_bks_linear_counts.tab")
}
names(input) = Samples
bks_linear_counts.tab.gz <-
 rbindlist(lapply(input, fread, data.table=T,showProgress=F),
 use.names=T, idcol="sample_id")
bks_linear_counts.tab.gz[, ':='(circ_id = sub('.*"([^"]+)".
*', "\cr1", V9))]
bks_linear_counts.tab.gz[, V1 := NULL]
```

3. Compose the host-gene expression matrix.
    (a) Remove strand info from circ_id if you have an unstranded library.

```
bks_linear_counts.tab.gz[, circ_id := sub(":[-+.]", "", cir-
c_id)]
```

    (b) Sum the linear reads that overlap the backsplice junction.

```
ciri_bks_linexp <-
 bks_linear_counts.tab.gz[, .(lin.reads=sum(V10)),
 by = .(sample_id, circ_id)]
Linear <- data.frame(dcast(circ.lin.xpr, formula=circ_id ~
sample_id, value.var="lin.reads", fill=0), row.names="cir-
c_id")
Linear$circ_id <- rownames(Linear)
Linear <- Linear[Circ$circ_id, ]
```

4. Run *Circ.test*. (*see* **Note 68**).

```
test <- Circ.test(Circ, Linear,
 group=coldata$condition,
 circle_description=1)
```

5. Result can be accessed from the summary table field contained in the "test" object.

```
test$summary_table
```

**3.4 CircRNA Characterization**

Several functions were described for circRNAs, mainly mediated by interactions with miRNAs and proteins, or linked to a specific coding potential. Public databases collect diverse functional data on circRNAs detected in published studies, including associations with diseases, circRNA sequence conservation and cell/tissue specificity (*see* **Note 69**).

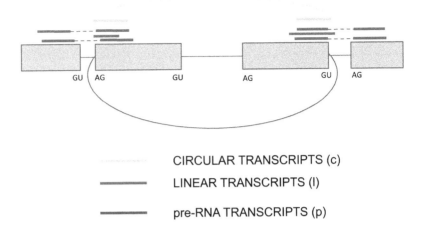

CIRCULAR TRANSCRIPTS (c)

LINEAR TRANSCRIPTS (l)

pre-RNA TRANSCRIPTS (p)

$$CLP = c/[c+(l+p)/2]$$

**Fig. 3** Circular to Linear proportion calculation. Circular RNA junction reads are shown in green. Host gene expression is estimated from the average read depth of linear-spliced reads (shown in red) and pre-RNA reads (shown in black) close to the backsplice junction at both flanking exons

Nevertheless, they lack information for newly identified circRNAs. Moreover, precalculated functional predictions may be limiting and reductive for the aim one is achieving (Fig. 4). Researchers willing to obtain more specific functional predictions can leverage several tools dedicated to circRNAs. Starting from the circRNA sequence, they will mainly predict miRNA binding sites (for instance miRanda [39] and PITA [40]), RNA binding protein (RBP) recognition motifs (e.g., beRBP [41], iDeepS [42]), and coding potential (e.g., ORFfinder, available online at https://www.ncbi.nlm.nih.gov/orffinder/, and CircCode [43]) (Fig. 4).

**3.5 CircRNA Function Databases**

For annotated circRNAs one should choose the circRNA information to retrieve (e.g., circRNA–miRNA interactions) and search in the appropriate public circRNA databases, for instance CSCD [44]; *see* **Note 69** for a description of the main types of circRNA databases. The backsplice junction coordinates or the host gene name must be given in input to the search form (*see* **Note 70**).

Downstream analysis typically requires to filter and prioritize the predictions based on the parameters/scores provided by the tools/databases queried, possibly giving priority to experimentally validated data.

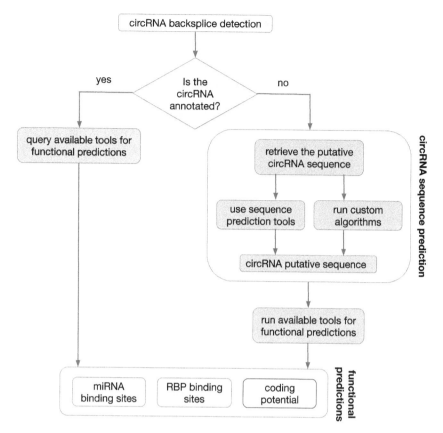

**Fig. 4** Schematic procedure for circRNA functional predictions

**3.6 CircRNA Custom Functional Predictions**

*3.6.1 CircRNA Sequence Reconstruction*

Various criteria can be used to predict circRNA sequence starting from the backsplicing coordinates (*see* **Note 71**). One approach is to consider only annotated exons included within the backsplice junction coordinates, or just the two backspliced exons. A handy solution is to use CIRI-AS, which infers the circRNA sequence from RNA-seq reads aligned to the backsplice (*see* **Note 72**):

1. Enter the directory where data are stored.

```
user@mypc:~$ cd data
```

2. Run CIRI-AS (*see* **Notes 73** and **74**).

```
user@mypc:data$ perl ../tools/CIRI-vis_v1.4/CIRI_AS_1.2.pl -S
bwa_out/SRR6674620_bwa.sam -C ciri_out/SRR6674620_ciri.out -O
SRR6674620_ciriAS -F Homo_sapiens.GRCh38.dna.primary_assem-
bly.fa -A Homo_sapiens.GRCh38.100.gtf
```

3. Use "SRR6674620_ciriAS.list" to get the coordinates of predicted circRNA exons. Convert the coordinates in BED format (*see* **Note 75**).

```
user@mypc:data$ cat SRR6674620_ciriAS.list | awk '{print $2,
$3-1,$4,$1,".",$5}' | sed -e 's/ /\t/g' > SRR6674620_ciriAS.
bed
```

4. Retrieve the sequence of each exon in FASTA format.

```
user@mypc:data$ bedtools getfasta -fi Homo_sapiens.GRCh38.dna.
primary_assembly.fa -bed SRR6674620_ciriAS.bed -fo
SRR6674620_ciriAS.fa -s -name
```

5. Use "SRR6674620_ciriAS_AS.list" to get the coordinates of circRNA predicted exons affected by alternative splicing within circRNA.

6. Join exon sequences of **step 4** to create a single FASTA sequence for each circRNA (use bedtools groupby), taking into account the possible different isoforms due to alternative splicing (**step 5**).

*3.6.2 Functional Predictions*

Once obtained the circRNA sequence (**step 6**), prediction of sequence recognition motifs for proteins and miRNAs and open reading frames can inform the potential circRNA interactions and functions. A well-known function of circRNAs is the ability to bind and sponge miRNAs. Several approaches can be followed to predict miRNA-binding sites of circRNAs, but no gold standard has been identified. The main shortcoming of all algorithms is the huge number of predicted binding sites for a single input sequence due to the limited length of the sequences involved in miRNA–circRNA pairing and on the fact that perfect complementarity is not required. Similarly, several tools are available for RBP binding site prediction, all suffering from low specificity.

Generally, downstream analyses to prioritize the most reliable prediction are needed. They include filters based on the tool parameters, the merging/intersection of predictions from more tools, and/or the incorporation of independent data (e.g., miRNA or protein expression data in the cell line/tissue analyzed, and/or information about miRNA–circRNA binding sites overlapping Ago protein peaks and/or about validated sites) [45].

Since circRNAs can be translated into peptides, the coding potential of circRNAs is another feature worth investigating, focusing particularly on the ORFs created by the backsplice and specific of circRNAs.

# 4  Notes

1. Having a larger number of CPU cores can speed up the analysis as most of the software for the analysis is highly parallelized.

2. The amount of RAM required depends also on the reference genome and methods used: larger genomes will require larger free slots of primary memory.

3. The required free disk space depends on the sample size and sequencing depth: the larger the number of samples and the deeper the sequencing depth, the larger the required free disk space.

4. If you cannot/do not want to install a Linux distribution on your workstation/server, you can use virtualized OS such as virtual machines or Docker images.

5. Older or more recent versions of this OS could raise errors because of unsupported software versions installed by default.

6. You will need to install the following packages from a fresh installation of Ubuntu 16.04: `user@mypc:~$ sudo apt install wget unzip lbzip2 build-essential zlib1g-dev libbz2-dev liblzma-dev libcurl4-openssl-dev libncurses5-dev python default-jre`. *wget* is required to download the packages; *unzip* and *libzip2* to decompress ZIP and BZ2 archives; install required packages–*build-essential, zlib1g-dev, libbz2-dev,* and *liblzma-dev*–to compile software such as bedtools and samtools. Some of the following tools might be available from the package manager. However, you should check which version would be installed, as often only old instances are available. You may need to run apt update in a docker image of Ubuntu 16.04 before installing the packages. By default, Ubuntu runs the *Bash* application to interpret the commands typed in the terminal window. Besides, other interpreters exist, such as *sh* or *zsh*, which can behave differently from *bash*. In the command prompt you can type `ps -p $$` to know which shell you are running on.

7. Since the analysis may take a long time, you should consider using virtual terminals such as screen or tmux. These programs allow to keep alive the terminal session, which runs in background, even when the user exits the display session or, if connected remotely to a server, for instance via SSH, to resume the terminal session if the connection fails. Mind that the virtual terminal should be started (and run) on the server. After opening the terminal and connecting to the server, run tmux (or screen) from the command line.

8. Linux terminal is case-sensitive and accepts only ASCII characters.

9. You can monitor the machine resources and usage from the command line with command line programs like ps, top, or htop.

10. Execution of a command can be interrupted by typing CTRL +C (i.e., press and hold the CTRL key while pressing the "c" key).

11. We chose CIRI2 as the circRNA detection tool to use in the sample analysis as it is one of the best performing methods.

12. Having a link to the main executable files into one directory simplifies the typing of paths when the commands are called.

13. BWA is required by the CIRI2 method.

14. BWA v0.7.12-r1039 is available from the Ubuntu 16.04 repository.

15. Precompiled BEDTools v2.25.0 is available from the Ubuntu 16.04 repository.

```
user@mypc:~$ sudo apt install bedtools
```

16. To compile from a fresh Ubuntu 16.04 you may need to install build-essential and zlib1g-dev, libbz2-dev, liblzma-dev packages. This will solve compilation errors like the following.

```
cram/cram_io.c:57:19: fatal error: bzlib.h: No such file or
directory
```

17. The installation considers the compilation of the executables files.

18. If the compiling process terminates with error messages like

```
hfile_libcurl.c:47:23: fatal error: curl/curl.h: No such file
or directory
```

you may need to install in your system the relative dependency library such as libcurl4-openssl-dev, libncurses5-dev and libncursesw5-dev (in Ubuntu).

19. Only obsolete samtools v0.1.19 is available from the Ubuntu 16.04 repository. Newer versions are recommended for higher performance.

20. HISAT2 is one of the fastest methods for spliced read alignment and its RAM usage is perhaps the lowest with respect to other tools.

21. You will need Python v2.7 installed on your system to run hisat2-build (as well as other tool scripts, as long as their code has not yet been ported to Python3):

```
user@mypc:~$ sudo apt install python
```

You might have a more recent default version of Python in your system, as Python2 is no longer supported since January 1st, 2020. To install and work with other versions of Python you can use virtualenv, a tool that generates a virtual environment with your preferred Python version and Python packages. Quick sample to create and start a virtual environment with python2.7 follows.

```
user@mypc:~$ sudo apt install virtualenv
user@mypc:~$ virtualenv -p /usr/bin/python2.7 venv
user@mypc:~$ source venv/bin/activate
```

Now, the default python environment refers to the venv (or whatever you named it) directory that has been created. To exit the virtual environment, type the following.

```
(venv) user@mypc:~$ deactivate
```

22. You need the Java runtime environment (JRE) on your system to run FASTQC:

```
user@mypc:~$ sudo apt install default-jre
```

23. If no files to process are specified on the command line then the program will start as an interactive graphical application.

24. This is only necessary if you are going to analyze data stored in SRA https://www.ncbi.nlm.nih.gov/sra.

25. Always use the most recent version of SRAToolkit. Check updates at https://trace.ncbi.nlm.nih.gov/Traces/sra/sra.cgi?view=toolkit_doc.

26. Prepend the new directory to the PATH variable as the search for the executable will begin from prepended directories.

27. The "export" command will affect only the current session. If you want persistent behavior (for your user only) you can add the export command to the .bashrc file in your home directory:

```
user@mypc:~$ echo "export PATH=$PWD:$PATH" >> ~/.bashrc
```

28. Many organisms' reference genome sequences in FASTA format can be found on the Ensembl FTP server (http://www.ensembl.org/info/data/ftp/index.html) or the UCSC database (https://genome.ucsc.edu/goldenPath/help/ftp.html).

29. Chromosome names in the annotation file must match the chromosome names of the genome file. For instance, UCSC chromosome sequences are identified with "chr" followed by the chromosome number for the human genome (chr1, chr2, ...), while Ensembl GTF annotation has not the chr prefix in the chromosome names. The chr prefix can be removed by means of the following command.

```
user@mypc:data$ sed -i "s/^>chr/>/" genomefile.fa
```

This command will modify the FASTA entry names in the file by removing the chr prefix. Moreover, the annotation file must be in the same version of the genomic reference file.

30. Data in the SRA are packaged in a compressed format (denoted by the .sra file name extension). RNA-seq analysis software, instead, generally require the sequence input data in the FASTQ (FASTA with Qualities) format.

31. Use the `--split-files` option only if your data is paired-end and you want to keep separate files for the mates.

32. A faster way is to prefetch, fastq-dump, and eventually compress, for instance, with a parallelized compression tool such as pigz.

```
user@mypc:data$ prefetch SRR6674620
user@mypc:data$ fastq-dump --split-files SRR6674620
user@mypc:data$ pigz *.fq
```

33. Package names are case-sensitive.

34. CircTest was designed to work with the output of DCC, but can also run on your own tables (e.g., refer here to "keep" tables obtained at point 6 and 7).

35. Comprehensive software pipelines have been developed to perform all the analysis steps automatically, such as CirCompara [46], FUCHS [47], circtools [48], circMETA [49], or CIRCexplorer3 [49, 50].

36. Results are summarized in HTML file(s) and you will need a web browser to open them.

37. You can oversee warning and error summary alerts and just inspect the read quality drop in the rightmost sequence, the read length, most common sequences and adapter contaminants to decide whether a read cleaning preprocessing should be performed (*see* **step 3**).

38. This procedure is recommended yet not essential, as low-quality reads can reduce the accuracy of backsplice prediction [22, 51]. Here, we used Trimmomatic to remove possible adapter sequences from the reads, as well as to trim low-quality stretches of reads. Other tools to clean reads can be Cutadapt or Trimgalore.

39. Use the -jar option to run the Trimmomatic Java archive (JAR). Differently from an executable script, you have to specify the full path to the jar file, as it is an argument of the java interpreter program.

40. HISAT2 will generate several files having the same prefix name "Homo_sapiens.GRCh38.dna.primary_assembly" but different extensions into the hisat2 directory.

41. With 4 CPUs, ~ 10GBytes RAM will be used.

42. If available, you can download a precomputed genome index for HISAT2. Check the genomes available at the tool website http://daehwankimlab.github.io/hisat2/download/. *Homo sapiens* GRCh38 is what we will use. Mind that you may want to match the genome reference and chromosome names of the genome FASTA you will use for chimeric alignments in the next steps if you are going to merge/compare linear and chimeric alignments.

```
user@mypc:data$ wget https://cloud.biohpc.swmed.edu/index.
php/s/grch38/download -O indexes/grch38.tar.gz
 user@mypc:data$ cd indexes
 user@mypc:data$ tar -xf grch38.tar.gz
 user@mypc:data$ cd ..
```

43. The same index files can also be reused for the analysis of additional samples.

44. Also for BWA, the same index files can also be reused for the analysis of additional samples.

45. Mind the parameters used that assure reads are aligned only collinearly.

46. Strandness parameters such as `--rna-strandness RF` specifies that read strandness was preserved during library preparation. RF value is suitable for dUTP library protocols like the Illumina Ribo-Zero rRNA Removal Kit. However, that parameter does not affect the resulting unmapped reads.

47. Use parameters to directly save unmapped reads into separate files. This will avoid the later extraction of unmapped reads from the alignment file.

48. To save space, you can redirect standard output into /dev/ null. The command will look like this.

```
user@mypc:hisat2_out$ ../../tools/hisat2 -x ../grch38/genome
--no-discordant --no-mixed -p 4 -1 ../SRR6674620_1.fastq.gz -2
../SRR6674620_2.fastq.gz --un-conc-gz unmapped_%.fq.gz 2>
SRR6674620_hisat2.log > /dev/null
```

However, we do not recommend this procedure as you will lose collinear alignments that could be used in downstream analysis, such as the computation of CLP.

49. Sorted (by chromosome and start coordinate) alignment files allow faster processing.

50. Once compressed into a BAM file, you can delete the SAM file as BAM format can be converted back into SAM without losing information.

51. You can concatenate the alignment and conversion commands to save a step and use less disk space by means of the pipe operator, which redirects the standard output of the command on the left into the standard input of the command on the right.

```
user@mypc:hisat2_out$ hisat2 -x ../indexes/hisat2/Homo_sa-
piens.GRCh38.dna.primary_assembly --no-discordant --no-mixed
-p 4 -1 ../SRR6674620_1.fastq.gz -2 ../SRR6674620_2.fastq.gz
2> SRR6674620_hisat2.log | samtools sort -m 768M -O 'bam' -@
4 -T hisat2_SRR6674620 > SRR6674620_hisat2.bam
```

52. The -f 12 option value will select unmapped and not concordantly mapped read mates (read unmapped $0 \times 4$ and mate unmapped $0 \times 8$). The -F 3328 option value will discard not primary alignment, PCR or optical duplicate and supplementary alignment reads. See https://broadinstitute.github.io/picard/explain-flags.html for further explanation of values representing SAM flags.

53. The singleton.fastq file should result empty.

54. If you want to process the reads as they were single-ended you can concatenate gzipped files.

```
user@mypc:data$ cat hisat2_out/unmapped_1.fq.gz hisat2_out/
unmapped_2.fq.gz > unmapped.fq.gz
user@mypc:data$ ../tools/bwa mem -t 6 -T 19 indexes/bwa/
Homo_sapiens.GRCh38.dna.primary_assembly unmapped.fq.gz >
bwa_out/SRR6674620_bwa.sam
```

55. CIRI2 output circRNA coordinates are 1-based, end included (as in GTF standard) as opposed to BED format, which is 0-based, end excluded.

56. Use less threads than in other tools because of memory usage (~10GB with 2 CPUs, ~7.5GB for single thread). With multiple threads you will need extra disk space for temporary files (−T 1 for single thread).

57. Linear spliced reads on backspliced junctions for CLP is the only way to reliably determine the relation with the linear expression of the parent gene.

58. Here we leverage the bedtools coverage method default behavior, which considers gapped/split alignments as single intervals (i.e., comprising the gap region). Otherwise, if the -split option was set, spliced reads spanning the backsplice junction flanking bases would not be counted.

59. DCC [38] provides a method to retrieve parent gene linear counts, as well.

60. Check that matrix is actually numeric and numbers are correctly read as it may happen that they are interpreted as characters, then converted into factors (which are represented as integers), eventually losing the right numeric value. Setting stringAsFactors = F in the read.table function should prevent the automatic conversion into factors.

61. Column names of the count matrix must match the order of the coldata rownames.

62. In general, filtering out low count circRNAs removes many false negative detections.

63. The estimation steps performed by this function are described in the manual page for?DESeq and in the Methods section of the DESeq2 publication [52].

64. CircRNA count matrices from ribodep RNA-seq is characterized by low values and for modeling data with low counts You might consider to set the following options in *DESeq* to better handle.
    - use test = "LRT" for significance testing, over the Wald test,
    - set the following *DESeq* arguments: useT = TRUE, minmu = 1e-6.

```
dds <- DESeq(dds, useT=TRUE, minmu=1e-6)
```

65. With no additional arguments to results, the log2 fold change and the test p value will refer to the last variable in the design formula, and if this is a factor, the comparison will be the last level of this variable over the reference level.

66. As a proportion measure, CLP has been demonstrated to follow a Beta-Binomial distribution [38]. In particular, we are interested in testing whether the mean of the marginal Beta-Binomial distribution for the $i$th circRNA differs between the respective conditions $j$:1, …,k.

67. These tables should have the same order, that is, circ[i,j] and linear[i,j] are read-counts for the same circRNA.

68. It is important that the grouping is correct (group) and the non–read count columns are specified (circle_description).

69. Many databases are publicly available, with different information about circRNAs. The main categories include [53] the following.
    - Tissue-specific databases: circRNAs are generally annotated as tissue-specific if they are detected in specific tissues or cell types, sometimes assessed by a specificity score.
    - Database reporting circRNA–miRNA interactions.
    - Database reporting circRNA–RBP interactions.

- Database about circRNA coding potential: databases report predicted internal ribosome entry sites (IRES) elements or predicted open reading frames (ORFs).

- Database about circRNA conservation: based on the idea that the conservation of a particular genomic sequence may hint at a functional role.

- Database about circRNA–disease associations: circRNAs are considered disease-specific when up- or downregulated in a particular disease sample, or if there is a link between the parental gene of the circRNA and a specific disease.

- Database with other information: some databases have unique annotation features, for instance, correlation between the circRNA host gene expression and the normalized backspliced junction read numbers, associations between drug response and circRNA expression, information about backsplicing involving two genes, functional predictions based on gene ontology enrichment analysis, and so on.

70. Some databases can be queried with the circRNA backsplice junction coordinates. Others allow searching only by the circRNA host gene name to return the whole list of annotated circRNAs of the host gene. Tip: as different databases use different genome versions to store circRNAs, use LiftOver (https://genome.ucsc.edu/cgi-bin/hgLiftOver) to convert genomic coordinates across genome versions.

71. Existing tools base circRNA sequence prediction on the position of the circRNA backsplice junction, providing full length circRNA sequences, so different isoforms from the same backsplice junction are not distinguished. Moreover, circRNA sequence is inferred based on the reference genome sequence.

72. CIRI-AS is applicable only to paired-end sequencing data.

73. Make sure you have installed Perl 5.12 or higher to use CIRI-AS.

74. Gene annotations are not mandatory. When annotation file is provided, CIRI-AS can calculate insert length and provide correction value of $\Psi$ for alternative spliced exons accordingly.

75. The file should have six columns: "`chr`", "`start`", "`end`", "`circRNA_id`", "`no_info`", "`strand`".

# References

1. Rybak-Wolf A, Stottmeister C, Glažar P et al (2015) Circular RNAs in the mammalian brain are highly abundant, conserved, and dynamically expressed. Mol Cell 58:870–885

2. Gaffo E, Boldrin E, Dal Molin A et al (2019) Circular RNA differential expression in blood cell populations and exploration of circRNA deregulation in pediatric acute lymphoblastic leukemia. Sci Rep 9:14670

3. Hansen TB, Jensen TI, Clausen BH et al (2013) Natural RNA circles function as efficient microRNA sponges. Nature 495:384–388

4. Schneider T, Hung L-H, Schreiner S et al (2016) CircRNA-protein complexes: IMP3 protein component defines subfamily of circRNPs. Sci Rep 6:31313

5. Rossi F, Legnini I, Megiorni F et al (2019) Circ-ZNF609 regulates G1-S progression in rhabdomyosarcoma. Oncogene 38:3843–3854

6. Legnini I, Di Timoteo G, Rossi F et al (2017) Circ-ZNF609 is a circular RNA that can be translated and functions in Myogenesis. Mol Cell 66:22–37.e9

7. Chekulaeva M, Rajewsky N (2019) Roles of long noncoding RNAs and circular RNAs in translation. Cold Spring Harb Perspect Biol 11:a032680

8. Pan Z, Cai J, Lin J et al (2020) A novel protein encoded by circFNDC3B inhibits tumor progression and EMT through regulating snail in colon cancer. Mol Cancer 19:71

9. Bonizzato A, Gaffo E, Te Kronnie G, Bortoluzzi S (2016) CircRNAs in hematopoiesis and hematological malignancies. Blood Cancer J 6:e483

10. Sadeghi H, Heiat M (2020) A novel circular RNA hsa_circ_0060927 may serve as a potential diagnostic biomarker for human colorectal cancer. Mol Biol Rep 47(9):6649–6655. https://doi.org/10.1007/s11033-020-05716-9

11. Chen P, Yao Y, Yang N et al (2020) Circular RNA circCTNNA1 promotes colorectal cancer progression by sponging miR-149-5p and regulating FOXM1 expression. Cell Death Dis 11:557

12. Xia B, Zhao Z, Wu Y et al (2020) Circular RNA circTNPO3 regulates paclitaxel resistance of ovarian cancer cells by miR-1299/NEK2 signaling pathway. Mol Ther Nucleic Acids 21:780–791

13. Zhang M, Zhao K, Xu X et al (2018) A peptide encoded by circular form of LINC-PINT suppresses oncogenic transcriptional elongation in glioblastoma. Nat Commun 9:4475

14. Dal Molin A, Bresolin S, Gaffo E et al (2019) CircRNAs are here to stay: a perspective on the recombinome. Front Genet 10:88

15. Wen J, Liao J, Liang J et al (2020) Circular RNA HIPK3: a key circular RNA in a variety of human cancers. Front Oncol 10:773

16. Papaioannou D, Volinia S, Nicolet D et al (2020) Clinical and functional significance of circular RNAs in cytogenetically normal AML. Blood Adv 4:239–251

17. Hirsch S, Blätte TJ, Grasedieck S et al (2017) Circular RNAs of the nucleophosmin (NPM1) gene in acute myeloid leukemia. Haematologica 102:2039–2047

18. Wu Z, Sun H, Liu W et al (2020) Circ-RPL15: a plasma circular RNA as novel oncogenic driver to promote progression of chronic lymphocytic leukemia. Leukemia 34:919–923

19. Jeck WR, Sorrentino JA, Wang K et al (2013) Circular RNAs are abundant, conserved, and associated with ALU repeats. RNA 19:141–157

20. Jeck WR, Sharpless NE (2014) Detecting and characterizing circular RNAs. Nat Biotechnol 32:453–461

21. Toubia J, Conn VM, Conn SJ (2018) Don't go in circles: confounding factors in gene expression profiling. EMBO J 37:e97945

22. Wang J, Liu K, Liu Y et al (2017) Evaluating the bias of circRNA predictions from total RNA-Seq data. Oncotarget 8:110914–110921

23. Gao Y, Zhang J, Zhao F (2018) Circular RNA identification based on multiple seed matching. Brief Bioinform 19:803–810

24. Li H (2013) Aligning sequence reads, clone sequences and assembly contigs with BWA-MEM

25. Quinlan AR (2014) BEDTools: the Swiss-Army tool for genome feature analysis. Curr Protoc Bioinformatics 47:11.12.1–11.1234

26. Li H, Handsaker B, Wysoker A et al (2009) The sequence alignment/map format and SAMtools. Bioinformatics 25:2078–2079

27. Kim D, Langmead B, Salzberg SL (2015) HISAT: a fast spliced aligner with low memory requirements. Nat Methods 12:357–360

28. Babraham Bioinformatics - FastQC A Quality Control tool for High Throughput Sequence Data. https://www.bioinformatics.babraham.ac.uk/projects/fastqc/. Accessed 18 Aug 2020

29. Leinonen R, Sugawara H, Shumway M, on behalf of the International Nucleotide Sequence Database Collaboration (2011) The sequence read archive. Nucleic Acids Res 39:D19–D21

30. Bolger AM, Lohse M, Usadel B (2014) Trimmomatic: a flexible trimmer for Illumina sequence data. Bioinformatics 30:2114–2120

31. Gao Y, Wang J, Zheng Y et al (2016) Comprehensive identification of internal structure and alternative splicing events in circular RNAs. Nat Commun 7:12060

32. Chen L, Wang C, Sun H et al (2020) The bioinformatics toolbox for circRNA discovery and analysis. Brief Bioinform. https://doi.org/10.1093/bib/bbaa001

33. Love M, Anders S, Huber W (2014) Differential analysis of count data--the DESeq2 package. Genome Biol 15:10–1186

34. Robinson MD, McCarthy DJ, Smyth GK (2010) edgeR: a Bioconductor package for differential expression analysis of digital gene expression data. Bioinformatics 26:139–140

35. Ritchie ME, Phipson B, Wu D et al (2015) Limma powers differential expression analyses for RNA-sequencing and microarray studies. Nucleic Acids Res 43:e47

36. Hardcastle TJ (2012) baySeq: empirical Bayesian analysis of patterns of differential expression in count data. R package version 2

37. Liang D, Tatomer DC, Luo Z et al (2017) The output of protein-coding genes shifts to circular RNAs when the pre-mRNA processing machinery is limiting. Mol Cell 68:940–954.e3

38. Cheng J, Metge F, Dieterich C (2016) Specific identification and quantification of circular RNAs from sequencing data. Bioinformatics 32:1094–1096

39. Enright AJ, John B, Gaul U et al (2003) MicroRNA targets in Drosophila. Genome Biol 5:R1

40. Kertesz M, Iovino N, Unnerstall U et al (2007) The role of site accessibility in microRNA target recognition. Nat Genet 39:1278–1284

41. Yu H, Wang J, Sheng Q et al (2019) beRBP: binding estimation for human RNA-binding proteins. Nucleic Acids Res 47:e26

42. Pan X, Rijnbeek P, Yan J, Shen H-B (2018) Prediction of RNA-protein sequence and structure binding preferences using deep convolutional and recurrent neural networks. BMC Genomics 19(1):511

43. Sun P, Li G (2019) CircCode: a powerful tool for identifying circRNA coding ability. Front Genet 10:981

44. Xia S, Feng J, Chen K et al (2018) CSCD: a database for cancer-specific circular RNAs. Nucleic Acids Res 46:D925–D929

45. Dori M, Bicciato S (2019) Integration of Bioinformatic predictions and experimental data to identify circRNA-miRNA associations. Genes (Basel) 10:642. https://doi.org/10.3390/genes10090642

46. Gaffo E, Bonizzato A, Kronnie GT, Bortoluzzi S (2017) CirComPara: a multi-method comparative bioinformatics pipeline to detect and study circRNAs from RNA-seq data. Noncoding RNA 3:8. https://doi.org/10.3390/ncrna3010008

47. Metge F, Czaja-Hasse LF, Reinhardt R, Dieterich C (2017) FUCHS-towards full circular RNA characterization using RNAseq. PeerJ 5:e2934

48. Jakobi T, Uvarovskii A, Dieterich C (2019) Circtools—a one-stop software solution for circular RNA research. Bioinformatics 35:2326–2328

49. Chen L, Wang F, Bruggeman EC et al (2020) circMeta: a unified computational framework for genomic feature annotation and differential expression analysis of circular RNAs. Bioinformatics 36:539–545

50. Ma X-K, Wang M-R, Liu C-X et al (2019) CIRCexplorer3: a CLEAR pipeline for direct comparison of circular and linear RNA expression. Genomics Proteomics Bioinformatics 17:511–521

51. Hansen TB (2018) Improved circRNA identification by combining prediction algorithms. Front Cell Dev Biol 6:20

52. Love MI, Huber W, Anders S (2014) Moderated estimation of fold change and dispersion for RNA-seq data with DESeq2. Genome Biol 15:550

53. Vromman M, Vandesompele J, Volders P-J (2020) Closing the circle: current state and perspectives of circular RNA databases. Brief Bioinform 22(1):288–297. https://doi.org/10.1093/bib/bbz175

# Chapter 23

# Study of Circular RNA Expression by Nonradioactive Northern Blot Procedure

## Eleonora D'Ambra and Mariangela Morlando

## Abstract

Circular RNAs (circRNAs) are covalently closed transcripts generated by back-splicing reaction. The lack of free ends endows these RNA molecules with high stability thus allowing them to accumulate in tissues and body fluids. They are widely expressed in most organisms, are modulated during development and display tissue-specific expression, resulting particularly enriched in the nervous system. Deregulation of circRNA expression has also been associated with several pathological conditions including neurological diseases and cancer.

Here we present a Northern blot procedure that allows the analysis of the expression of bona fide circRNAs through the use of a digoxigenin-labeled RNA probe and the immunodetection of the signals.

**Key words** circRNA, Northern Blot, RNA electrophoresis, Noncoding RNA, Digoxigenin, RNA probe, Immunodetection

## 1 Introduction

Circular RNA (circRNAs) belong to a new class of noncoding RNAs characterized by a covalently closed circular structure. They are produced through a noncanonical splicing event, the back-splicing (BS), of the host linear messenger RNAs (mRNAs) involving one or more exons [1, 2]. The BS occurs in a reverse orientation with respect to the canonical splicing thus joining a downstream 5' splice site with an upstream 3' splice site. This inverted splicing junction is called back-splicing junction (BSJ) and it is the unique region which allows the circRNAs to be discriminated from their linear counterparts. An additional distinctive feature of circRNAs is their high stability when compared to linear RNAs as they are not sensitive to exoribonuclease treatments [3–5].

CircRNAs are conserved in evolution and show tissue specific expression, being particularly abundant in the nervous system [6–8]. They are involved in many biological processes acting as sponges/scaffolds for microRNAs and proteins, as regulators of

Alfons Navarro (ed.), *Long Non-Coding RNAs in Cancer*, Methods in Molecular Biology, vol. 2348,
https://doi.org/10.1007/978-1-0716-1581-2_23, © Springer Science+Business Media, LLC, part of Springer Nature 2021

transcription and alternative splicing and as potential source for new protein isoforms when being translated [4, 9–16]. Because of their high stability, they accumulate in body fluids where they can be detected and quantified, pointing to their use as biomarkers in the field of molecular diagnosis [17].

In the last few years, increasing evidence supporting the importance of circRNAs in cellular metabolism links their altered expression with the initiation and progression of many diseases including cancer [13, 18–21]. In this regard, numerous examples of circRNAs participating in cellular processes related to proliferation, migration and invasion as well as drug resistance and treatment response have been described. These findings indicate that they can be considered potential therapeutic targets as well as diagnostic and prognostic biomarkers for various types of cancers [21–23].

Different molecular biology techniques used to detect linear RNAs have been adapted to investigate or validate the expression of circular molecules in biological samples [24].

Among them the Northern blot represents the gold standard method to analyze and quantify circRNAs. Although it is less sensitive than reverse transcription PCR (RT-PCR) it avoids to detect artifacts derived from the amplification of the target: linear RNAs containing an inverted splicing junction derived from other sources (trans-splicing events or genomic duplications) and long cDNAs containing concatemers of exons arising from the rolling-circle RT phenomenon hampering the identification and quantification of circRNAs (Fig. 1).

Nevertheless, the sensitivity of Northern blot can be increased by the use of highly specific antisense RNA probes, positively charged nylon membranes and eventually removal of linear RNAs through RNase R treatment. This latter limits the hybridization specifically to circRNAs and, at the same time, allows to validate the circularity of the molecule.

In this method chapter, we describe an approach for detecting circRNAs by Northern blot which uses a nonradioactive RNA probe; this latter is synthetized in vitro in presence of digoxigenated rUTP and is revealed by immunodetection. The RNA probe can target the BSJ, for circRNA detection only, or, alternatively, a region shared by both the linear and circular molecules thus allowing to analyze the expression of both transcripts [16, 25].

## 2    Materials

### 2.1    Reagents, Buffers, and Solutions

1. DNA and RNA samples.
2. Distilled $H_2O$.
3. RNase-free milliQ $H_2O$.
4. RNase AWAY® decontamination reagent for RNase (Sigma).

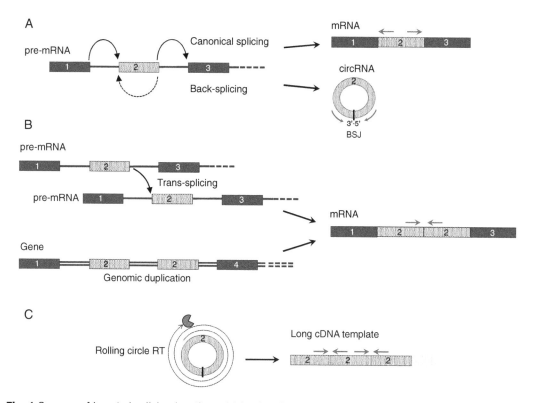

**Fig. 1** Sources of inverted splicing junctions. (**a**) back-splicing event gives rise circRNAs containing a BSJ, a productive substrate for PCR amplification using divergent primers (red arrows), while canonical splicing produces linear transcripts that cannot generate any PCR product. (**b**) Trans-splicing reaction and genomic duplication events can produce linear RNAs with inverted splicing junctions that can be amplified by PCR. However, they represent false positive products since they do not derive from circRNAs. (**c**) long cDNAs are generated by Rolling-circle RT reaction occurring on circRNAs. These long cDNAs are concatemers of exon/s thus containing several BSJs. Therefore, many PCR products can be created from a single cDNA molecule

5. Agarose powder.

6. NorthernMax™-Gly Sample Loading Dye (Invitrogen).

7. RNA Markers.

8. NorthernMax buffer (Invitrogen).

9. DIG Luminescent Detection Kit (Roche).

10. T7 RNA polymerase (T7 Ribomax, Promega).

11. DIG-RNA labeling mix (Roche).

12. RNase Inhibitor.

13. 40% acrylamide–bis-acrylamide 29:1 (Sigma).

14. $N,N,N',N'$-Tetramethyl-ethylenediamine (TEMED).

15. Ammonium persulfate (APS).

16. Ethidium bromide 10 mg/mL (EtBr).

17. RNA Gel Loading Dye (2×) (Thermo Scientific).

18. Phenol–chloroform–isoamyl alcohol (PCA).

19. Glycogen RNA grade 20 mg/mL.

20. Ethanol.

21. 1M Tris–HCl pH 8.0 and pH 7.5 solutions: dissolve 121.14 g of Tris base in 700 mL distilled $H_2O$; use HCl to adjust to pH 8.0 or 7.5; fill to 1000 mL with and sterilize by autoclave.

22. 0.5 M EDTA pH 8 solution: dissolve 73.06 g of EDTA in 300 mL of distilled $H_2O$; use NaOH to adjust to pH 8; fill to 500 mL and sterilize by autoclave.

23. 3 M Na Acetate pH 5.5 solution: dissolve 123.05 g of Sodium Acetate in 300 mL of distilled $H_2O$; use HCl to adjust to pH 5.5; fill to 500 mL and sterilize by autoclave.

24. 30% (w/v) APS: dissolve 3 g of APS in 6 mL of distilled $H_2O$; fill to 10 mL. Store at 4 °C for up to 6 months.

25. 10× MOPS buffer: to prepare 10× stock solution dissolve 21 g of MOPS, 10 mL of 0.5M EDTA ph:8 and 8.3 mL of 3M Na Acetate ph:5.5 in 400 mL distilled $H_2O$; use NaOH to adjust to pH 7; fill to 500 mL and sterilize by filtering.

26. 10× SSC stock buffer: to prepare 10× stock buffer dissolve 175.3 g of NaCl and 88.2 g of Na3citrate in 700 mL deionized-distilled $H_2O$; fill to 1000 mL and sterilize by autoclave.

27. SSC 2X-SDS wash buffer: dilute SSC 10× to 2× in distilled $H_2O$ and add 0.1% of SDS.

28. SSC 0.2X-SDS wash buffer: dilute SSC 10× to 0.2× in distilled $H_2O$ and add 0.1% of SDS.

29. 5× TB buffer: to prepare 5× stock solution (*see* **Note 1**) dissolve 54 grams of Tris base, 27.5 grams of boric acid and 20 mL of 0.5 M EDTA pH 8 in 700 mL distilled $H_2O$; fill to 1000 mL and sterilize by autoclave.

30. Elution Buffer: 0.3 M Na Acetate, 0.1 mM EDTA ph 8, 0.2% SDS, 1:100 of Phenol; 40 mg/mL of glycogen in RNase-free milliQ $H_2O$.

*2.2 Equipment*

1. Agarose and Acrylamide Gels Electrophoresis apparatus (*see* **Note 2**).

2. Power supply.

3. Hybond N + membrane (GE Healthcare).

4. Whatman paper.

5. Towel paper.

6. Plastic wrap.

7. UV cross-linker (Stratalinker-Stratagene or similar).

8. UV-transilluminator.

9. Hotplate stirrer.

10. Rotating wheel.

11. Microwave.

12. Block heaters.

13. Parafilm.

14. UV/Vis spectrophotometer.

15. Hybridization bottle.

16. Rotary oven.

17. ChemiDoc XRS+ System (Bio-Rad) or similar.

18. Image Lab software or similar.

## 3  Methods

### 3.1  Agarose Gel Electrophoresis

1. Wash the gel apparatus including the gel-casting chamber (7x8 cm) and comb with distilled $H_2O$ and treat them with RNase AWAY decontamination reagent for RNase. Assemble the apparatus following the manufacturer's instructions.

2. Mix 0.6 g of agarose in 45 mL of deionized-distilled $H_2O$ and boil in a microwave. Let it cool down to 60 °C, and then add 5 mL of $10\times$ MOPS and fill the gel-casting chamber. Insert the comb and allow the gel to solidify for 40 min.

3. Remove the comb and fill the Gel tank with $1\times$ MOPS buffer (*see* **Note 3**).

4. Mix 10µg of total RNA samples (*see* **Note 4**) and 2µg of a RNA Marker with NorthernMax™-Gly Sample Loading Dye (1:1) and incubate in a block heater for 30 min at 50 °C to allow denaturation of RNA secondary structures.

5. Load the samples and the RNA Marker into the gel wells.

6. Run the agarose gel at 60 V for 2 h.

7. In a clean RNase-free plastic box soak gel with RNase-free milliQ $H_2O$ for 20 min, with gentle agitation.

8. Check the gel on ChemiDoc XRS+ System (UV light) and save the file on the gel-documentation system (*see* **Note 5**).

9. In the plastic box soak gel with $10\times$ SSC buffer for 20 min, with gentle agitation.

### 3.2  Transfer of RNA from Gel to Membrane Using Capillary Blotting

All the steps for setting up the capillary transfer are schematized in Fig. 2a

1. Prepare a plastic tank containing $10\times$ SSC buffer and place a support in the middle.

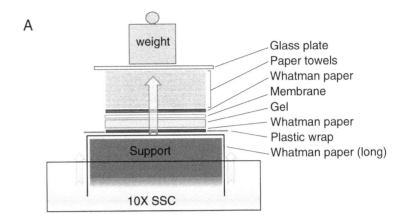

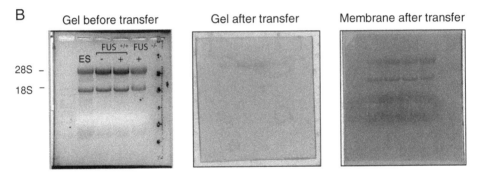

**Fig. 2** Northern Blot Transfer. (**a**) Schematic representation of the blotting apparatus for agarose gel. All the components are indicated on the side. Arrows indicate the transfer direction. (**b**) Left panel: image obtained under the UV light of agarose electrophoresis of 10μg of total RNA extracted from mouse embryonic stem cells (ES), GFP negative (−) and GFP positive (+) cell population obtained during an in vitro motor neurons differentiation of WT (FUS$^{+/+}$) and FUS knock out (FUS$^{−/−}$) ES cells (reproduced from ref. 25 which is licensed under the Creative Commons Attribution 4.0 International License). The original image has been modified as follows: the dimension of the image has been reduced and the position of the two rRNAs has been added. Middle panel: image obtained under the UV light of the agarose gel (left panel) after overnight capillary blotting. Right panel: image obtained under the UV light of Hybond N + membrane after overnight capillary blotting of the agarose gel described in the left panel

2. Cut a long piece of Whatman paper, soak it in 10× SSC buffer and place it on the support in a way that the paper's sides can soak up the buffer.

3. Cut the Hybond N+ membrane and 6 pieces of Whatman paper to the size of the gel and soak the membrane in 10× SSC buffer.

4. Soak 3 pieces of Whatman paper in 10× SSC buffer and place them on top of each other on the long Whatman paper, air trapped between the sheets are removed (*see* **Note 6**).

5. Lay the gel with the top side facing down, crop the gel eliminating the wells part and cover the area around the gel with plastic wrap (*see* **Note 7**).

6. Place the Hybond N+ membrane on the top of the gel without trapping any air.

7. Soak 3 left pieces of Whatman paper in 10× SSC buffer and place them on top of each other on the membrane; remove the air bubbles.

8. Lay at least 8 cm of cut-to-size paper towels on the top of Whatman paper.

9. Place a glass plate with a balanced weight on top of the paper towels.

10. Allow the capillary transfer of the RNA from the gel to the membrane for 16 h.

11. At the end of the transfer, remove the weight and paper towels (*see* **Note 8**); mark the back of the membrane with lead pencil, turn over the gel with the membrane, discard the gel and cut off the upper left corner so that the gel orientation and sample order can be identified later (*see* **Note 9**).

12. Fix the RNA to the membrane, with the RNA side facing upward, using the UV crosslinker ($1200 \times 100 \mu J/cm^2$) (*see* **Note 10**).

13. Place the membrane in a hybridization bottle and bake it in 50 mM Tris–HCl pH:8 in the rotary oven at 45 °C for 20 min (*see* **Note 11**).

14. Store the membrane in a plastic wrap at 4° until hybridization.

**3.3 Probe Preparation and Purification**

To prepare digoxigenin labeled probe, 3 µg of PCR T7 containing fragments are required (*see* **Note 12**) (Fig. 3a).

1. Mix 3 µg of PCR fragments with 10µL of RiboMAX™ Express T7 2× Buffer, 2 µL DIG RNA labeling mix 10×, 40 units of RNase Inhibitor and 40 units of T7 RNA polymerase; add RNase-free milliQ $H_2O$ up to 20 µL and incubate for 2 h at 37° C in a block heater.

2. While the reaction incubates, prepare a 6% denaturing Acrylamide gel as follows: mix 1.5 mL of 40% acrylamide–bis-acrylamide 29:1, 2.8 g of Urea, 2 mL of 5× TB, add distilled $H_2O$ up to 10 mL and warm to 50 °C on a hotplate stirrer until urea dissolves.

3. Add 33.2µL of APS and 4µL of TEMED, mix well and pour the gel rapidly into the assembled gel plates ($8.6 \times 6.8$ cm × 0.75 mm) and insert a 10-well gel comb without introducing air bubbles.

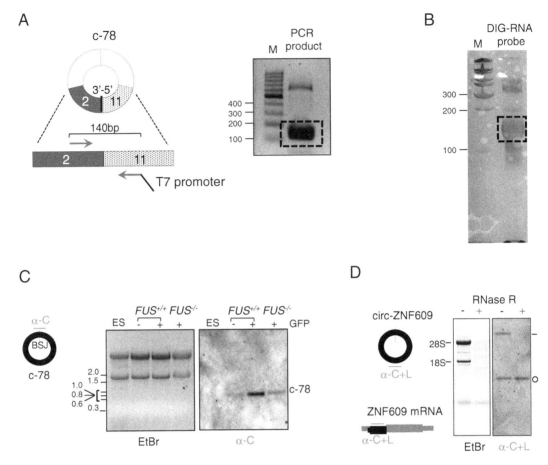

**Fig. 3** Digoxigenated probe preparation and Northern blot analyses (**a**) Left panel: schematic representation of c-78 circRNA identify by Errichelli et al. and of the region used as template to obtain 140 bp PCR product containing T7 promoter sequence. Primers are indicated by red arrows; the reverse primer is equipped with T7 promoter sequence. Right Panel: agarose electrophoresis of the PCR amplification products performed with primers indicated in the left panel and cDNA obtained by reverse transcription of total RNA from Embryoid bodies [26]. Dashed box indicates the gel band that will be excised with a razor blade and will undergo purification (*see* **Note 12**); marker of molecular weights is also indicated (M). (**b**) Polyacrylamide electrophoresis of the 140 nt antisense digoxigenated RNA probe (DIG RNA probe). Dashed box indicates the gel band that will be excised with a razor blade and will undergo purification; marker of molecular weights is also indicated (M). (**c**) Northern blot analysis (right) of RNA samples described in Fig. 2b together with the EtBr staining of the agarose gel (left) (reproduced from ref. 25 which is licensed under the Creative Commons Attribution 4.0 International License). Marker of molecular weights is indicated. The original image has been modified as follows: (1) a different scheme of c-78 is shown together with the position of the probe spanning the BSJ (α-C). This probe allowed the detection of the circRNA only; (2) RQ values under the Northern blot (right) have been removed and replaced with "α-C"; (3) "EtBr" indication has been added under panel showing EtBr staining of the agarose gel. (**d**) Left: schematic representation depicting circ-ZNF609 and ZNF609 mRNA together with the position the digoxigenated RNA probe (αC + L). This latter targets a region in common between the circular and linear ZNF609 RNAs. Right: Northern blot analysis of 20μg of total RNA from primary myoblasts untreated (−) or treated (+) with the exoribonuclease RNase R. The symbols "−" and "o" indicate the linear and the circular RNA forms, respectively. EtBr staining of the agarose gel is also shown where the migration of the rRNAs is indicated. The Northern analysis clearly shows that ZNF609 mRNA, as well as the rRNAs (EtBr panel), is degraded by the RNase R while circ-ZNF609 is highly resistant (reproduced from ref. 16 with permission from Elsevier)

4. Precipitate the RNA transcript by adding 10μL of Na Acetate 3 M pH 5.3, 70μL of RNase-free milliQ $H_2O$ and 300μL of prechilled 100% ethanol (3 volumes). Incubate at $-20$ °C for 1 h.

5. After centrifugation (15,000 $\times$ $g$ for 30 min at 4 °C) wash the pellet by adding 500μL of prechilled 80% ethanol and centrifuge at 15,000 $\times$ $g$ for 5 min at 4 °C. Air dry the pellet.

6. Resuspend the pellet in 4 μL of RNase-free milliQ $H_2O$ and add 4 μL of RNA Gel Loading Dye (2$\times$); boil the samples and 2 μg of RNA Marker (with 2 μL of loading dye) at 95 °C for 3 min in a block heater and then chill on ice for 2 min.

7. Remove the comb from the gel, cast it into an empty running tank and fill with 1$\times$ TB to cover the wells. Use a syringe with needle to clean wells from the urea.

8. Load the sample and the RNA marker into wells and run the Acrylamide gel at 100 V until the Bromophenol Blue (present in the loading dye) is on the bottom.

9. Disassemble the apparatus and separate the two plates gently; put the gel in 1$\times$ TB containing ethidium bromide (1μL per 100 mL) and shake gently for 15 min.

10. Wash the gel with RNase-free milliQ $H_2O$ for 10 min by gently shaking.

11. Place the gel on UV-transilluminator and excise the RNA band with a razor blade (Fig. 3b).

12. Place the gel slice in a microcentrifuge tube with 500μL of gel Elution buffer, seal the tube with parafilm and allow the RNA elution overnight on a rotating wheel at room temperature.

13. Recover the supernatant and extract the RNA with 1 volume of PCA. Precipitate the RNA with 2 volumes of 100% ethanol as described in point 4 and 5 of this section (*see* **Note 13**).

14. Resuspend the pellet in 5–10μL of RNase-free milliQ $H_2O$ and quantify by A260 using a Spectrophotometer (*see* **Note 14**).

*3.4  Hybridization and Signal Detection*

1. Prewarm NorthernMax buffer in the rotary oven at 68 °C until clear.

2. Place the membrane in a hybridization bottle (RNA side upward) and prehybridize it with prewarmed NorthernMax buffer (10 mL are sufficient for 7 $\times$ 8 cm membrane). Incubate in the rotary oven at 68 °C for 30 min.

3. Boil 500 ng of RNA probe at 95 °C for 3 min in a block heater and add it directly into the hybridization bottle. Incubate overnight in the rotary oven at 68°C (*see* **Note 15**).

4. Prewarm SSC 2X-SDS and SSC 0.2X-SDS at 68 °C.

5. Discard the hybridization solution and add prewarmed washing buffers into the hybridization bottle.

   (a) Wash twice with SSC 2X-SDS wash buffer (20 mL each) for 30 min at 68 °C;

   (b) Wash with 20 mL of SSC 0.2X-SDS wash buffer for 30 min at 68 °C;

   (c) Wash with 20 mL of SSC 0.2X-SDS wash buffer for 1 h at 68 °C.

6. Perform the immunological detection of the signal using DIG Luminescent Detection Kit following the manufacturer's instructions with minor modifications (*see* **Note 16**).

7. Detect the luminescence using ChemiDoc XRS+ System or similar, record images at different time points and stored them in gel-documentation system (Fig. 3b, c).

8. Verify the size of the target RNA by using the Image Lab software that allows to merge the gel file (3.1 point 8), containing the RNA marker bands, with one of the images recorded as in the previous point.

# 4    Notes

1. It is also possible to use more concentrated stock solutions of TB (10×), However, 5× stock solution is more stable because the solutes do not precipitate during storage.

2. All the volumes and dimensions mentioned in this method chapter are referred to: Thermo Scientific™ Owl™ EasyCast™ B1A Mini Gel and Mini-PROTEAN® Tetra Vertical Electrophoresis Cell (Bio-Rad) for agarose and acrylamide gel electrophoresis respectively.

3. Gel should be covered by at least 0.5 cm of 1× MOPS buffer.

4. High quality RNA samples can be obtained from mammalian cells using RNeasy Mini Spin columns, TRIreagent, and TRIzol.

5. The two ribosomal RNAs (rRNAs) 28S and 18S are visible under the UV light since the NorthernMax™-Gly Sample Loading Dye contains EtBr (Figs. 2b and 3b, c). They act as markers to verify the integrity of the RNA samples (sharp signals with the 28S band being almost twice in intensity compared to the 18S band) and to verify that equal amounts of total RNA have been loaded.

6. Roll a Stripette over the gel "sandwich" to eliminate bubble air. Trapped bubble air will impair completely the transfer and will eventually result in a blank patch in the signals.

7. The plastic wrap will ensure that any contact occurs between the Whatman paper under the gel and paper towel avoiding short circuits that would impair the transfer.

8. When the capillary blot apparatus is disassembled there should some dried towel paper on the top. This means that towel paper used was sufficient to complete the transfer.

9. Marking the back of the membrane will allow to orientate the RNA side upward in the UV crosslinker and in the hybridization bottle. Labeling with lead pencil is important as ink is removed by the hybridization buffer.

10. The efficiency of the transfer after 16 h can be checked by visualization of the rRNAs on the gel and on the membrane using UV transilluminator or the ChemiDoc XRS+ System (UV light). As shown in Fig. 2b after 16 h transfer almost all the rRNA signals are exclusively on the membrane.

11. This step is required for removal of glyoxal adducts from the RNA. The baking time can be extended up to 1 h.

12. Antisense RNA probe should be 140 nucleotides to obtain an efficient and specific hybridization with the circRNA target. The corresponding DNA template is produced by PCR amplification on cDNA using a primer containing the T7 promoter sequence ( TAATACGACTCACTATAGG ) at its 5′ end (Fig. 3a). Purification of the PCR products using PCR cleanup columns (Macherey-Nagel 740609.50 or similar) is preferred otherwise, in presence of unspecific amplification products, a gel purification is required (Fig. 3a).

13. The addition of Na Acetate and glycogen is not required since they are already included in the Elution buffer.

14. NanoDrop Microvolume Spectrophotometer (Thermo Fisher) is preferred since it is fast (does not require preparation of the samples) and very sensitive ($0.4$–$15,000$ nanograms/µL).

15. In our hands, $68\ °C$ is the best temperature for almost all RNA probes we used (Fig. 3b, c) [16, 25]. However, for AU-rich probes the temperature can be lowered to $65$–$60\ °C$. In this case cross-hybridization with rRNAs might occur.

16. Maleic acid was replaced by Tris–HCl, pH 7.5. Differently from the manufacturer's procedure the Blocking solution was prepared at lower concentration ($1\times$) since, in our hands, $10\times$ Blocking solution was very difficult to dissolve. 1X Blocking solution was prepare as follows: 1% Blocking reagent (w/v) was dissolved in maleic acid buffer and mixed on hotplate stirrer for 1 h at $40$–$50\ °C$. Moreover, incubation time of the membrane with Blocking and Antibody solution was increased up to 45 min.

## Acknowledgments

The authors would like to thank Lorenzo Errichelli and Ivano Legnini for the images in Fig. 3, panels c and d (reproduced respectively from ref. 25 which is licensed under the Creative Commons Attribution 4.0 International License and from ref. 16 with permission from Elsevier).

## References

1. Guo JU, Agarwal V, Guo H et al (2014) Expanded identification and characterization of mammalian circular RNAs. Genome Biol 15:409

2. Zhang XO, Dong R, Zhang Y et al (2016) Diverse alternative back-splicing and alternative splicing landscape of circular RNAs. Genome Res 26:1277–1287

3. Jeck WR, Sorrentino JA, Wang K et al (2013) Circular RNAs are abundant, conserved, and associated with ALU repeats. RNA 19:141–157

4. Memczak S, Jens M, Elefsinioti A et al (2013) Circular RNAs are a large class of animal RNAs with regulatory potency. Nature 495:333–338

5. Enuka Y, Lauriola M, Feldman ME et al (2016) Circular RNAs are long-lived and display only minimal early alterations in response to a growth factor. Nucleic Acids Res 44:1370–1383

6. Wang PL, Bao Y, Yee MC et al (2014) Circular RNA is expressed across the eukaryotic tree of life. PLoS One e90859:9

7. Rybak-Wolf A, Stottmeister C, Glažar P et al (2015) Circular RNAs in the mammalian brain are highly abundant, conserved, and dynamically expressed. Mol Cell 58:870–885

8. You X, Vlatkovic I, Babic A et al (2015) Neural circular RNAs are derived from synaptic genes and regulated by development and plasticity. Nat Neurosci 18:603–610

9. Hansen TB, Jensen TI, Clausen BH et al (2013) Natural RNA circles function as efficient microRNA sponges. Nature 495:384–388

10. Ashwal-Fluss R, Meyer M, Pamudurti NR et al (2014) circRNA biogenesis competes with pre-mRNA splicing. Mol Cell 56:55–66

11. Du WW, Fang L, Yang W et al (2017) Induction of tumor apoptosis through a circular RNA enhancing Foxo3 activity. Cell Death Differ 24:357–370

12. Rossi F, Legnini I, Megiorni F et al (2019) Circ-ZNF609 regulates G1-S progression in rhabdomyosarcoma. Oncogene 38:3843–3854

13. Liu CX, Li X, Nan F et al (2019) Structure and degradation of circular RNAs regulate PKR activation in innate immunity. Cell 177:865–880

14. Chen N, Zhao G, Yan X et al (2018) A novel FLI1 exonic circular RNA promotes metastasis in breast cancer by coordinately regulating TET1 and DNMT1. Genome Biol 19:218

15. Pamudurti NR, Bartok O, Jens M et al (2017) Translation of CircRNAs. Mol Cell 66:9

16. Legnini I, Di Timoteo G, Rossi F et al (2017) Circ-ZNF609 is a circular RNA that can be translated and functions in myogenesis. Mol Cell 66:22

17. Memczak S, Papavasileiou P, Peters O et al (2015) Identification and characterization of circular RNAs as a new class of putative biomarkers in human blood. PLoS One 10: e0141214

18. Greene J, Baird A-M, Brady L et al (2017) Circular RNAs: biogenesis, function and role in human diseases. Front Mol Biosci 4:38

19. D'Ambra E, Capauto D, Morlando M (2019) Exploring the regulatory role of circular RNAs in neurodegenerative disorders. Int J Mol Sci 20:5477

20. Aufiero S, Reckman YJ, Pinto YM et al (2019) Circular RNAs open a new chapter in cardiovascular biology. Nat Rev Cardiol 16:503–514

21. Liu J, Zhang X, Yan M, Li H (2020) Emerging role of circular RNAs in cancer. Front Oncologia 10:663

22. Kristensen LS, Hansen TB, Veno MT et al (2018) Circular RNAs in cancer: opportunities and challenges in the field. Oncogene 37:555–565

23. Lei B, Tian Z, Fan W et al (2019) Circular RNA: a novel biomarker and therapeutic target for human cancers. Int J Med Sci 16:292–301

24. Barrett SP, Salzman J (2016) Circular RNAs: analysis, expression and potential functions. Development 143:1838–1847

25. Errichelli L, Dini Modigliani S, Laneve P et al (2017) FUS affects circular RNA expression in murine embryonic stem cell-derived motor neurons. Nat Commun 14741:8

26. Wichterle H, Peljto M (2008) Differentiation of mouse embryonic stem cells to spinal motor neurons. Curr Protoc Stem Cell Biol 223:1H.1.1–1H.1.9

# Correction to: Methods Used to Make Lipid Nanoparticles to Deliver LNA Gapmers Against lncRNAs into Acute Myeloid Leukemia (AML) Blasts

## Chun-Tien Kuo, Robert J. Lee, and Ramiro Garzon

**Correction to: Chapter 11 in: Alfons Navarro (ed.),** *Long Non-Coding RNAs in Cancer: Methods and Protocols,* **Methods in Molecular Biology, vol. 2348,**
https://doi.org/10.1007/978-1-0716-1581-2_11

In the original version of this book, Chapter 11 was published with incorrect author name and affiliation. It has now been updated in the revised version of this book.

---

The updated online version of this chapter can be found at:
https://doi.org/10.1007/978-1-0716-1581-2_11

Alfons Navarro (ed.), *Long Non-Coding RNAs in Cancer*, Methods in Molecular Biology, vol. 2348,
https://doi.org/10.1007/978-1-0716-1581-2_24, © Springer Science+Business Media, LLC, part of Springer Nature 2021

# INDEX

Lightning Source UK Ltd.
Milton Keynes UK
UKHW051812280622
405096UK00002B/4